Therapeutic Strategies

DIABETES

Edited by

Coen D. A. Stehouwer
Nicolaas Schaper

CLINICAL PUBLISHING

OXFORD

Clinical Publishing
an imprint of Atlas Medical Publishing Ltd

Oxford Centre for Innovation
Mill Street, Oxford OX2 0JX, UK
Tel: +44 1865 811116
Fax: +44 1865 251550
Email: info@clinicalpublishing.co.uk
Web: www.clinicalpublishing.co.uk

Distributed in USA and Canada by:
Clinical Publishing
30 Amberwood Parkway
Ashland OH 44805 USA
Tel: 800-247-6553 (toll free within USA and Canada)
Fax: 419-281-6883
Email: order@bookmasters.com

Distributed in UK and Rest of World by:
Marston Book Services Ltd
PO Box 269
Abingdon
Oxon OX14 4YN, UK
Tel: +44 1235 465500
Fax: +44 1235 465555
Email: trade.orders@marston.co.uk

© Atlas Medical Publishing Ltd 2009

First published 2009

A catalogue record for this book is available from the British Library.

ISBN 13   978 1 904392 87 3
ISBN e-book 978 1 84692 609 9

The publisher makes no representation, express or implied, that the dosages in this book are correct. Readers must therefore always check the product information and clinical procedures with the most up-to-date published product information and data sheets provided by the manufacturers and the most recent codes of conduct and safety regulations. The authors and the publisher do not accept any liability for any errors in the text or for the misuse or misapplication of material in this work.

Project manager: Gavin Smith, GPS Publishing Solutions, Hertfordshire, UK
Typeset by Mizpah Publishing Services Private Limited, Chennai, India
Printed by Marston Book Services, Abingdon, Oxon, UK

Therapeutic Strategies

DIABETES

Contents

Editors

COEN D.A. STEHOUWER, MD, PhD, Professor of Medicine, Chair, Department of Internal Medicine, Maastricht University Medical Centre, Maastricht, The Netherlands

NICOLAAS C. SCHAPER, MD, PhD, Professor of Diabetology, Head, Division of Endocrinology, Department of Internal Medicine, Maastricht University Medical Centre, Maastricht, The Netherlands

Contributors

GEREMIA B. BOLLI, MD, Professor of Internal Medicine, Consultant Cardiologist and Rheumatologist, Department of Internal Medicine, Endocrinology and Metabolism, University of Perugia, Perugia, Italy

ANDREW J.M. BOULTON, MD, DSc (Hon), FRCP, Professor of Medicine and Consultant Physician, University of Manchester and Manchester Royal Infirmary, Manchester, UK; Visiting Professor of Medicine, University of Miami, Miami, Florida, USA

JOHN A. COLWELL, MD, PhD, Emeritus Professor of Medicine, Division of Endocrinology, Diabetes and Medical Genetics, Medical University of South Carolina, Charleston, South Carolina, USA

CAROLYN F. DEACON, PhD, DMSc, Senior Lecturer, Department of Biomedical Sciences, The Panum Institute, University of Copenhagen, Copenhagen, Denmark

MARC EVANS, MD, MRCP, Consultant Diabetologist, Department of General Medicine, Diabetes and Endocrinology, Cardiff and Vale NHS Trust, Llandough Hospital, Penarth, Wales, UK

MILES FISHER, MD, FRCP, MBChB, Consultant Physician, Diabetes Clinic, Glasgow Royal Infirmary, Glasgow, UK

ANDRIES J. GILDE, PhD, Post-doctoral Fellow, INSERM U545, Department of Atherosclerosis, Institut Pasteur de Lille, Lille, France

JENS JUUL HOLST, MD, DMSc, Professor, Department of Biomedical Sciences, The Panum Institute, University of Copenhagen, Copenhagen, Denmark

FILIP K. KNOP, MD, PhD, Physician and Clinical Researcher, Diabetes Research Division, Department of Internal Medicine, Gentofte Hospital, University of Copenhagen, Copenhagen, Denmark

SØREN SØGAARD LUND, MD, Steno Diabetes Center, Gentofte, Denmark

GILLIAN E. MARSHALL, MBChB, MRCP, PhD, Specialist Registrar in Cardiology, Department of Cardiology, Glasgow Royal Infirmary, Glasgow, UK

JOHN A. MCKNIGHT, MB, BCh, BAO, MD, FRCP (Ed), Consultant Physician, Metabolic Unit, Western General Hospital; Honorary Reader, University of Edinburgh, Edinburgh, UK

PAUL L. PADFIELD, MB, BCh, FRCP (Edin), MBA, Professor of Hypertension, Consultant Physician, Metabolic Unit, Western General Hospital, Edinburgh, UK

RAJESH PETER, MD, MRCP, Consultant Diabetologist, Department of General Medicine, Diabetes and Endocrinology, Neath Port Talbot Hospital, Port Talbot, West Glamorgan, Wales, UK

JOHN P. D. RECKLESS, DSc, MD, FRCP, Consultant Endocrinologist, Department of Endocrinology, Royal United Hospital, Bath; Honorary Reader in Medicine, School of Health, University of Bath, Bath, UK

ERIC RENARD, MD, PhD, Professor of Endocrinology, Diabetes and Metabolic Diseases, Senior Medical Practitioner in Endocrinology, Diabetes and Metabolic Diseases, Department of Endocrinology, Montpellier University Hospital; UMR CNRS 5232, University of Montpellier, Montpellier, France

LUIS M. RUILOPE, MD, PhD, Nephrologist, Hypertension Unit, Department of Nephrology, Hospital 12 de Octubre, Madrid, Spain

ELEANNA SALGAMI, MD, PhD, Clinical Research Fellow, Department of Medicine, University of Manchester, Manchester, UK

JULIÁN SEGURA, MD, PhD, Nephrologist, Hypertension Unit, Department of Nephrology, Hospital 12 de Octubre, Madrid, Spain

YVO M. SMULDERS, MD, PhD, Internist, Department of Internal Medicine, VU University Medical Center, Amsterdam, The Netherlands

BART STAELS, PhD, Professor of Pharmacy and Group Leader, Department of Atherosclerosis, Unit 545 INSERM, Institut Pasteur, University of Lille 2, Lille, France

MARK W. J. STRACHAN, BSc (Hons), MBChB (Hons), MD, FRCP (Ed), Consultant Physician, Metabolic Unit, Western General Hospital; Honorary Senior Lecturer, University of Edinburgh, Edinburgh, UK

ALLAN ARTHUR VAAG, MD, PhD, DMSc, Endocrinologist, Steno Diabetes Center, Gentofte, Denmark; Chief Physician and Adjunct Professor of Metabolism and Clinical Diabetes Research, Lund University, Sweden

COEN VAN GULDENER, MD, PhD, Internist, Department of Internal Medicine, Amphia Hospital, Breda, The Netherlands

TINA VILSBØLL, MD, DMSc, Physician, Diabetes Research Division, Department of Internal Medicine, Gentofte Hospital, University of Copenhagen, Copenhagen, Denmark

FRANK L. J. VISSEREN, MD, PhD, Professor in Vascular Medicine, Epidemiologist, Department of Vascular Medicine, University Medical Center Utrecht, The Netherlands

Preface

We are witnessing a global epidemic of diabetes and obesity, and, in their wake, of cardio-vascular and renal disease. Prevention and treatment will require an in-depth understanding of therapeutic options. It is therefore timely and appropriate that this book has been dedicated to the topic of therapeutic strategies in diabetes and its cardiovascular complications. It is meant for all physicians who care for individuals with diabetes.

In many parts of the world, individuals with diabetes are treated by physicians who received their primary training either in diabetology (and often feel less familiar with cardiovascular treatment options), or by physicians who received their primary training in cardiovascular disease (and often feel less familiar with metabolic treatments). This book specifically aims to provide a bridge between these traditions.

As editors, we are fortunate to have persuaded leading authorities in the field to provide detailed discussions of current concepts and challenges. We have deliberately sought a balance between the metabolic and the cardiovascular perspectives. Accordingly, we have divided the book in two parts, with chapters on metabolic and cardiovascular treatment options, respectively.

In the first part, the opening chapter, by Marc Evans and Rajesh Peter, gives an overview of glucose lowering strategies, both old and new, and their rationale. As a variety of blood glucose lowering drugs are now available, with different modes of actions and safety profiles, the treatment of type 2 diabetes is rapidly gaining in complexity. This chapter sets the stage for the next five chapters. The first two of these provide in-depth discussions of the use of insulin analogues by Geremia Bolli and of specific novel ways of insulin administration (continuous subcutaneous insulin infusion, continuous intraperitoneal insulin infusion, and inhaled insulin administration) by Eric Renard. In the next chapter, Allan Vaag and Søren Lund discuss old and new uses of arguably the most important oral antidiabetic drug available, namely metformin. Andries Gilde and Bart Staels discuss the somewhat contentious issue of the use of glitazones (rosiglitazone and pioglitazone), which are PPARγ agonists, and of a new class of PPAR activators, the glitazars, which are agonists of both PPARα (like fibrates) and of PPARγ (like glitazones). In the final chapter of this section, Tina Vilsbøll and co-workers discuss the exciting development of incretin hormone mimetics as a treatment for type 2 diabetes. These drugs are either activators of the receptor for glucagon-like peptide-1 (GLP-1), or inhibit the breakdown of endogenous GLP-1 (so-called DPP-4 inhibitors), and appear to ameliorate many important aspects of the pathophysiology of type 2 diabetes.

One of the most important lessons learnt in the past decade is that what works for primary and secondary prevention of cardiovascular disease in individuals without diabetes, works as well, if not better, in individuals with diabetes. Thus, in the second part of this book, John Reckless, Frank Visseren, and Gillian Marshall and co-workers discuss the appropriate use of statins and other lipid-lowering treatments; John McKnight and colleagues, and Julián Segura and Luis Ruilope summarize the management of high blood pressure both from a cardiovascular and a renal perspective; and John Colwell explains how and when to use antiplatelet therapy in diabetes.

Are other options on the horizon? Hyperhomocysteinaemia is a particularly strong risk factor for cardiovascular disease in diabetes. Coen van Guldener and Yvo Smulders explain that homocysteine levels can be reduced by folic acid, but that the jury is still out on whether such treatment will reduce cardiovascular disease risk.

The final chapter of this book, by Eleanna Salgami and Andrew Boulton, is on the treatment of symptomatic diabetic neuropathy. Although strictly speaking this is not a cardiovascular disease, we have included it here because it often is an extremely distressing complication of diabetes, and because all practitioners who treat individuals with diabetes need to be aware of the available treatment options.

We hope that you will enjoy reading these chapters, as we have, and that you will find them both practical and thought-provoking.

Coen D.A. Stehouwer
Nicolaas Schaper

Part 1

Metabolic considerations

1

Blood glucose lowering therapies

M. Evans, R. Peter

INTRODUCTION

The results of the randomised, multicentre United Kingdom Prospective Diabetes Study (UKPDS) confirmed the importance of long-term glycaemic control in limiting the complications associated with type 2 diabetes [1]. Indeed the long-term benefits of intensive blood glucose control were demonstrated by the UKPDS follow-up analysis in which despite a loss of glycaemic differences between the intensive and standard therapy groups on completion of the randomised phase of the study, emergent risk reductions for mortality and myocardial infarction during 10 years of post-trial follow-up [2]. Hence tight glucose control early in the natural history of type 2 diabetes appears to confer long-term benefits, even if control deteriorates, while the benefits of blood pressure control are only apparent as long as control is maintained [2]. Such data drives current clinical practice in which treatment is directed towards the attainment of near normal glycaemia (glycosylated haemoglobin [HbA1c] concentrations <7%). While such targets maybe difficult to attain for many patients there is clear consensus that chronic hyperglycaemia should be optimally managed, weighing safety and quality of life considerations on an individual basis. The safety considerations of glycaemic control were highlighted by the recent Action to Control Cardiovascular Risk in type 2 Diabetes (ACCORD) study in which intensive glycaemic control (HbA1c 6.4%) was associated with an increased risk of all cause mortality compared with conventional control (HbA1c 7.4%) [3]. Such an observation may at least in part be attributable to hypoglycaemia, indeed hypoglycaemia is a major consideration in the management of blood glucose in patients with type 2 diabetes. Symptomatic hypoglycaemia is reported by up to 38% of patients with type 2 diabetes taking oral glucose lowering medications, being associated with detrimental effects on quality of life, treatment satisfaction and therapy adherence [4]. Glycaemic control is just one aspect of the overall management plan of patients with type 2 diabetes; which should also encompass effective blood pressure and lipid management. The benefits of intensive multiple risk factor intervention on vascular complications have been shown to be both clinically and cost-effective in reducing morbidity and mortality [5] and has given rise to the genesis blood pressure and cholesterol treatment targets in patients with type 2 diabetes, as outlined by the recent Joint British Societies' (JBS) 2 Guidelines [6]. While evidence of the clinical effectiveness of such inter-

Marc Evans, MD, MRCP, Consultant Diabetologist, Department of General Medicine, Diabetes and Endocrinology, Cardiff and Vale NHS Trust, Llandough Hospital, Penarth, Wales, UK.

Rajesh Peter, MD, MRCP, Consultant Diabetologist, Department of General Medicine, Diabetes and Endocrinology, Neath Port Talbot Hospital, Port Talbot, West Glamorgan, Wales, UK.

ventions is available the translation of this approach into population based therapy presents a considerable challenge.

Insulin resistance along with defective insulin secretion are the cardinal metabolic features of type 2 diabetes, with subtle abnormalities of both being evident even at the earliest stages of glucose intolerance. Whilst insulin resistance is highly prevalent, linked to obesity and physical inactivity, near normal glucose tolerance can be maintained as long as β-cell insulin secretion is maintained. The development of glucose intolerance and thus type 2 diabetes is therefore dependent on progressive β-cell dysfunction. The initial management of a newly diagnosed person with type 2 diabetes involves advice and education relating to the potential benefits of dietary modification and lifestyle change. The objectives of this being to improve metabolic control through reductions in body weight that may help improve insulin sensitivity. The majority of patients will, however, require pharmacological therapy in the medium to long term. In UKPDS only 25% of patients maintained an HbA1c level <7% after 9 years without either oral agents or exogenous insulin [7]. Not only was drug therapy required but the need for escalating polypharmacy was also clearly demonstrated. This phenomenon was further illustrated in the A Diabetes Outcome Progression Trial (ADOPT) study, in which only 21.9%, 21% and 16.5% respectively of patients treated with either rosiglitazone, metformin or glyburide monotherapy demonstrated sustained blood glucose control after 4 years of treatment [8].

Gradual decline in β-cell function is held to be the major determinant of this progressive hyperglycaemia. Other factors such as weight gain and concordance failure with therapy or lifestyle modification may also contribute.

The selection of initial pharmacotherapy is based on the clinical and biochemical characteristics of the patient. Safety considerations must always be carefully considered since few, if any, oral hypoglycaemic agents are completely devoid of risk. Patients presenting with weight loss or failing to respond rapidly to oral hypoglycaemic therapy, despite optimum compliance with both treatment and lifestyle advice, usually signals the need for early insulin initiation. Exogenous insulin is otherwise usually reserved for patients who fail to respond oral therapies, or in whom safety considerations dictate its use as the agent of choice.

Several classes of oral hypoglycaemic agents are currently available with considerable expansion in recent years. Based on data from UKPDS [9], metformin is currently accepted as the initial oral pharmacotherapy of choice in the management of overweight people with type 2, the addition of further hypoglycaemic agents being indicated once glycaemic control is suboptimal (HbA1c concentration >7%) despite maximally tolerated initial oral therapy. This so called step-wise approach to the glycaemic management of people with type 2 diabetes has resulted in the genesis of both national and international treatment guidelines (Figure 1.1).

The current therapies available for the management of blood glucose in type 2 diabetes maybe divided according to their principle mode of action:

- Those agents that increase insulin secretion (insulin secretagogues).
- Those agents that improve insulin sensitivity.
- Drugs that facilitate weight loss.
- Drugs that delay the rate of digestion and absorption of carbohydrates.
- Drugs that mimic the physiological effects of gut hormones (incretin mimetics).

In this chapter we reflect on the mode of action, pharmacokinetics, indications and contraindications, efficacy, safety, tolerability and current place in management of these classes of drugs.

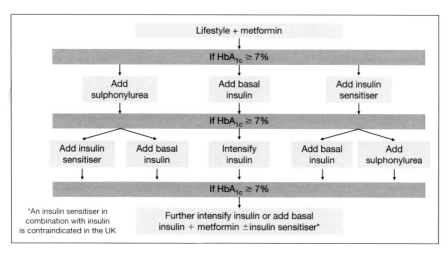

Figure 1.1 US and European guidelines demonstrating a step-wise approach to glycaemic management in people with type 2 diabetes.
HbA1c = glycosylated haemoglobin.

INSULIN SECRETAGOGUES

SULPHONYLUREAS

Sulophonylureas have been used extensively for treating type 2 diabetes for over 50 years. They exert blood glucose lowering effects primarily by stimulating insulin secretion from β-cells. By the 1960s several different agents were available including tolbutamide, tolaz-amide and chlorpropamide. Doubts about safety were raised in the 1970s, but a review of the available literature provides little in the way of convincing evidence of cardiovascular toxic-ity and the UKPDS demonstrated no increased risk of myocardial infarction among patients treated with sulphonylureas compared with patients randomised to insulin as monotherapy [1], while the benefits of glucose lowering with sulphonylureas in the STENO-2 study are clearly apparent [5]. More potent second generation sulphonylureas emerged in the 1970s and 80s including glimepiride, glibenclamide, gliclazice and glipizide. The ADVANCE study (Action in Diabetes and Vascular Disease: Preterax and Diamicron MR Controlled Evaluation) study has demonstrated the utility of these agents in limiting microvascular complications but no impact on cardiovascular outcomes has been demonstrated [10].

Mode of action

Sulphonylureas bind to the β-cell sulphonylurea receptor (SUR1), which is part of a trans-membrane complex, the activation of which results in closure of K^+ ATP channels reducing cellular potassium efflux, thus favouring membrane depolarisation [11] (Figure 1.2). As a consequence, voltage-dependent calcium channels open resulting in an influx of calcium thus activating calcium-dependent proteins, which control the release of insulin. When sul-phonylureas bind to the SUR1, a prompt release of pre-formed insulin takes place adjacent to the plasma cell membrane – the so-called first phase of insulin release [12]. Sulphonylyreas also increase the extended or second phase of insulin release, which begins approximately 10 minutes later as insulin granules are translocated to the membrane from within the β-cell [12]. A protracted stimulation of the second phase of insulin release involves the secretion of newly formed insulin granules, which continues while there is ongoing drug stimulation, provided there are sufficient β-cell reserves. Sulphonylureas can thus cause hypoglycaemia

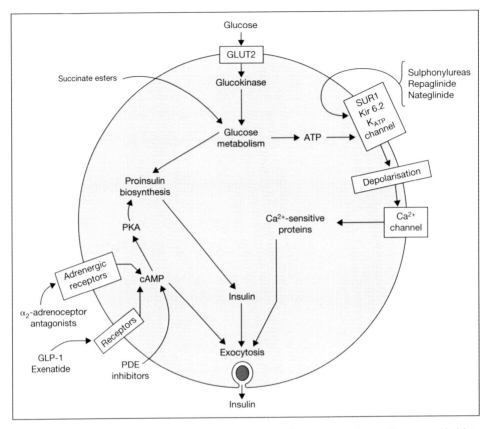

Figure 1.2 The insulin releasing effects of sulphonylureas and other agents acting on the pancreatic islet cell.
ATP = adenosine triphosphate; cAMP = cyclic AMP; GLP-1 = glucagon-like peptide-1; GLUT2 = glucose transporter 2; PDE = phosphodiesterase; PKA = protein kinase A; SUR1 = sulphonylurea receptor 1.

since insulin release is initiated even when glucose concentrations are below the normal threshold for glucose-stimulated insulin secretion (<5 mmol/l).

The principle distinguishing feature between individual sulphonylureas is their pharmacokinetic profile, with duration of action varying from <12 h for tolbutamide to >24 h for chlorpropamide [13]. This arises as a result of differences in rates of metabolism, activity of metabolites and rates of elimination. These properties have important implications for the risk of sulphonylurea-associated hypoglycaemia. All sulphonylureas are well absorbed, reaching peak plasma concentrations within 2–4 h. They are all primarily metabolised in the liver, although metabolites and subsequent routes of elimination vary. Since all sulphonylureas are highly plasma protein bound they have the potential to interact with other drugs sharing this banding, for example salicylates, sulphonamides and warfarin. Displacement from circulating proteins has been implicated in cases of severe sulphonylurea-induced hypoglycaemia.

Indications and contraindications
Since metformin is considered as the first-line oral hypoglycaemic for the majority of patients, sulphonylureas are a commonly used second-line agent. They may also be used as a first-line therapy; customarily, they are preferred for patients who are not overweight since

weight gain is an associated feature of sulphonylurea therapy [13]. Sulphonylureas are commonly used in combination therapy with agents from other treatment classes, with the exception of other insulin secretagogues. Daytime sulphonylurea treatment may also be used in combination with bedtime insulin and may reduce insulin requirement by up to 50% [14]. Sulphonylureas should be introduced at a low dose, increased over 2–4 weeks until glycaemic targets are achieved. If hypoglycaemia ensues it is advisable to return to the previous dose. Improved β-cell capacity resulting from alleviation of glucose toxicity and fatty acid toxicity may contribute to an increased risk of hypoglycaemia in some patients, In general, patients achieving a lesser degree of fasting hyperglycaemia following diet and exercise are more likely to develop hypoglycaemic symptoms than those with more marked fasting hyperglycaemia [13]. The maximal blood glucose lowering effect of sulphonylurea therapy is usually achieved at doses below the recommended maximum, probably reflecting the fact that maximum β-cell stimulation occurs at submaximal doses.

Efficacy

When used as monotherapy, sulphonylureas can reduce fasting plasma glucose by 2–4 mmol/l, accompanying a 1–2% reduction in HbA1c, although individual responses may vary. Since the hypoglycaemic effects of sulphonylureas relates to increased insulin secretion, the effectiveness of these agents is dependent on adequate β-cell reserve. The rate of decline of β-cell function appears to be the main determinant of loss of sulphonylurea efficacy and this may be greater with sulphonylurea than with insulin sensitising therapy [8]. The deterioration in glycaemic control associated with sulphonylureas is occasionally termed 'secondary sulphonylurea failure' and occurs at a rate of approximately 15% of patients per annum [8]. In essence, this is a reflection of disease progression rather than a true therapeutic failure.

The plasma insulin concentration achieved during sulphonylurea therapy does not usually extend beyond the normal physiological range observed in non-diabetic individuals. Consequently, the suggestion that sulphonylurea-induced hyperinsulinaemia may increase the detrimental insulin-related effects on the cardiovascular system remains largely unsubstantiated.

Sulphonylureas usually have modest effects on lipid profiles with small decreases in plasma triglyceride levels, most likely linked to improved glycaemic control. When a sulphonylurea is used in combination with another oral hypoglycaemic agent, the glucose lowering efficacy of both agents is additive, with the response again being dependent on the preservation of adequate β-cell function. Thus, following monotherapy failure, early use of combination therapy is a key approach to the maintenance of optimal glycaemic control.

Adverse events

Hypoglycaemia, whether subclinical, minor, or occasionally life-threatening, is the most common and serious adverse effect of sulphonylureas. The reported incidence of sulphonylurea hypoglycaemia in clinical studies ranges from 10–40% [8, 15]. Patients thus receiving sulphonylurea therapy should receive education on the recognition and prevention of hypoglycaemia. Severe protracted hypoglycaemia is more likely with longer acting sulphonylureas such as glibenclamide, while shorter acting agents such as gliclazide have a lower risk. Patient specific factors may also influence hypoglycaemia risk including irregular eating habits, excessive alcohol consumption and in those with tight glycaemic control as a manifest by HbA1c concentrations within or just above the non-diabetic range. More severe hypoglycaemia (i.e. requiring assistance) has been estimated to occur in about 1% of sulphonylurea treated patients (0.2–2.5 episodes per 1000 patient-years) with a mortality risk from such severe episodes being calculated at between 0.014–0.033 per 1000 patient-years, with longer-acting agents appearing to carry the greater mortality risk [16]. The development of new onset sulphonylurea-related hypoglycaemia should alert the clinician to the possibility of other confounding factors such as occult malignancy, renal failure or hepatic impairment. Severe episodes of sulphonylurea-induced hypoglycaemia require treatment with intravenous dextrose infusions, while diazoxide and somatostatin may also be of benefit.

Other potential adverse events related to sulphonylureas include uncommon hypersensitivity reactions, which are usually transient. Fever, jaundice, blood dyscrasias and acute porphyria in predisposed individuals are also recognised rare adverse events. Weight gain is recognised as a class-related side-effect in sulphonylurea therapy ranging from 1–4 kg in the first six months of treatment and stabilising thereafter.

The issue of cardiovascular safety relating to the sulphonylureas was raised by the discovery of isoforms of the sulphonylurea receptor on both cardiac and vascular smooth muscle (SUR2A, 2B). Sulphonylureas containing a badenzamido group (gliclazide, glibenclamide, glipizide and glimepiride) can bind to these receptors where as those without demonstrate very little interaction [17]. The effects of the K^+ channel-opening nicorandil are blocked by such badenzamido-containing sulphonylureas, however, the clinical implications of these observations remain unclear. Indeed, in two recent megatrials, namely ADOPT and RECORD no increased adverse cardiovascular signal was seen in association with sulphonylurea therapy [8, 18]. However, very high concentrations of sulphonylureas may cause contraction of cardiac and vascular muscle, although this is thought unlikely to be of any clinical significance at the therapeutic drug concentrations.

RAPID-ACTING PRANDIAL INSULIN RELEASERS

The first phase of glucose-stimulated insulin secretion is diminished early in the natural history of type 2 diabetes [19]. Early phase insulin secretion is important for postprandial glucose regulation and it is increasingly recognised that postprandial hyperglycaemia precedes fasting hyperglycaemia [20]. Furthermore, the contribution of postprandial glucose is the predominant contributor to excess glycaemia relatively well controlled (HbA1c <7.3%) patients, while the contribution of fasting glucose increases as glycaemia deteriorates [20]. Postprandial blood glucose excursions would thus appear to be a relevant therapeutic target. Rapid-acting prandial insulin releasers are available, which are taken orally immediately before a meal and produce rapid, but short-lived, insulin secretion. These agents, meglitinide derivatives, (netaglinide, repaglinide) are promoted as prandial glucose regulators but in fact also impact to a lesser extent on fasting hyperglycaemia.

Mode of action
These agents bind to the SUR1 in the β-cell membrane at a site distinct from the sulphonylurea binding site (Figure 1.2). Since the K^+ ATP channel is closed when either the sulphonylurea binding site or the meglitanide binding site is occupied by its respective agonist, there is no advantage in combining a prandial insulin releaser with a sulphonylurea. The short half-life of these meglitanide agents results in enhancement of first phase and early second phase insulin secretion, which is less sustained than that seen with sulphonylureas.

Pharmacokinetics
Repaglinide is rapidly and almost completely absorbed following oral administration with peak plasma concentrations at around 1 h [21]. It is rapidly metabolised in the liver, with its metabolites excreted in bile. When taken around 15 minutes before a meal, repaglinide produces a prompt insulin release, which is limited to a period of around 3 h. Netaglinide has a slightly faster onset and shorter duration of action with its binding to target receptors lasting only a matter of seconds.

Indications and contraindications
These agents maybe used as monotherapy or in combination with agents other than sulphonylureas. Suitable candidates include individuals with irregular eating patterns, while the lower risk of hypoglycaemia makes repaglinide an attractive option for individuals at risk of hypoglycaemia. The need for multiple daily dosing is a potential disincentive while the dosing regimen may also be confusing. Repaglinide should be ideally taken 15–30 minutes prior to a meal, starting at the lowest dose of 0.5 mg before each meal with dose titration over a subsequent 2–4 week period to a maximum of 4 mg before each meal according to response. Unlike some sulphonylureas and metformin, repaglinide is suitable for patients with moderate renal impairment, although careful dose titration and glucose monitoring is still required [21].

Efficacy
Overall reductions in HbA1c are similar in order of magnitude to those observed in sulphonylureas (1–2%). When used in combination with metformin, reductions in HbA1c of a similar order of magnitude are observed.

Adverse events
The overall incidence of hypoglycaemia is lower than with sulphonylureas. Sensitivity reactions, usually transient, may occur. Small increases in body weight maybe expected but these are minimal when compared to sulphonylurea therapy and there is little effect seen on weight when these agents are used in combination with metformin.

ALPHA-GLUCOSIDASE INHIBITORS

Inhibitors of intestinal α-glucosidase enzymes reduce the rate of carbohydrate ingestion, thereby providing an alternative means to reducing postprandial glucose levels [22]. Acarbose is the only agent licensed in the UK and does not cause weight gain, can reduce postprandial hyperinsulinaemia and has lowered plasma triglyceride concentrations in some studies [22].

Mode of action
These agents inhibit the activity of α-glucosidase enzymes in the brush border lining the intestinal villi. This prevents the cleaving of polysaccharide substrates into monosaccharides prior to absorption. This defers the completion of carbohydrate digestion until further along the intestinal tract, consequently causing glucose absorption to be delayed. The displacement of glucose absorption more distally along in the intestinal tract alters glucose-dependent release of intestinal hormones that enhance nutrient induced insulin secretion.

Pharmacokinetics
Acarbose is absorbed only to a trivial degree (<2%) and is degraded by amylases in the small intestine. Some of these products may be absorbed and are eliminated in the urine over a period of about 24 h.

Indications and contraindications
Acarbose maybe a useful first-line treatment in patients who have only slightly raised fasting glucose concentrations and more marked postprandial hyperglycaemia; the STOP-NIDDM study confirmed the utility of acarbose in delaying progression from impaired glucose tolerance to type 2 diabetes [23]. These agents maybe used either as monotherapy

or in combination with other oral agents and when starting treatment it is important to ensure a patient's diet is rich in complex carbohydrates rather than simple sugars. Acarbose should be taken before meals, commencing with low dose (15 mg/day) with slow titration over several weeks, with a maximum dose often being limited by gastrointestinal (GI) symptoms. Intuitively, therefore, patients experiencing gastrointestinal adverse effects with metformin may not be the optimum candidates for such an agent, while a history of chronic intestinal disorders may also theoretically represent a contraindication to acarbose. As with all other hypoglycaemic agents, pregnancy and breast-feeding are traditionally regarded to be contraindications, mainly due to a lack of safety data rather than evidence of detrimental effects.

Efficacy
Used in patients who comply with dietary modification, acarbose will typically reduce prandial glucose concentrations by 1–4 mmol/l. As with prandial glucose regulators, there also appear to be small reductions in fasting glycaemia of up to 1 mmol/l. The decrease in HbA1c is usually around 0.5–1% providing that a sufficient dose of the drug is tolerated and dietary compliance is maintained.

Adverse effects
The most commonly reported adverse effect of acarbose is gastrointestinal upset occurring with a frequency of up to 31% in the STOP-NIDDM trial [23]. If the dosage of drug is too high relative to the amount of complex dietary carbohydrate, undigested oligosaccharides pass into the large bowel and become fermented by intestinal flora causing flatulence, abdominal discomfort and diarrhoea. Hypolgycaemia is only likely to be encountered in combination with either a sulphonylurea or insulin and no clinically significant drug interactions have been reported.

INSULIN SENSITISERS

Insulin resistance is a prominent metabolic abnormality in many patients with type 2 diabetes and therefore represents an attractive therapeutic target. The biguanides and thiazolidenidiones are regarded as insulin sensitising drugs [24].

BIGUANIDES

Metformin is currently the only available biguanide and since it is both the least expensive oral hypoglycaemic, combined with data suggesting cardiovascular benefits in overweight patients with type 2 diabetes [8], it is now considered as the first-line agent for the majority of patients.

Mode of action
Metformin has a variety of metabolic effects (Table 1.1), many of which extend beyond glucose lowering. The true molecular mechanism of metformin action is, however, not fully understood. At the cellular level, metformin may improve insulin sensitivity via postreceptor signalling pathways for insulin [25]. Recent data have also suggested that adenosine V monophosphate activated protein kinase (AMPK) is a possible intracellular target for metformin, which, via phosphorylation pathways, acts as a regulator of cellular energy metabolism [26]. Metformin does not stimulate insulin release and small reductions in fasting insulin concentrations are often observed. The predominant glucose-lowering effect of metformin appears to be the reduction of excess hepatic glucose release (Figure 1.3). Metformin attenuates gluconeogenesis by increasing hepatic sensitivity to insulin and

Table 1.1 Summary of metabolic and vascular effects of metformin

Antihyperglycaemic action
– Suppresses hepatic glucose production
– Increase insulin mediated glucose utilisation
– Decrease fatty acid oxidation
– Increase splanchnic glucose turnover
Weight stabilisation or reduction
Improved lipid profile
– Reduction in plasma triglyceride
– Reduction in plasma fatty acids
Improved insulin sensitivity
Vascular effects
– Improved endothelial function
– Increased fibrinolysis

decreasing hepatic extraction of certain gluconeogenic substrates such as lactate. Hepatic glycogenolysis is also reduced, while insulin-stimulated glucose uptake in skeletal muscle may also be increased to some extent [25]. Metformin also acts in an insulin-dependent manner to suppress the oxidation of fatty acids, thus reducing triglyceride levels and further reducing the energy supply for hepatic gluconeogenesis [25]. Glucose metabolism in the splanchnic bed may also be increased by metformin in an insulin-dependent fashion. This may further contribute to blood glucose lowering effects and also aid in the prevention of weight gain.

Pharmacokinetics
Metformin is a hydrophilic biguanide that is completely absorbed and eliminated unchanged in the urine. Consequently, renal impairment represents a contraindication to metformin as sufficient renal function is required to avoid accumulation of the drug. Renal clearance is achieved more by tubular secretion than by glomerular filtration. Metformin is not metabolised and therefore does not interfere with co-administered drugs. It is widely distributed, being retained in the walls of the gastrointestinal tract, providing a reservoir from which plasma concentrations are maintained. Peak plasma metformin concentrations are, however, short-lived – in patients with normal renal function, the half-life for metformin is 2–5 h, with 90% of an administered dose being eliminated within 12 h [25].

Indications and contraindications
Metformin is the first-line therapy of choice for obese patients with type 2 diabetes and may be equally effective in patients of normal weight. Metformin may be used in combination with any other oral hypoglycaemic agent or with insulin. The drug is contraindicated in patients with impaired renal function (serum creatinine >150 μmol/l, glomerular filtration rate [GFR] <60 ml/min). Conditions predisposing to tissue hypoxia also represent a contraindication, along with severe liver disease, alcohol abuse and a history of metabolic acidosis. Metformin may be used in the elderly, provided that renal insufficiency and other exclusions are not present. The improvement in insulin sensitivity may also cause ovulation to resume in cases of polycystic ovarian syndrome and it has been used in this condition (unlicensed) to enhance fertility. Metformin should be taken with meals or immediately before eating in order to minimise gastrointestinal side-effects. Treatment should be commenced ordinarily at a dose of 500 mg once or twice daily with slow dosage increase (one tablet at a time) at intervals of around 2–3 weeks until a target level of glycaemic control is achieved. The maximal effective dosage appears to be around

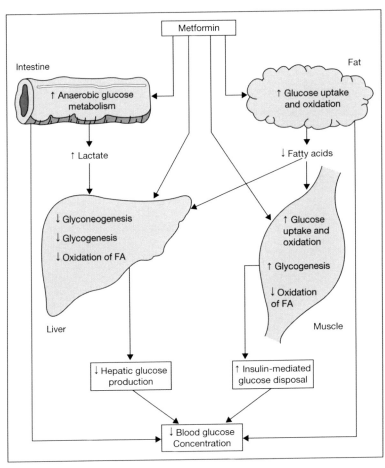

Figure 1.3 Metabolic actions of metformin – primarily related to inhibition of hepatic glucose production. FA = fatty acid.

2 g/day given in divided doses, the maximum being 3000 g/day. A slow-release formulation of metformin is available and is said to have fewer in the way of gastrointestinal side-effects. During long-term treatment with metformin, it is advisable to monitor patients for the development of contraindications, in particular renal dysfunction. Metformin may also reduce gastrointestinal absorption of Vitamin B_{12}: while anaemia is very rare, an annual haemoglobin measurement and B_{12} assessment is prudent. It is advisable to stop metformin treatment temporarily during intravenous radiographic contrast administration, surgery and any other inter-current situation that may invoke the exclusion criteria, in particular renal dysfunction.

Efficacy

As monotherapy, or in combination therapy, metformin typically reduces fasting plasma glucose levels by 2–4 mmol/l with a corresponding decrease in HbA1c of between 1–2%. The effect is largely independent of body weight, age and duration and diabetes, however, given the progressive nature of type 2 diabetes, metformin monotherapy alone is often insufficient to maintain adequate glycaemic control with data from the recent ADOPT study suggesting an annual failure rate of up to 10% [8]. Metformin is unlikely to cause significant hypoglycaemia, body weight tends to stabilise or decrease slightly, while small improvements in lipid profiles maybe observed with reductions in plasma triglyceride concentrations, fatty acid levels and low-density lipopoprotein cholesterol levels and high-density lipoprotein (HDL) cholesterol tends to increase, all of which appear to be independent of blood glucose lowering. These attributes may contribute to the putative cardiovascular benefits of metformin [9], although no clear dose response relationship is evident, suggesting that patients who can only tolerate low doses of metformin may benefit in terms of cardiovascular outcomes from continuing with the drug, even if other agents need to be added to optimise glycaemic control. Detracting from the generally favourable notion of cardiovascular benefits related to metformin there was evidence of an initially greater mortality when metformin was added to sulphonylurea therapy in a UKPDS substudy [9]. Longer term follow up has, however, demonstrated that the cardiovascular benefits of metformin were maintained, with one potential explanation being at least in part a spuriously low mortality rate in the comparator sulphonylurea monotherapy group. Similar findings of an increased cardiovascular mortality have been suggested in observational studies assessing combination metformin and sulphonylurea therapy [27]. However, data from large US studies and a variety of patient source databases have provided considerable reassuring evidence for the cardiovascular safety of metformin–sulphonylurea combination therapy [28, 29]. Consistent with the insulin sensitising action of metformin, it is now common practice to add metformin to ongoing insulin therapy, which may reduce exogenous insulin dose requirements, attenuates weight gain associated with exogenous insulin and the potential reductions in hypoglycaemia risk due to reduced exogenous insulin requirements. This approach is now widespread and includes combination with all insulin regimens including once daily, twice daily and basal bolus. Metformin has, in the US Diabetes Prevention Programme, also been shown to reduce the incidence of progression from impaired glucose tolerance to frank type 2 diabetes in overweight and obese patients by 33% compared with an intensive lifestyle regimen reduction of 58%. Younger, more obese individuals demonstrate the most substantial responses to metform therapy.

Adverse effects

Abdominal discomfort and various adverse gastrointestinal effects are the most common tolerability issues related to metformin therapy. These symptoms may remit if the dose is reduced or titration occurs slowly, however, around 10% of patients cannot tolerate metformin at any dose. The most serious and feared adverse event associated with metformin is lactic acidosis. The occurrence is rare (0.03 cases per 1000 patient-years), but the mortality rate is high. The majority of cases of lactic acidosis that have been reported in association with metformin have been due to inappropriate prescription of the drug, primarily in the context of significant renal insufficiency. Metformin increases lactate, particularly in the splanchnic bed, which may be aggravated by any hypoxic condition or in the context of impaired liver function. Hyperlactataemia occurs in cardiogenic shock and other conditions associated with tissue hypoperfusion and thus metformin is often an innocent bystander in cases of lactic acidosis caused by other severe illnesses. However, in the absence of any reliable data to the contrary, metformin should be discontinued immediately in all cases of suspected or proven lactic acidosis, regardless of cause or in any conditions that may result in tissue hypoperfusion. Lactic acidosis is typically characterised by elevated serum lactate (>5 mmol/l), decreased arterial pH and reduced bicarbonate concentrations with a high ion gap (>15 mmol/l). Presentation is often non-specific but frequently includes hyperventilation, malaise and abdominal discomfort. Bicarbonate is the therapy of choice, but evidence of its efficacy is limited.

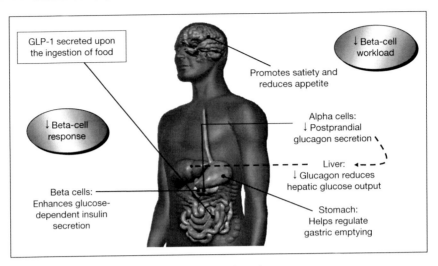

GLP-1 secreted upon
the ingestion of food

↓ Beta-cell
workload

Promotes satiety and
reduces appetite

↓ Beta-cell
response

Alpha cells:
↓ Postprandial
glucagon secretion

Liver:
↓ Glucagon reduces
hepatic glucose output

Beta cells:
Enhances glucose-
dependent insulin
secretion

Stomach:
Helps regulate
gastric emptying

Figure 1.4 Summary of the glucoregulatory effects of the incretin system.
GLP-1 = glucagon-like peptide-1.

THE INCRETIN HORMONES

Factors released from the gastrointestinal tract have the potential to lower blood glucose [30] (Figure 1.4). The entero-insular axis is a concept that was developed to describe the regulation of pancreatic islet cell hormone secretion by signals from the gastrointestinal tract [31]. This idea was based on the observation that for equivalent levels of glycaemia, oral glucose stimulates considerably more insulin than intravenous glucose, referred to as the 'incretin effect'. This incretin effect is not limited to glucose, since an augmented release of insulin is observed in response to oral as compared with parenteral administration of lipids and amino acids [32, 33]. This incretin effect is predominantly based on the insulinotropic effect of two hormones, gastric inhibitory polypeptide (GIP) and glucagon-like peptide-1 (GLP-1) [34, 35], accounting for up to 60% of postprandial insulin secretion in healthy individuals [35].

GLP-1

GLP-1 is a product of the glucagon gene [36]. It is produced from proglucagon in the enteroendocrine L-cells in the distal ileum and colon. Proglucagon is cleaved, not to produce glucagon as in the islets, but to release from its C-terminal part the two glucagon-like peptides GLP-1 and GLP-2, both exhibiting approximately 50% amino acid identity to pancreatic glucagon. GLP-1 has 30 amino acids and is rapidly secreted from the distal gut within minutes of food being ingested via a combination of neural and endocrine stimulatory factors. It is now well established that the pancreatic β-cell expresses the GLP-1 and GIP receptors. These receptors are members of the glucagon/secretin family of G-protein coupled receptors. Activation of the incretin receptors by ligand binding stimulates the generation of cAMP and through the guanine nucleotide exchange factor II pathway insulin exocytosis from the β-cell occurs [37]. The insulinotropic effect of the incretins is dependent on acute elevations in ambient glucose and is only minimally apparent at basal glucose concentrations. GLP-1 contains an NH_2-terminal alanine at position 2, rendering it a substrate for cleavage by the endovascular serine protease enzyme dipeptidyl peptidase (DPP)-4. Both enzymatic action and renal clearance contribute to the short half-life for native GLP-1. Inactivation of GLP-1 by the enzyme DPP-4 leads to the generation of the metabolite GLP-1(9-36) amide, which does not activate the GLP-1 receptor [38] and may even antagonise the actions of intact GLP-1 [39].

In addition to stimulation of glucose-dependent insulin secretion, GLP-1 has been shown to improve insulin sensitivity, delay gastric emptying, induce satiety with resultant reduction in calorie intake and also suppress glucagon secretion [40]. GLP-1 reduces excess glucagon secretion from islet α-cells without having an impact on its protective effect on hypoglycaemia. The effect of GLP-1 on gastric emptying and satiety also offers the potential for weight reduction. GLP-1 also has extrametabolic effects on the cardiovascular, pulmonary and hypothalamic–pituitary systems [41]. However, its most interesting effect is on the suppression of apoptosis and proliferation of β-cells in animal studies. GLP-1 increases β-cell mass in rodent models – treatment for between 2 days and 2 weeks leads to a 1.4- to 6.2-fold increase in β-cell mass [41] with β-cell hyperplasia being responsible for this increase in mass [42]. Should this effect be demonstrated in humans, it would be a key milestone in treatment aimed at reversing the inevitable decline in β-cells seen in type 2 diabetes.

Due to the fact that *in vivo* GLP-1 only remains active for 1–2 minutes it has to be administered as a continuous infusion. Longer-acting GLP-1 analogues that resist inactivation by the enzyme DPP-4 are now commercially available. Exendin-4, which has 50% homology with human GLP-1, a compound isolated from the saliva of the Gila monster resists inactivation by DPP-4. Exenatide (synthetically produced exendin-4) the first incretin mimetic to become available was a granted a licence in Europe in 2006. It is administered by subcutaneous (SC) injections of 5 μg bd for 4 weeks, increased to 10 μg bd thereafter. This dose titration is to avoid its most common side-effect of nausea, which is prevalent in 36–39% at 5 μg bd and 45–50% with 10 μg bd [43].

Exenatide has been assessed as adjunctive therapy in three trials of similar design, including > 1400 obese patients with type 2 diabetes uncontrolled with metformin [44], sulfonylurea (SU) [45], or both [46]. After 30 weeks, average reductions in HbA1c levels with the high-dose of exenatide (10 μg bd) were approximately 0.8 and 1.0% compared with baseline and placebo, respectively. Similar reductions in HbA1c values were reported in a smaller trial (n = 232) of shorter duration (16 weeks), in which exenatide was evaluated as add-on therapy in patients with type 2 diabetes suboptimally controlled on a thiazolidenedione (TZD) and metformin [47]. At the end of the previous five trials, the average proportions of subjects who achieved HbA1c value of ≤ 7.0%, were 45 and 10% in the exenatide and placebo groups, respectively, an observation that relates both to drug efficacy and baseline HbA1c. In subgroup analysis of subjects with baseline HbA1c >9% compared with <9%; greater reductions were seen with exenatide (5 μg dose, –0.8% vs. –0.4%, respectively; and 10 μg, –1.5% vs. –0.6%)

Exenatide was compared with insulin glargine in 549 patients with type 2 diabetes (baseline HbA1c 8.3%) on a background therapy of SU plus metformin [48]. After 26 weeks, HbA1c was reduced by 1.1% in both groups. In another trial, exenatide was compared with biphasic insulin aspart (formed of 30% short-acting insulin aspart and 70% intermediate-acting insulin) as adjunctive therapy in patients with type 2 diabetes (n = 501) inadequately controlled on metformin plus SU (mean baseline HbA1c 8.6%) [49]. After 52 weeks, no significant differences in HbA1c reductions were found between the exenatide and biphasic insulin aspart groups: 1 and 0.9%, respectively. At 52 weeks, significantly more subjects achieved an HbA1c <7 % in the exenatide group (32%) vs. the biphasic aspart group (24%). In both studies, better postprandial control was achieved with exenatide (difference –0.7 to –1.7 mmol/l).

In the previous two studies, the mean daily doses of insulin glargine and biphasic insulin aspart at the study ends were 26 and 24 units, respectively, suggesting that exenatide efficacy (10 μg bd) may be equivalent to mean daily insulin doses close to that range. However, more studies are needed to examine the benefits and risks of switching from insulin to exenatide therapy. Until these studies become available, such a strategy is not recommended, particularly in patients whose diabetes is not controlled on relatively high-doses of insulin.

For instance, in an exploratory study of 49 subjects with type 2 diabetes having mean baseline HbA1c values of approximately 8.1% while receiving insulin doses > 40 units/day, the substitution of exenatide for insulin resulted in further deterioration of glycemic control in 40% of patients, and lack of improvement in the remaining 60% of patients [50]. Open label long-term extension data has demonstrated a sustained reduction in HbA1c and progressive weight loss (Figures 1.3 and 1.4), with reductions in HbA1c of 1.1% achieved after 12 weeks being maintained after 3 years [51].

In clinical studies, exenatide was associated with progressive and dose-dependent weight loss. After 30 weeks, subjects receiving 10 µg bd exenatide had lost more weight than those receiving placebo (mean 1.6 kg or 2.8 kg) compared with 0.3 and 0.9 kg for placebo. There was no correlation between reported nausea and weight loss. Weight loss was progressive throughout the study period and persisted through the 104 week open label completer analysis. In this study there was progressive reduction in body weight of 1.6, 2.4 and 4.7 kg at weeks 12, 30 and 104, respectively. A similar pattern of weight loss was seen in an 82 week open label completer analysis study (2.9 kg at 30 weeks, 5. 3 kg at 82 weeks) [52]. At week 156, patients completing 3 years of exenatide treatment (n = 217) continued to loose body weight (–5.3 ± 0.4 kg; 95% confidence interval [CI]: –6.0 to –4.5 kg; P <0.0001) [28]. In both insulin comparator trials, weight change favoured exenatide after only 2 weeks.

Significant reductions in Apo B (–5.2 mg/dl) and triglycerides (-73 mg/dl), and increases in high-density lipoprotein-cholesterol (HDL-C) (+4.5 mg/dl) have been seen compared to placebo [52]. Total and low-density lipoprotein-cholesterol (LDL-C) were also reduced (-7.3 mg /dl and –4.4 mg/dl), while LDL-C/HDL-C and TC/HDL-C ratios both fell (–0.37 and –0.73, respectively). Systolic and diastolic blood pressures were also reduced using exenatide for 82 weeks by 6.3 mm.Hg and 4.1 mm.Hg, respectively.

Safety and tolerability of exenatide

The main reported adverse events are gastrointestinal, occurring in a dose-dependent manner in 39% and 48% of subjects receiving 5 µg or 10 µg exenatide, respectively. Symptoms peaking after 8 weeks and declining thereafter and resulting in study withdrawal in only 2% (5 µg) and 4% (10 µg) of subjects, respectively.The etiology of nausea is not fully clear, but may be related to the delay in gastric emptying. Nausea did not seem to be the predominant factor in the weight loss induced by exenatide, as there was no significant correlation between change in body weight and the duration of nausea.

Consistent with the glucose-dependent insulinotropic effect of exenatide, hypoglycemia caused by the drug is generally uncommon and mild-to-moderate in severity. Studies in healthy volunteers suggest that glucagon and other hormonal counter-regulatory responses to hypoglycemia are preserved with short-term administration of exenatide [53]. In clinical trials using metformin alone as background treatment, the frequency of hypoglycemia in the exenatide and placebo groups was similar. However, hypoglycemia was more frequent with exenatide compared with placebo in trials that included a SU as background therapy. The incidence and severity of hypoglycemia with exenatide treatment were similar when compared with insulin glargine and biphasic insulin aspart, which may be due in part due to the moderate insulin doses used in these studies. Nocturnal hypoglycaemia was, however, lower with exenatide compared with either glargine or biphasic insulin (–1.6 and –0.9 events per patient-year).

Anti-exenatide antibodies were present in 41% to 49% of subjects receiving exenatide, although the clinical significance is unclear [54]. The antibodies were generally in low titre and were not predictive of glycaemic control or adverse events.

In the post-marketing period, 30 cases of pancreatitis possibly caused by exenatide were reported from the date of the drugs approval through to 31 December 2006 [55], although the frequency of pancreatitis did not appear to be significantly greater than that observed in the background population of patients with type 2 diabetes.

GLP1 – Analogues under development

Liraglutide is another GLP-1 analog with a long duration of action (half-life of around 12 h) owing to its stability against DPP-4, albumin-binding acylated side chain, and self-association, resulting in slow absorption from subcutaneous tissue [56] . It is given by a single daily SC injection [56], and is currently under evaluation in Phase III trials. In the largest randomised trial published to date, Liraglutide Effect and Action in Diabetes 3 (LEAD) [57], 746 patients with early type 2 diabetes were randomly assigned to once daily liraglutide (1.2 mg [*n* = 251] or 1.8 mg [*n* = 247]) or glimepiride 8 mg (*n* = 248) for 52 weeks, with the primary outcome being change in HbA1c. At 52 weeks, HbA1c decreased by 0.51% with glimepiride, compared with 0.84% with liraglutide 1.2 mg (difference –0.33%; 95%CI –0.53 to –0.13, *P* = 0.0014) and 1.14% with liraglutide 1.8 mg (-0.62; –0.83 to –0.42, *P* <0.0001). Five patients in the liraglutide 1.2 mg, and one in 1.8 mg groups discontinued treatment because of vomiting, whereas none in the glimepiride group did so, while subjects receiving liraglutide 1.8 mg od had a reduction in body weight of 3.5 kg as opposed to 0.8 kg weight gain in the glimeparide group.

The effects of a long-acting release (LAR) formulation were assessed in a 15 week placebo-controlled study [58] in which exenatide LAR was given once weekly at doses of 0.8 mg and 2.0 mg suboptimally controlled with metformin and / or diet and exercise with mean duration of diabetes of around 5 years and mean baseline HbA1c 8.5%. From baseline to week 15, exenatide LAR reduced mean HbA1c by –1.4 +/– 0.3% (0.8 mg) and –1.7 +/– 0.3% (2.0 mg), compared with +0.4 +/– 0.3% with placebo LAR (*P* <0.0001 for both). HbA1c of < or =7% was achieved by 36 and 86% of subjects receiving 0.8 and 2.0 mg exenatide LAR, respectively, compared with 0% of subjects receiving placebo LAR. Fasting plasma glucose was reduced by –2.4 +/– 0.9 mmol/l (0.8 mg) and –2.2 +/– 0.5 mmol/l (2.0 mg) compared with +1.0 +/– 0.7 mmol/l with placebo LAR (*P* <0.001 for both). Exenatide LAR reduced self-monitored postprandial hyperglycemia. Subjects receiving 2.0 mg exenatide LAR had body weight reductions (-3.8 +/– 1.4 kg) (*P* <0.05), whereas body weight was unchanged with both placebo LAR and the 0.8-mg dose. Mild nausea was the most frequent adverse event, with no subjects withdrawing from the study. Thus based on these early results both liraglutide and exenatide LAR appear to be promising therapeutic entities.

DPP-4 INHIBITORS

DPP-4 is the key enzyme responsible for the degradation of GLP-1 and GIP. Hence the inhibition of this enzyme augments endogenous plasma concentrations of GLP-1 and GIP [59]. Although the precise substrates important for DPP-4 action in subjects with type 2 diabetes remains unclear, disruption of GLP-1 and GIP receptors in mice completely eliminates the glucose-lowering properties of DPP-4 inhibitors [60]. Treating diabetic rodents with DPP-4 inhibitors improves islet survival and maintains β-cell mass and islet function [61]. These agents are administered orally and metabolised either by hydrolysis in the liver (vildagliptin) or primary clearance via the kidneys (sitagliptin). These agents are reported to have no impact on satiety or body weight.

In addition to its impact on GLP-1 and GIP, inhibition of DPP-4 is non-specific and may potentially affect other peptides including peptide tyrosine tyrosine (YY), endomorphin, neuropeptide Y, growth hormone releasing hormone, GLP-2, vasoactive intestinal polypeptide as well as paracrine chemokines, stromal cell-derived factor, eotaxin and macrophage-derived chemokine that are involved in regulatory systems [62]. It is also recognised that DPP-4 is a membrane-associated molecule on the surface of T-cells (where it is also known as CD26) and has a function in the immune system by contributing to T-cell activation and proliferation [63]. It has been suggested that GLP-2 acts as an intestinal growth factor [64]. Although DPP-4 inhibition is likely to cause a lesser increase in the concentration of active GLP-2 than that observed for GLP-1, DPP-4 inhibitors may thus also have effects on intestinal proliferation.

Sitagliptin is currently available in the UK at a dose of 100 mg od orally and licensed for use as an add-on therapy to either metformin or a sulphonylurea. Clinical studies have shown it to reduce HbA1c, by around 0.7%, as well as reducing postprandial fasting plasma glucose and proinsulin–insulin ratio [65]. Vildagliptin has also recently been licensed for use in the UK at a dose of 100 mg daily and demonstrates similar effects on HbA1c and glucose homesostasis [66].

The two available DPP-4 inhibitors have not been compared directly, but both appeared to lower HbA1c similarly compared with placebo (–0.74% vs. –0.73% for sitagliptin and vildagliptin respectively).

DPP-4 INHIBITORS IN COMPARISON WITH EXISTING THERAPY

Sulphonylureas

In a non-inferiority trial, sitagliptin was compared with glipizide as add-on therapy in > 1000 patients with inadequate glycemic control on metformin [67]. After 52 weeks, both groups had similar reductions in HbA1c values of approximately 0.7% versus baseline. However, the mean daily dose of glipizide was submaximal (around 10 mg), and withdrawal rates due to lack of efficacy were higher with sitagliptin compared with glipizide: 86 of 588 patients (15%) versus 58 of 584 (10%) patients [67]. On the other hand, sitagliptin was associated with lower rates of hypoglycemia (5 vs. 32% of patients), and weight loss of 1.5 kg compared with 1.1 kg of weight gain with glipizide [67].

Metformin

In a non-inferiority trial, vildagliptin (50 mg bd) was compared with metformin (1000 mg bd) in 780 drug-naïve patients. After 52 weeks, the average reductions in HbA1c values from baseline were significantly greater with metformin compared with vildaglitin: 1.4 and 1.0%, respectively [68]. In another trial of 24-week duration, the placebo-subtracted reductions in HbA1c values with sitagliptin (100 mg once daily), metformin (500 mg bd) and metformin (1000 mg bd) were 0.8, 1.0, and 1.3%, respectively. In these studies there was no significant difference in hypoglycaemia or weight between metformin and DPP-4 inhibitor treated groups, however, GI side-effects were significantly greater with metformin.

Thiazolidinediones

In drug-naïve patients with type 2 diabetes, vildagliptin (50 mg bd) and rosiglitazone (8 mg once daily) decreased HbA1c values by 1.1 and 1.3%, respectively, after 24 weeks, meeting the statistical criterion of non-inferiority of vildagliptin relative to rosiglitazone. Patients on rosiglitazone had an average weight gain of 1.6 kg, while vildagliptin had no effect on weight [69]. In another trial including patients with type 2 diabetes inadequately controlled on metformin (mean HbA1c 8.4%), additional treatment with vildagliptin (50 mg bd) was compared with pioglitazone given in submaximal doses (30 mg/day) [70]. After 24 weeks, the reductions in mean HbA1c values were similar in the vildagliptin and pioglitazone groups: 0.9 and 1.0%, respectively. Mean weight gain was significantly greater in the pioglitazone group compared with the vildagliptin group – 1.9 and 0.3 kg, respectively.

SAFETY OF DPP-4 INHIBITORS

Both sitagliptin and vildagliptin appear to be well tolerated. Withdrawal rates in patients randomised to either agent being similar to placebo. A recent meta-analysis suggested that the commonest adverse effects reported in slightly higher proportions of patients receiving sitagliptin or vildagliptin were nasopharyngitis (6.4 vs. 6.1% vs. comparator, risk ratio 1.2), urinary tract infection (3.2 vs. 2.4% with placebo, risk ratio 1.5) and headache (5.1 vs. 3.9% with placebo, risk ratio 1.4) [66]. Available data suggest that DPP-4 inhibitors may be better tolerated than metformin, glipizide and acarbose [66]. There was no difference in reported mild to moderate hypoglycemia between DPP-4 inhibitors and a comparator group (1.6% vs 1.4%, respectively; risk ratio 1.0). Hypoglycemia did become more evident when DPP-4 inhibitors were used in conjunction with SU, with the proportions of patients reporting hypoglycemia being 12% (27 of 222) and 1.8% (4 of 219) in patients receiving sitagliptin plus glimepiride versus patients receiving glimepiride plus placebo, respectively [71].

ROLE OF INCRETIN THERAPIES IN CLINICAL PRACTICE

There is no doubt that incretin-based drugs represent a useful addition to the existing arma-mentarium of antidiabetic drugs. These agents have several advantages. First, because of their distinct mechanism of action, they generally exert a beneficial effect on glycemic con-trol, irrespective of the type of background oral agents. Second, by targeting postprandial hyperglycemia more than fasting or pre-meal hyperglycemia, they complement the action of metformin, TZD, and long-acting SU, which act mainly by lowering fasting plasma glu-cose. A third advantage is the progressive weight loss caused by exenatide, and the weight-neutral effect of the DPP-4 inhibitors. Fourth, the use of incretin-related agents is uncommonly associated with severe hypoglycemia. Moreover, the use of DPP-4 inhibitors is simple, with once or twice-daily oral dosing irrespective of meal intake.

Meanwhile, exenatide and current DPP-4 inhibitors have important limitations. First, it should be emphasized that 50% of patients in clinical trials failed to achieve HbA1c levels < 7.0%. Second, exenatide has to be injected twice daily, and is associated with high rates of nausea, although tolerance to nausea appears to develop over time and a dose escalation protocol for exenatide appears to minimise the gastrointestinal adverse effects. Third, while the short-term (≤ 1 year) safety profile of two DPP-4 inhibitors – sitagliptin and vildaglitin – is reassuring, there are still some unresolved issues related to their safety. For instance, the enzyme DPP-4 plays an important role in the immune system, being a T-cell co-stimulator [72]; this raises concern about possible immune suppression as result of DPP-4 inhibition. In addition to GLP-1 and GIP, DPP-4 inhibits the degradation of other peptides *in vitro*, such as substance P [50]. Thus, there is a possibility that serum levels of such peptides may rise with the use of DPP-4 inhibitors leading to potential undesired effects. There are also two other enzymes, DPP-8 and DPP-9, structurally related to DPP-4 but with largely unknown functions [72]. Although *in-vitro* data suggest that DPP-4 inhibitors display high selectivity for DPP-4, no *in-vivo* data are available.

In individual studies, DPP-4 inhibitors showed no characteristic pattern of adverse effects. However, a recent meta-analysis showed an increased risk of infections, such as urinary tract infection and nasopharyngitis. Although the observed relative risk was small, its impli-cations in clinical practice are unclear and longer term evaluation is required. Potential skin toxicity also remains a consideration with DPP-4 inhibitors with a few serious cases of hypersensitivity reactions being reported possibly related to sitagliptin, including anaphy-laxis, angio-oedema and Stevens-Johnson syndrome.

On balance, incretin-based therapies, with modest glucose lowering effects, favourable weight profile, low hypoglycaemia risk and potentially positive effects on cardiovascular risk factors for exenatide, represent a useful alternative to and may offer an advantage over currently available hypoglycaemic agents. Hypoglycemia may still be an issue, especially if incretin therapy is combined with an insulin secretagogue; therefore, when incretin therapy is co-administered with such agents, the dose of the latter should be adjusted to minimise hypoglycemia.

Metformin will remain the drug of choice for initial treatment of type 2 diabetes due to its long-term safety, efficacy and low cost [73]. Meanwhile, based on the available data, and while longer term efficacy, safety and cost-effectiveness evaluation is awaited, incretin-based therapies may be of particular benefit in specific situations:

Exenatide / GLP-analogue therapy

The most recent blood glucose lowering guidelines from the National Institute for Clinical Excellence (NICE) in the UK [74] suggest that such agents may be considered for use in patients with suboptimal glycaemic control, with ongoing metformin / sulphonylurea combination therapy if a person is:

- Obese (a body mass index (BMI) ≥ 35 kg/m^2) in those of European descent, with appropriate adjustment for other ethnic groups and other specific psychological or medical problems associated with high body weight.
- Overweight (BMI < 35 kg/m^2) and for whom initiation of insulin therapy would have significant occupational implications, or where weight loss would benefit other significant comorbidities such as sleep apnoea.
- Therapy should be only be continued following an appropriate assessment of efficacy and safety, e.g. 1% reduction in HbA1c at 6 months and 5% weight loss after 1 year.

The above approach to the use of these agents, while providing some useful guidance, may be considered as somewhat over prescriptive in nature. Given their high cost and subcutaneous method of administration, it is unlikely that they would gain widespread support for second-line use following metformin monotherapy failure. However, such agents would make a sensible second-line therapy choice for people in who weight loss is a crucial therapeutic priority (e.g. obstructive sleep apnoea and non-alcoholic steatohepatosis).

When considering stipulations around discontinuation of therapy, this is an area where the effects of therapy on both weight and glycaemic control should be assessed on an individual patient basis with the decision to continue treatment or otherwise based on the overall clinical picture, including an evaluation of the potential limitations of alternative therapy options.

The most recent American Diabetes Association / European Association for the Study of Diabetes (ADA / EASD) consensus algorithm for the management of blood glucose in type 2 diabetes [75], suggests that exenatide should only be considered when weight loss is a major consideration and the HbA1c level close to target (<8%). This suggested approach is based on reductions in HbA1c of 0. 5–1% seen in clinical trials with exenatide. It is, however, noteworthy that greater reductions in HbA1c have been noted (1–1.5%) in patients with higher baseline HbA1c levels and that these reductions may be maintained for up to 82 weeks of therapy. Thus to define the clinical indication for such agents based on the minimal reported glucose lowering effects set in the context of a population-based glycaemic target approach as opposed to a more individualised approach may lead to significant numbers of patients who would otherwise gain benefit either in terms of weight and glucose reduction being denied treatment.

When deciding between the use of GLP-analogue therapy and insulin, the progression of type 2 diabetes along with the expected improvement in HbA1c as compared with the individualised patient glycaemic are important considerations. In particular if hyperglycaemia is sufficiently pronounced that the addition of GLP-analogue therapy is unlikely to achieve the desired HbA1c target then insulin would be a more appropriate therapy choice.

DPP-4 inhibitors

The relatively high cost, limited long-term safety data and modest glucose lowering efficacy means that DPP-4 inhibitors should not generally replace a sulphonylurea as second-line therapy at this time. These agents may, however, be considered as an alternative to a sulphonylurea in a range of circumstances. These include people for who hypoglycaemia and / or weight gain are of particular concern, although there is insufficient data currently available to define a threshold BMI above which the use of a DPP-4 inhibitor would be particularly appropriate. Rather the potential weight / hypoglycaemia benefits of these agents should be evaluated on an individual patient basis. When considering the use of second-line oral agents in patients with suboptimal glycaemic control on metformin monotherapy, a DPP-4 inhibitor may be more appropriate than a TZD in patients where fracture risk or congestive cardiac failure are a concern or in who further weight gain would exacerbate psychological or medical problems associated with a high body weight. A DPP-4 inhibitor may be considered as add-on therapy to patients with suboptimal glucose control receiving sulphonylurea monotherapy, where the person does not tolerate metformin or it is contraindicated.

If metformin in combination with a sulfonylurea does not adequately control blood glucose (HbA1c ≤ 7.5%) and injection-based therapies such as insulin or GLP-1 analogues are inappropriate then a DPP-4 inhibitor is an appropriate third-line therapy alternative to a TZD based on the considerations outlined above.

The most recent ADA / EASD consensus guidance on the management of blood glucose in type 2 diabetes [75] do not include DPP-4 inhibitors based on their limited clinical data and relative expense. While the absence of long-term data will currently preclude the widespread adoption of this class as a preferred second-line therapy, it is important to remember that these agents have been studied in a wide variety of clinical scenarios over periods of up to 1 year. Furthermore, in an era of ever tighter glycaemic targets there is not only considerable patient morbidity but also cost implications associated with managing hypoglycaemia, weight gain and congestive heart failure risk associated with achieving HbA1c targets of < 7% with more established therapies such as sulphonylureas and TZDs.

The decision to continue DPP-4 inhibitor therapy should be based on an individual patient assessment and not simply guided by the achievement of a prespecified Hba1c reduction, taking into consideration the individualized HbA1c target, comorbid conditions and the limitations of alternative therapy options.

SUMMARY

Type 2 diabetes is a complex and progressive disorder that is difficult to effectively treat in the long term. The majority of patients are obese or overweight and find difficulty is sustaining glycaemic control without multiple oral therapies, with a sizeable proportion requiring exogenous insulin. This characteristic need for therapeutic escalation reflects progressive loss of β-cell function combined with obesity-related insulin resistance. The management of type 2 diabetes has never before been so complex, with a variety of differing classes of hypoglycaemic therapies comprising heterogeneous modes of action, safety and tolerability profiles. These classes include agents that stimulate insulin secretion (sulphonylureas, insulin secretagogues and incretin mimetics), agents that reduce hepatic glucose output (biguanides), and agents that improve insulin sensitivity (thaizolidinediones) The UKPDS (United Kingdom Prospective Diabetes Study) demonstrated the benefits of intensive blood glucose control on microvascular complications, while metformin was demonstrated to improve macrovascular outcomes in obese patients. The STENO-2 study demonstrated that a target driven multifactorial approach based around a sulphonylurea was associated with improved macrovascular and microvascular outcomes. Recent studies using thiazolidinediones have suggested improved cardiovascular outcomes with pioglitazone and benefits around sustained glycaemic control with rosiglitazone, although safety concerns have been raised around potential cardiovascular adverse events with rosiglitazone and an increased fracture risk with the class as a whole. The selection of initial monotherapy is based on both clinical and biochemical patient factors, insulin may be the treatment of choice where non-pharmacological intervention has failed. Oral therapies should be initiated at low dose and titrated according to glycaemic response. The average glucose lowering effects of the individual agents is broadly similar (1–2% reduction in HbA1c). Doses are gradually increased according to response, although maximal glucose lowering effects occur at between 50–75% of the recommended maximum daily dose. With an increasing recognition of the benefits of intensive glucose reduction combination therapy is required in the majority of patients.

Considerable advances have been made over the last few years in understanding the endocrine connections that link the gastrointestinal tract and the pancreatic islet. New therapies that enhance the incretin effect will increasingly become more widely available to both clinicians and patients in day-to-day practice. The possibility of a once weekly preparation of some of these agents in the future holds much promise. DPP-4 inhibitors as oral preparations may have advantages over the parenterally administered GLP-1 analogues. However, they are weight neutral and it must be remembered that DPP-4 is a ubiquitous enzyme with the potential to inhibit various other peptides and there is much more to learn about the long-term side-effects of these agents. Having said that, the potential for these agents to improve β-cell mass, durability and function is an exciting prospect for a metabolic condition that inevitably progresses in spite of optimum treatment.

REFERENCES

1. UK prospective diabetes study group. Intensive blood glucose control with sulphonylureas or insulin compared with conventional treatment and risk of complications in patients with type 2 diabetes (UKPDS 33). *Lancet* 1998; 352:837–853.
2. Holman RR, Paul SK, Bethel MA, Matthews DR, Neil HA. 10 year follow up of intensive blood glucaoe control in type 2 diabetes. *N Engl J Med* 2008; 359:1577–1589.
3. Gerstein HC, Miller ME, Byington RP *et al*. Effects of intensive blood glucose lowering in type 2 diabetes. Action to Control Cardiovascular Risk in Diabetes Study Group. *N Engl J Med* 2008; 358:2545–2559.
4. Alvarez-Guisasola F *et al*. Hypoglycaemic symptoms, treatment satisfaction, adherence and their associations with glycaemic goal in patients with type 2 diabetes mellitus: findings from the Real-Life Effectiveness and Care Patterns of Diabetes Management (RECAP-DM) Study. *Diabetes Ob Metab* 2008; 10(suppl 1):25–32.
5. Gaede P, Vedel P, Larsen N *et al*. Multifactorial intervention and cardiovascular disease in patients with type 2 diabetes. *N Engl J Med* 2003; 348:385–393.
6. Rajagopalan S, Alemao E, Finch L, Yin D. Impact of new Joint British Societies' (JBS 2) guidelines on prevention of cardiovascular disease: evaluation of serum total cholesterol goal achievement in UK clinical practice. *Curr Med Res Opin* 2007; 23:2027–2034.
7. Turner RC, Cull CA, Frighi V *et al*. Glycaemic control with diet, sulphonylureas, metformin or insulin in patients with type 2 diabetes: progressive requirements for multiple therapies. *JAMA* 1999; 281:2005–2012.
8. Khan SE, Haffner SM, Heise MA *et al*, ADOPT Study Group. Glycaemic durability of rosiglitazone, metformin, or glyburide monotherapy. *N Engl J Med* 2006; 355:2427–2443.
9. UK prospective diabetes study group. Effect of intensive blood glucose control with metformin on complications in overweight patients with type 2 diabetes. (UKPDS 34). *Lancet* 1998; 352:854–865.
10. Patel A, MacMahon S, Chalmers J *et al*, ADVANCE Collaborative Group. Intensive blood glucose control and cardiovascular outcomes in type 2 diabetes. *N Engl J Med* 2008; 358:2560–2572.
11. Ashcroft FM, Gribble FM. ATP sensitive K+ channels and insulin secretion: their role in health and disease. *Diabetologia* 1999; 42:903–919.
12. Rosrsman P, Renstrom E. Insulin granule dynamics in pancreatic beta cells. *Diabetologia* 2003; 46:1029–1045.
13. Rendell M. The role of sulphonylureas in the management of type 2 diabetes. *Drugs* 2004; 64:1339–1358.
14. Yki-Jarvinen H. Combination therapies with insulin in type 2 diabetes. *Diabetes Care* 2001; 24:756–767.
15. Bailey CJ, Day C. Antidiabetic drugs. *Br J Cardiol* 2003; 10:128–136.
16. Krentz AJ, Bailey CJ. Oral antidiabetic agents – current role in type 2 diabetes. *Drugs* 2006; 65:385–411.
17. Gribble FM, Reiman F. Pharmacological modulation of KATP channels. *Biochem Soc Trans* 2002; 46:1029–1045.

18. Rosiglitazone evaluated for cardiovascular outcomes – an interim analysis; Home PD on behalf of the RECORD study investigators. *N Engl J Med* 2007; 357.
19. Weyer C, Bogardus C, Mott DM, Pratley RE. The natural history of insulin secretory dysfunction and insulin resistance in the pathogenesis of type 2 diabetes mellitus. *J Clin Invest* 1999; 104:787–794.
20. Monnier L, Lapinski H, Colette C. Contributions of fasting and postprandial plasma glucose increments to the overall diurnal hyperglycaemia of type 2 diabetic patients: variations with increasing levels of HbA_{1c}. *Diabetes Care* 2003; 26:881–885.
21. Landgraf R. Meglitinide analogues in the treatment of type 2 diabetes. *Drugs Aging* 200; 17:411–425.
22. Lebowitz HE. Alpha glucosidae inhibitors in the treatement of diabetes. *Diabetes Rev* 1998; 6:132–145.
23. Chiasson J-L, Cull CA, Gomis R *et al*. Acarbosr and the risk of hypertension and cardiovascular disease in patients with impaired glucose tolerance. The STOP-NIDDM Trial Research Group. *JAMA* 200; 290:486–494.
24. Reaven GM. Role of insulin resistance in health and disease. *Diabetes* 1998; 37:1595–1607.
25. Cusi K, DeFronzo RA. Metformin: a review of its metabolic effects. *Diabetes Rev* 1998; 6:89–131.
26. Winder WW, Hardie G. AMP-activated protein kinase, a metabolic master switch: possible roles in type 2 diabetes. *Am J Physiol* 1999; 277:E1–E10.
27. Hermann LS, Lindberg G, Lindblad U *et al*. Efficacy, effectiveness and safety of sulphonylurea-metformin combination therapy in patients with type 2 diabetes. *Diabetes Obese Metab* 2002; 4:296–304.
28. De-Fronzo RA. Pharmacologic therapy for type 2 diabetes mellitus. *Ann Intern Med* 1999; 131:281–303.
29. Johnson JA, Majumdar SR, Simpson SH. Decreased mortality associated with sulphonylurea monotherapy in type 2 diabetes. *Diabetes Care* 25; 2244–2248.
30. Moore B, Edie ES, Abram JH. On the treatment of diabetes mellitus by acid extract of duodenal mucous membrane. *Biochem J* 1906; 1:28–38.
31. Kieffer TJ, Habener JF. The glucagon-like peptides. *Endocr Rev* 1999; 20:876–913.
32. Ebert R. Gut signals for islet hormone release. *Eur J Clin Invest* 1990; 20(suppl 1):S20–S26.
33. Fieseler P, Bridenbaugh S, Nustede R *et al*. Physiological augmentation of amino acid induced insulin secretion by GIP and GLP-1 but not by CCK-8. *Am J Physiol* 1995; 268(5 Pt 1):E949–E955.
34. Creutzfeldt W, Nauck M. Gut hormones and diabetes mellitus. *Diabetes Metab Rev* 1992; 8:149–177.
35. Nauck MA, Homberger E, Siegel EG *et al*. Incretin effects of increasing glucose loads in man calculated from venous insulin and C-peptide responses. *J Clin Endocrinol Metab* 1986; 63:492–498.
36. Bell GI, Sanches-Pescador R, Laybourn PJ *et al*. Exon duplication and divergence in the human preproglucagon gene. *Nature* 1983; 304:368–371.
37. Kashima Y, Miki T, Shibasaki T *et al*. Critical role of cAMP-GEF-II-Rim 2 complex in incretin-potentiated insulin secretion. *J Biol Chem* 2001; 276:46046–46053.
38. Vahl TP, Paty BW, Fuller BD *et al*. Effects of GLP-1 (7-36) NH_2, GLP-1 (7-37), and GLP-1 (9-36) NH_2, on intravenous glucose tolerance and glucose induced insulin secretion in healthy humans. *J Clin Endocrinol Metab* 2003; 88:1772–1779.
39. Wettergren A, Wojdemann M, Holst JJ. The inhibitory effect of GLP-1 (7-36) amide on antral motility and is antagonised by its N-terminally truncated primary metabolite GLP-1 (9-36) amide. *Peptides* 1998; 19:877–882.
40. Levy JC. Therapeutic intervention in the GLP-1 pathway in type 2 diabetes. *Diabetic Medicine* 2006; 23(suppl 1):14–19.
41. Kieffer TJ, Habener JF. The glucagon-like peptides. *Endocr Rev* 1999; 20:876–913.
42. Xu G, Stoffers DA, Habener JF *et al*. Exendin-4 stimulates both beta cell replication and neogenesis, resulting in increased beta cell mass and improved glucose tolerance in diabetic rats. *Diabetes* 1999; 48:2270–2276.
43. Munro N, Levy J, Gayar HE *et al*. New therapies for diabetes: incretin mimetics and gliptins. *Diabetes and Primary Care* 2007; 9:72–80.
44. DeFronzo RA, Ratner RE, Han J *et al*. Effects of exenatide (Exendin-4) on glycemic control over 30 weeks in metformin-treated patients with type 2 diabetes. *Diabetes Care* 2005; 28:1092–1099.
45. Buse JB, Henry RR, Han J *et al*. Effects of exenatide (Exendin-4) on glycemic control over 30 weeks in sulfonylurea-treated patients with type 2 diabetes. *Diabetes Care* 2004; 27:2628–2635.
46. Kendall DM, Riddle MC, Rosenstock J *et al*. Effects of exenatide (Exendin 4 on glycemic control over 30 weeks in patients with type 2 diabetes treated with metformin and a sulfonylurea. *Diabetes Care* 2005; 28:1083–1091.
47. Zinman B, Hoogwerf BJ, Garcia SD *et al*. The effect of adding exenatide or a thiazolidinedione in suboptimally controlled type 2 diabetes. *Ann Intern Med* 2007; 146:477–485.

48. Heine RJ, Van Gaal LF, Johns D et al, GWAA Study Group. Exenatide versus insulin glargine in patients with suboptimally controlled type 2 diabetes. A randomized trial. *Ann Intern Med* 2005; 143:559–569.

49. Nauck MA, Duran S, Kim D et al. A comparison of twice-daily exenatide and biphasic insulin aspart in patients with type 2 diabetes who were suboptimally controlled with sulfonylurea and metformin: a non-inferiority trial. *Diabetologia* 2007; 50:259–267.

50. Davis SN, Johns D, Maggs D et al. Exploring the substitution of exenatide for insulin in patients with type 2 diabetes treated with insulin in combination with oral antidiabetes agents. *Diabetes Care* 2007; 30:2767–2772.

51. Klonoff DC, Buse JB, Nielsen LL et al. Exenatide effects on diabetes, obesity, cardiovascular risk factors and hepatic biomarkers in patients with type 2 diabetes treated for at least 3 years. *Curr Med Res Opin* 2008; 24:275–286.

52. Ratner RE, Maggs D, Nielsen LL et al. Long-term effects of exenatide therapy over 82 weeks on glycaemic control and weight in over-weight metformin-treated patients with type 2 diabetes mellitus. *Diabetes Obes Metab* 2006; 8:419–428.

53. Degn KB, Brock B, Juhl CB et al. Effect of intravenous infusion of exenatide (synthetic exendin-4) on glucose-dependent insulin secretion and counterregulation during hypoglycemia. *Diabetes* 2004; 53:2397–2403.

54. Cvetković RS, Plosker GL. Exenatide: a review of its use in patients with type 2 diabetes mellitus (as an adjunct to metformin and/or a sulfonylurea). *Drugs* 2007; 67:935–954.

55. Ahmad SR, Swann J. Exenatide and rare adverse events [letter]. *N Engl J Med* 2008; 358:1970–1972.

56. Harder H, Mscodont LN, Thi TDT, Drmedski AA. The effect of liraglutide, long-acting glucagon-like peptide 1 derivative, on glycemic control, body composition, and 24 h energy expenditure in patients with type 2 diabetes. *Diabetes Care* 2004; 27:1915–1921.

57. Garber A, Henry R, Ratner R et al.; LEAD-3 (Mono) Study Group. Liraglutide versus glimepiride monotherapy for type 2 diabetes (LEAD-3 Mono): a randomised, 52-week, phase III, double-blind, parallel-treatment trial. *Lancet* 2009; 373:473–481.

58. Kim D, McConnell L, Zhunag D et al. Effects of once-weekly dosing of a long-acting release formulation of exenatide on glucose control and body weight in subjects with type 2 diabetes. *Diabetes Care* 2007; 30:1487–1493.

59. Holst JJ, Deacon CF. Inhibition of the activity of dipeptidyl-peptidase IV as a treatment for type 2 diabetes. *Diabetes* 1998; 47:1663–1670.

60. Hansotia T, Baggio LL, Delmeire D et al. Double incretin receptor knockout (DIRKO) mice reveal an essential role for the enteroinsular axis in transducing the glucoregulatory actions of DPP IV inhibitors. *Diabetes* 2004; 53:1326–1335.

61. Reimer MK, Holst JJ, Ahren B. Long term inhibition of dipeptidyl peptidase IV improves glucose tolerance and preserves islet function in mice. *Eur J Endocrinol* 2002; 146:717–727.

62. Mentlein R. Dipeptidyl-peptidase IV (CD26)-role in the inactivation of regulatory peptides. *Regul Pept* 1999; 85:9–24.

63. Fleischer B. CD26: a surface protease involved in T-cell activation. *Immunol Today* 1994; 15:180–184.

64. Drucker DJ, Ehrlich P, Asa SL et al. Induction of intestinal epithelial proliferation by glucagon-like peptide 2. *Proc Natl Acad Sci USA* 1996; 93:7911–7916.

65. Aschner P, Kipnes MS, Lunceford JK et al. Effect of the dipeptidyl peptidase-4 inhibitor sitagliptin as monotherapy on glycaemic control in patients with type 2 diabetes. *Diabetes Care* 2006; 29:2632–2637.

66. Rosenstock J, Zinman B. Dipeptidyl peptidase-4 inhibitors and the management of type 2 diabetes mellitus. *Curr Opin Endocrinol Diabetes Obes* 2007; 14:98–107.

67. Nauck MA, Meininger G, Sheng D et al, Sitagliptin Study 024 Group. Efficacy and safety of the dipeptidyl peptidase-4 inhibitor, sitagliptin compared with the sulfonylurea, glipizide, in patients with type 2 diabetes inadequately controlled on metformin alone: a randomized, double-blind, non-inferiority trial. *Diabetes Obes Metab* 2007; 9:194–205.

68. Schweizer A, Couturier A, Foley JE, Dejager S. Comparison between vildagliptin and metformin to sustain reductions in HbA(1c) over 1 year in drug-naïve patients with type 2 diabetes. *Diabet Med* 2007; 24:955–961.

69. Rosenstock J, Baron MA, Dejager S et al. Comparison of vildagliptin and rosiglitazone monotherapy in patients with type 2 diabetes. *Diabetes Care* 2007; 30:217–223.

70. Bolli G, Dotta F, Rochette E, Cohen SE. Efficacy and tolerability of vildagliptin vs. pioglitazone when added to metformin: a 24-week, randomized, double-blind study. *Diabetes Obes Metab* 2008; 10:82–90.

71. Hermansen K, Kipnes M, Luo E *et al*, Sitagliptin Study 035 Group. Efficacy and safety of the dipeptidyl peptidase-4-inhibitor, sitagliptin, in patients with type 2 diabetes inadequately controlled on glimepiride and metformin. *Diabetes Obes Metab* 2007; 9:733–745.

72. Barnett A. DPP-4 inhibitors and their potential role in the management of type 2 diabetes. *Int J Clin Pract* 2006; 60:1454–1470.

73. Bolen S, Feldman L, Vassy J *et al*. Systemic review: comparative effectiveness and safety of oral medications for type 2 diabetes mellitus. *Ann Intern Med* 2007; 147:386–399.

74. NICE blood glucose lowering guidelines May 2008

75. Nathan D, Buse JB, Davidson MB *et al*. Medical management of hyperglycaemia in type 2 diabetes: a consensus algorithm for the initiation and adjustment of therapy. *Diabetes Care* 2008; 31:1–11.

2

Insulin analogues

G. B. Bolli

INTRODUCTION

The modern goals of insulin replacement in type 1 and type 2 diabetes mellitus are the long-term maintenance of glycosylated haemoglobin (HbA1c) <6.5–7.0% whilst at the same time preventing hypoglycaemia (as well as the unawareness of the patient to their hypoglycaemia). In addition to appropriate education and motivation of diabetic subjects, the use of insulin analogues, both rapid- and long-acting, is critical to achieve these goals. The benefits of rapid-acting analogues (lispro, aspart and glulisine have similar pharmacodynamic effects and can therefore be used interchangeably) when compared with human unmodified regular insulin are:

■ Lower postprandial blood glucose.
■ Lower risk of late postprandial hypoglycaemia.
■ Better quality of life.

However, in type 1 diabetes, rapid-acting analogues improve HbA1c only by the extent to which replacement of basal insulin is optimised at the same time. This can be done either by multiple daily Neutral Protamine Hagedorn (NPH) insulin administrations or continuous subcutaneous insulin infusion, or the use of the long-acting insulin analogues glargine or detemir. In type 2 diabetes, rapid-acting insulin analogues reduce the 1- and 2-hour postprandial blood glucose, but systematic studies are needed to examine the long-term effects on HbA1c. The benefits of long-acting insulin analogues when compared with traditional NPH insulin are:

■ Lower risk of hypoglycaemia in the interprandial state (especially at night).
■ Lower variability of blood glucose.

When optimally combined, rapid- and long-acting insulin analogues maintain HbA1c at <7.0% over the long term better than human insulin with less hypoglycaemia, and preserve a better quality of life. In type 1 diabetes this regimen, based on insulin analogues, is not inferior to continuous subcutaneous insulin infusion (CSII) in terms of the goals of HbA1c preservation and prevention of hypoglycaemia.

> *'… in the end, I do not invent … instead I find it ready-made in nature, though I still have to extract it …'*
>
> Vincent Van Gogh, 1888

Geremia B. Bolli, MD, Professor of Internal Medicine, Consultant Cardiologist and Rheumatologist, Department of Internal Medicine, Endocrinology and Metabolism, University of Perugia, Perugia, Italy.

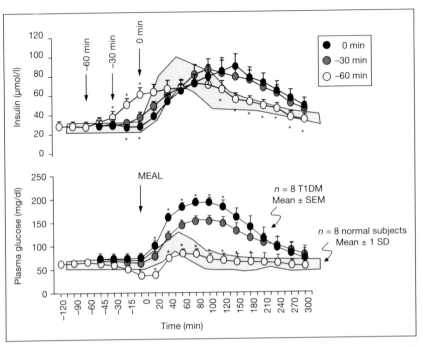

Figure 2.1 Effect of different time intervals between subcutaneous injection of human regular insulin and meal ingestion (0, 30, 60 min) on postprandial blood glucose control in subjects with type 1 diabetes mellitus (with permission from [8]).
SD = standard deviation; SEM = standard error of the mean; T1DM = type 1 diabetes mellitus.

More than 85 years after the discovery of insulin by Nicolae Paulescu in 1921 [1] and its subsequent and independent extraction from animal pancreata and use in humans for the first time in Toronto in 1922 [2, 3], the replacement of insulin in diabetes mellitus requiring insulin remains one of the major challenges in medicine. Insulin-treated subjects with type 1 diabetes mellitus continuously drift between hyper- and hypoglycaemia. If the former prevails, and the percentage of HbA1c remains elevated over the years, devastating long-term complications likely appear and unavoidably progress [4]. On the other hand, the condition of frequent, recurrent hypoglycaemia is not only dangerous and unpleasant for the patient, but may over time lead to the syndrome of hypoglycaemia unawareness [5]. In turn, hypoglycaemia unawareness is the major risk factor for subsequent episodes of severe hypoglycaemia [6, 7].

There are several reasons why it has been (and remains) so difficult to replace insulin in people with diabetes. Firstly, insulin is replaced in the wrong location, i.e. in the subcutaneous tissue (instead of the intravascular space), which drains into the peripheral rather than the portal circulation. This is responsible for slow insulin absorption at mealtimes, accompanied by an excessive increase in postprandial plasma glucose concentration (Figure 2.1) [8]. In addition, subcutaneous insulin delivery induces the systemic hyperinsulinaemia necessary to match the plasma portal physiological insulin concentrations, which are about 1.5–2 times greater than those found in the periphery [9]. Such a hyperinsulinaemia in the peripheral plasma concentration is itself a risk factor for hypoglycaemia, despite peripheral insulin resistance [10]. Secondly, insulin is injected at a time prior to eating and at a dose that cannot be ideal in terms of calculation of insulin absorption/peak and insulin sensitivity, despite optimal knowledge of the pharmacokinetics and pharmacodynamics of insulin preparations and despite carbohydrate counting [11].

Combining the above observations, it is no surprise that the current state of insulin replacement in people with diabetes is far from perfect. On the contrary, it is surprising that such a 'primitive' method of replacing insulin (subcutaneously), which is, after all, not that different from the method initiated in the early 1920s, indeed makes it possible to maintain HbA1c <7.0%, the level at which it protects from onset and/or progression of long-term complications [4].

At present, insulin analogues contribute to improving the outcome of the still imperfect method of subcutaneous insulin substitution by lowering the 1- and 2-hour postprandial blood glucose while minimising hypoglycaemia. In turn, this prevents and/or reverses unawareness of hypoglycaemia while still maintaining good glycaemic control (HbA1c <7.0%). This is in contrast to the early finding by the Diabetes Control and Complications Trial (DCCT) in 1993, where the lowering of HbA1c was associated with an approximately three-fold increase in risk for severe hypoglycaemia [4]. Thus, by reducing the risk of hypoglycaemia in intensive therapy, insulin analogues do a remarkable job in the good treatment of diabetes by maintaining intensive treatment over time in a large number of people who, on human insulin, would otherwise give up treatment because of frequent, intolerable hypoglycaemia.

In order to be successful, insulin replacement in people with diabetes should be based on the following criteria:

- Education of subjects by *educated doctors*.
- Use of modern insulin replacement regimens and insulin analogues.
- Awareness of the goals of treatment by both diabetic subjects and doctors.

In this chapter, the importance of the use of insulin analogues as a key tool in achieving good glycaemic control and prevent hypoglycaemia is emphasised.

PHYSIOLOGY OF PLASMA GLUCOSE HOMEOSTASIS

Normal, non-diabetic subjects maintain their plasma glucose below 100 mg/dl when fasting, and below 135 mg/dl in the postprandial period, even after a carbohydrate-rich meal [12]. In the fasting state, maintenance of normoglycaemia is possible because of the continuous release of insulin from the pancreas, which results in a flat, peak-free, steady plasma insulin concentration, which in turn restrains hepatic glucose production and prevents fasting hyperglycaemia. At mealtimes, the normal pancreas releases insulin very early in response to meal ingestion as indicated by the early and elevated peak in peripheral plasma. It can be estimated that the corresponding 'portal' plasma insulin concentrations of the prandial peaks seen in Figure 2.2 are nearly twice as elevated. This is what prevents postprandial hyperglycaemia. Equally important is the prompt decrease of plasma insulin 60–90 minutes after meal ingestion, which prevents hypoglycaemia in the postprandial state. Finally, the fact that between-meal plasma insulin is flat and peak-free as stated above helps preventing interprandial and fasting hypoglycaemia, especially during the nocturnal fasting hours.

Thus, nature's model of insulin dynamics should be mimicked whenever insulin is replaced in subjects with absent endogenous insulin secretion (type 1 diabetes), but also taken into consideration in those with impaired insulin response (type 2 diabetes).

In the fasting state, insulin should be replaced with a preparation of 'basal' insulin, reproducing a flat, peak-free concentration (Figure 2.2). In contrast, any basal insulin preparation that resulted in a peak in the fasting state would likely induce hypoglycaemia and any basal insulin that 'waned' during fasting would result in hyperglycaemia.

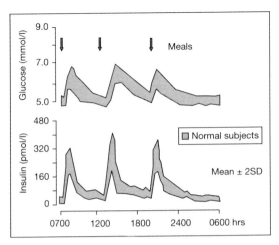

Figure 2.2 Physiology of glucose homeostasis in normal, non-diabetic subjects (with permission from [12]). SD = standard deviation.

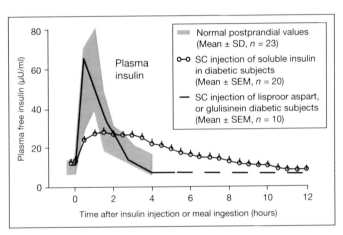

Figure 2.3 Pharmacokinetics following subcutaneous injection of regular, unmodified human insulin, and rapid-acting insulin analogues (data taken with permission from [13]).
SC = subcutaneous; SD = standard deviation; SEM = standard error of the mean.

At mealtimes, a bolus injection of rapid-acting insulin is needed to reproduce the early and elevated peak plasma insulin that coincides with carbohydrate ingestion. Ideally, the faster the time-to-peak of the injected prandial insulin preparation, the lower the increase in the postprandial hyperglycaemia. After meals, plasma insulin should then rapidly return to baseline levels. If plasma insulin remains elevated at the time at which carbohydrate absorption is completed, hypoglycaemia unavoidably develops. These are the theoretical considerations to bear in mind when comparing the superiority of insulin analogues (rapid-acting) with unmodified human insulin.

SUPERIORITY OF ANALOGUE VERSUS HUMAN UNMODIFIED INSULIN

In the early 1980s, human insulin was introduced with great emphasis on the belief that diabetic subjects would now be treated with the insulin secreted 'naturally' by the human body

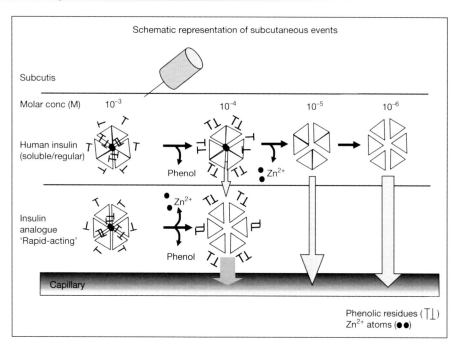

Figure 2.4 Slow and fast dissociation of hexamers of human insulin and insulin analogues in the subcutaneous tissue (with permission from [14]).

(in contrast with animal insulin). Better glycaemic control was expected in people with diabetes using human as compared to animal insulin. However, this was not the case, since no single advantage could be proved for human versus (purified) animal insulin, with the exception of the relevance of the innovation in production technology using the recombinant deoxyribonucleic acid (DNA) technique. Ironically, immediately after introducing human insulin, major efforts began to modify the human insulin molecule and develop 'analogues' (insulin designers) for administration to diabetic subjects. Thus, several insulin analogues were generated that, within a few years' time, replaced human insulin in the treatment of diabetes mellitus. The simple explanation of the short-lived popularity of human insulin is, of course, that human insulin works perfectly if delivered into the bloodstream as it occurs in people without diabetes (who secrete it into the portal system), but is much less efficient when injected into the subcutaneous tissue. Soluble human insulin should be 'rapid acting' in its action, but in reality this is not the case (Figure 2.3) [13]. This is due to the slow dissociation of hexamers into monomers in the subcutaneous tissue (Figure 2.4) [14], which delays the appearance of insulin in the plasma until *after* the absorption of carbohydrates and development of hyperglycaemia. This is the reason for hyperglycaemia soon after meal ingestion with subcutaneous injection of human insulin, combined (possibly) with late postprandial hypoglycaemia due to continuing absorption of insulin subsequent to absorption of the meal (Figure 2.1).

RAPID-ACTING INSULIN ANALOGUES

At present, there are three different rapid-acting insulin analogues, lispro, aspart and glulisine. All of these analogues are obtained using the technique of recombinant DNA, substituting or deleting one or more amino acids in regions of the insulin molecule that are not crucial for binding to the insulin receptor. These changes introduce repulsive electrical

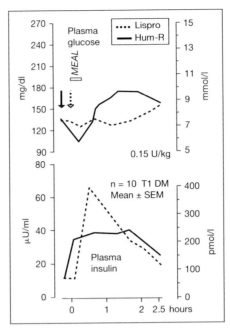

Figure 2.5 Better postprandial blood glucose after subcutaneous rapid-acting insulin analogue (lispro) versus regular, unmodified human insulin (with permission from [17]).
Hum-R = human regular insulin; SEM = standard error of the mean; T1DM = type 1 diabetes mellitus.

charges between monomer molecules, thus weakening the association forces within the hexamer when compared with human insulin. As a consequence, at the diluted concentrations found in the subcutaneous tissue, the hexamers of these analogues dissociate faster than those of unmodified human insulin, and appear in plasma with earlier and greater insulin peaks (Figures 2.3 and 2.4). Although lispro, aspart and glulisine are different molecules in terms of primary structure [15, 16], they exhibit similar pharmacokinetic and pharmacodynamic characteristics when compared with unmodified human regular insulin. Upon subcutaneous injection, all three of these rapid-acting analogues reach the status of monomeric insulin earlier than human regular insulin and are absorbed more rapidly, with no major differences between the three analogues. The earlier and greater plasma insulin peak achieved with these analogues controls postprandial plasma glucose more effectively than unmodified human soluble insulin (Figure 2.5) [17].

The advantages of rapid-acting analogues can be summarised as follows. Firstly, with the still 'primitive' injection of insulin into the subcutaneous tissue, it is nevertheless possible to mimic nature in terms of peak prandial insulin, and therefore to reduce postprandial hyperglycaemia when compared with human soluble insulin. Secondly, because of the early waning, insulin analogues reduce the risk of postprandial hypoglycaemia when compared with human soluble insulin. Thirdly, and perhaps most importantly, rapid-acting insulin analogues improve quality of life, since people with diabetes who require insulin can now 'inject and eat'. This is a great advantage when compared to previous years when diabetic people had to wait 15–45 minutes between injection of human (or animal) soluble insulin and meal ingestion, with the longest interval corresponding to the maximal improvement in postprandial blood glucose but also, of course, to a greatest risk of hypoglycaemia before or during the meal (Figure 2.1) [8].

At present, rapid-acting analogues are the *gold standard* of mealtime insulin replacement in people with diabetes. They should substitute human soluble insulin in all diabetic subjects, provided they are combined with optimal replacement of basal insulin (see below). Under these conditions, rapid-acting analogues lower the percentage of HbA1c and reduce the risk of hypoglycaemia [15]. The former goal reduces the risk of long-term complications [4], whereas the latter reduces the risk of hypoglycaemia unawareness [5]. The same question can be rephrased in different terms. At present, is there any role left for the use of soluble (rapid-acting) human insulin in people with diabetes? The answer is 'no' as long as the administration of insulin is in the subcutaneous tissue. The sole indication for the use of soluble (rapid-acting) human insulin remains intravenous administration since, using this route, rapid-acting analogues are not superior to human insulin.

Finally, comment should be made of the recently expressed view that rapid-acting insulin analogues should not be used in place of human soluble insulin since they would not 'improve glycaemic control' as measured by the percentage of HbA1c. This concept has been reiterated in three different publications by the same group of authors [18–20]. However, these papers [18–20] may be misleading and should be viewed with caution by diabetologists concerned about the good treatment of their patients. In fact, those authors [18–20] appear to confuse 'better glycaemic control' with 'lower HbA1c'. The reality is that rapid-acting insulin analogues on the one hand reduce the frequency of hypoglycaemia, and on the other reduce HbA1c *provided that basal insulin is optimally replaced* [15]. If basal insulin is not optimised, HbA1c does not decrease, but hypoglycaemia is still prevented [15]. Thus, firstly, rapid-acting insulin analogues always improve glycaemic control even in absence of changes in HbA1c levels. Secondly, when rapid-acting insulin analogues were introduced to the market in 1996, long-acting insulin analogues were not available and it was therefore also difficult to immediately optimise the replacement of basal insulin in the treatment of the general population with diabetes requiring insulin. However, it was soon demonstrated that rapid-acting analogues decreased HbA1c levels when used in pumps for CSII [21], the gold standard of basal insulin replacement. This was also demonstrated when replacement of basal insulin was optimised with multiple daily NPH administrations [22, 23]. Of course, it has really been seen with the recent introduction of glargine that the important beneficial effect of analogues on HbA1c has been proven [24, 25]. Nobody today would use a rapid-acting insulin analogue in the absence of its long-acting partner, whether it be glargine or detemir insulin. Thus, the claim that rapid-acting analogues are not superior to human regular insulin [18–20] is simply not the case, as witnessed by the fact that both rapid- and long-acting analogues, not rapid-acting analogues alone, are now used.

LONG-ACTING INSULIN ANALOGUES

NPH insulin, the first prolonged-acting insulin preparation invented by Hans Hagedorn in 1936 [26], reached the market in 1946. Since then, NPH has been the best-selling 'basal' insulin. However, when NPH is analysed with the glucose clamp technique [27] (Figure 2.6), it appears far from mimicking the flat, peak-free basal insulin of normal physiology that one would wish to replicate in people with diabetes (Figure 2.2). NPH has a peak 5–6 h after injection and wanes few hours later (Figure 2.6). Thus, when injected in the evening, the peak action of NPH increases the risk of hypoglycaemia after midnight. On the other hand, the relatively short duration of action of NPH makes it quite difficult to achieve near-normoglycaemia in the fasting state without increasing the risk of nocturnal hypoglycaemia. This is especially true in people with reduced or absent secretion of endogenous insulin (type 1 diabetes), who exhibit impaired glucose counter-regulation and reduced defences against hypoglycaemia, but also in many people with type 2 diabetes with a long duration of disease who have lost most of their endogenous insulin secretion. Finally, since NPH is an insoluble preparation that needs to be re-suspended prior to subcutaneous injection, it has an absorption that is quite variable, resulting in different fasting blood glucoses from one day to another. Taken together, these reasons indicate why NPH should no longer be

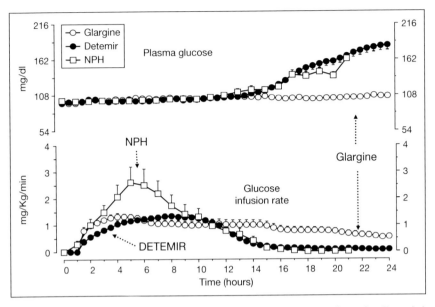

Figure 2.6 Comparison of pharmacodynamics following subcutaneous injection of NPH insulin and the long-acting insulin analogues glargine and detemir in subjects with type 1 diabetes (data taken with permission from [27, 31]).
NPH = Neutral Protamine Hagedorn.

used in people with type 1 diabetes mellitus and should be used only with caution in those with type 2 diabetes when the target is normoglycaemia of intensive therapy. Only long-acting insulin analogues (glargine, detemir) or the technique of CSII should be used to replace basal insulin in people with type 1 diabetes mellitus. Glargine or detemir should be preferred to NPH in the intensive treatment of type 2 diabetes mellitus.

Glargine
Glargine is a soluble long-acting insulin analogue, peak-free when compared with NPH, with a duration of action of 24 h or more [27, 28]. The mechanism of action of glargine is based on its modified isoelectric point (pH at which a protein is less soluble), which has been shifted from the acidic value of human insulin to one close to neutrality. After subcutaneous injection, the change in pH from acidic in the vial (where glargine is therefore soluble and 'clear') to the neutral value of subcutaneous tissue, causes microprecipitation of glargine insulin into microcrystals with subsequent slow absorption. Because it is soluble, it is by definition more reproducible than NPH [15, 29]. The more physiological pharmacokinetic/pharmacodynamics properties of insulin glargine versus NPH translate into the clinical advantage of lower risk for nocturnal hypoglycaemia with similar or lower HbA1c levels [15]. Glargine should be given as a once-daily evening injection, either before or after dinner. Some subjects with type 1 diabetes mellitus present an elevation in pre-dinner blood glucose despite optimal postprandial blood glucose [30]. However, this phenomenon is not explained by duration of action of glargine (<24 h), since glargine at steady state generally has duration of action >24 h [28, 31]. In all likelihood, the pre-dinner hyperglycaemia is caused by delayed absorption of the meal beyond the end of action of rapid-acting insulin given at lunchtime [30]. Therefore, administration of twice-daily glargine is not the solution to the problem of the 'afternoon phenomenon'; rather a dual bolus of rapid-acting insulin analogue should be given at lunchtime (before and 3 h after the meal: the latter should consist of 1–3 units with no snack) [32] (Figure 2.7).

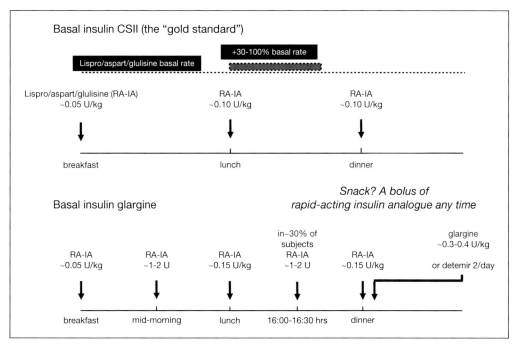

Figure 2.7 Modern regimens of insulin delivery in type 1 diabetes mellitus. Upper panel: continuous subcutaneous insulin infusion (minipumps). Lower panel: multiple daily insulin injections of insulin analogues (either lispro or aspart or glulisine are used at mealtime; glargine once daily, or detemir twice daily are given as basal insulin supplementation).
CSII = continuous subcutaneous insulin infusion; RA-IA = rapid-acting insulin analogues.

Detemir

Detemir is a soluble, long-acting insulin analogue that is also more reproducible than NPH [29]. When compared to therapeutic doses of glargine, detemir is similarly peak-free, but exhibits a shorter duration of action with an earlier increase in free fatty acids and plasma ketones during fasting [31]. Thus, in the majority of people with type 1 diabetes, detemir should be given every 12 h. In theory, twice-daily detemir administration should achieve good glycaemic control similar to that reported with glargine once daily [24, 25]. However, in the only study prospectively comparing glargine and detemir in people with type 1 diabetes, HbA1c did not reach the targets of intensive therapy with either of the two basal insulins [33]. Thus, additional studies are needed to determine the best method of using detemir in type 1 diabetes mellitus to improve HbA1c, specifically to establish the titration of detemir in the evening as well as in the morning, along with the titration of doses of the rapid-acting insulin analogue at mealtimes.

A peculiar characteristic of detemir, which is not shared either by NPH or by glargine, is that its long-term use is associated with less weight gain (0.5–1.0 kg) when compared with the other basal insulins such as NPH or glargine [34].

TYPE 1 DIABETES – REGIMENS OF MULTIPLE DAILY INJECTIONS AND CSII

In the NPH era, CSII has been shown to be superior to multiple daily injections (MDI) [35] because the 'basal' insulin delivered by CSII is soluble (either regular or rapid-acting analogue insulin), whereas that of MDI was insoluble, and therefore more variable [15]. In the era of soluble long-acting analogues, MDI is no longer inferior to CSII in terms of HbA1c and frequency of hypoglycaemia [36, 37]. CSII has the theoretical advantage of lower variability when compared with MDI [37], but this has so far been difficult to prove [36]. Thus, in the 'general' diabetic population, the choice between MDI and CSII is based on the preference of the individual person with type 1 diabetes, rather than a real medical indication. However, in special subgroup populations, such as subjects with long diabetes duration and /or low daily insulin requirements, and/or hypoglycaemia unawareness, CSII might prove an easier tool to reach the goal of HbA1c <7.0% while preventing hypoglycaemia. Needless to say, the insulin of choice to be used in CSII is a rapid-acting analogue, with no proven difference between lispro, aspart and glulisine.

TYPE 2 DIABETES – HOW TO START AND ADJUST INSULIN TREATMENT

The modern concept is to initiate insulin treatment in type 2 diabetes mellitus when HbA1c remains above the goal (7.0%) despite lifestyle changes and the use of metformin [38]. This is the concept of the 'early' use of insulin, in the hope of improving glycaemic control sooner and therefore to avoid complications. This contrasts with the old view of starting insulin late, long after the failure of oral agents and when complications have already become apparent. Insulin should be initiated as a single daily administration of basal preparation [38]. NPH has been proven to be as effective as glargine or detemir in reducing HbA1c to 7.0%, but to also result in a higher risk for nocturnal hypoglycaemia [39]. What it is important, however, is the active and continuing titration of basal insulin to fasting normoglycaemia, which results in HbA1c of <7.0%, even with cheap NPH insulin [39, 40]. If appropriate titration is not performed, for example in the 4T (Treating To Target in Type 2 diabetes) study recently published from the UK and Ireland, HbA1c does not decrease to the target level but remains elevated despite the use of the insulin analogue detemir [41]. Clearly, in the 4T study, either the dose of detemir had to be increased and/or it had to be given twice-daily to reduce HbA1c to 7.0%, as was successfully achieved in other studies using detemir [40].

In subjects with type 2 diabetes in whom fasting blood glucose is at the target level with basal insulin but HbA1c remains above 7.0%, treatment with a rapid-acting insulin analogue should be started whenever a carbohydrate-rich meal is eaten. This flexible regimen ultimately implies the use of basal insulin (always) and mealtime insulin (once-, twice- or thrice-daily) depending on the individual meal habits of the type 2 diabetic patient.

SUMMARY

When combined with appropriate education and motivation of people with type 1 diabetes, insulin regimens based on insulin analogues (either MDI or CSII) (Figure 2.7) successfully reach the glycaemic targets of the DCCT if the insulin dose is titrated to target, thus protecting against the risk of onset of long-term complications. At the same time, these regimens minimise the frequency of hypoglycaemia, prevent hypoglycaemia unawareness and improve quality of life. In type 2 diabetes, insulin is initially given as basal preparation. Although NPH remains an option, preference should be given to the long-acting analogues that make it possible to reduce HbA1c without increasing the risk of hypoglycaemia. However, basal insulin should be titrated aggressively to normalise fasting blood glucose in order to significantly reduce HbA1c. The second step in type 2 diabetes is to add prandial insulin (at each carbohydrate-rich meal) when HbA1c is not at the target level despite fasting normoglycaemia.

REFERENCES

1. Paulescu NC. Recherche sur le rôle du pancréas dans l'assimilation nutritive. *Arch Int Physiol* 1921; 17:85–109.
2. Banting F, Best CH, Collip JB, Campbell WR, Fletcher AA. Pancreatic extracts in the treatment of diabetes mellitus: preliminary report. *Can Med Ass J* 1922; 12:141–146.
3. Bliss M. *The discovery of insulin.* Chicago, University of Chicago Press, 1982
4. The effect of intensive treatment of diabetes on the development and progression of long-term complications in insulin-dependent diabetes mellitus. The Diabetes Control and Complications Trial Research Group. *N Engl J Med* 1993; 329:977–986.
5. Bolli GB. Treatment and prevention of hypoglycemia and its unawareness in type 1 diabetes mellitus. *Rev Endocr Metab Dis* 2003; 4:335–341.
6. Gold AE, MacLeod KM, Frier BM. Frequency of severe hypoglycemia in patients with type I diabetes with impaired awareness of hypoglycemia. *Diabetes Care* 1994; 17:697–703.
7. Zisman A, Miller M, Taneberg R. Relationship between prior mild-moderate hypoglycaemic events and the risk of subsequent severe hypoglycaemia in patients with type 2 diabetes mellitus treated with basal insulin according to fasting BG targets: a time-dependent covariate analysis. *Diabetologia* 2007; 50(Suppl 1):S82.
8. Dimitriadis G, Gerich J. Importance of timing of preprandial subcutaneous insulin administration in the management of diabetes mellitus. *Diabetes Care* 1985; 6:774–777.
9. Bolli GB. From physiology of glucose counterregulation to prevention of hypoglycaemia in type 1 diabetes mellitus. *Diab Nutr Metab* 1990; 4:333–349.
10. DeFronzo RA, Simonson D, Ferrannini E. Hepatic and peripheral insulin resistance: a common feature of type 2 (non-insulin-dependent) and type 1 (insulin-dependent) diabetes mellitus. *Diabetologia* 1982; 23:313–319.
11. Kelley DE. Sugars and starch in the nutritional management of diabetes mellitus. *Am J Clin Nutr* 2003; 78:858S–864S.
12. Ciofetta M, Lalli C, Del Sindaco P *et al.* Contribution of postprandial versus interprandial blood glucose to HbA$_{1c}$ in type 1 diabetes on physiologic intensive therapy with lispro insulin at mealtime. *Diabetes Care* 1999; 22:795–800.
13. Bolli GB, Dimitriadis GD, Pehling GB *et al.* Abnormal glucose counterregulation after subcutaneous insulin in insulin-dependent diabetes mellitus. *N Engl J Med* 1984; 310:1706–1711.
14. Brange J, Owens DR, Kang S, Vølund A. Monomeric insulins and their experimental and clinical implications. *Diabetes Care* 1990; 13:923–954.
15. Bolli GB, Di Marchi R, Park G, Pramming S, Koivisto VA. Insulin analogues and their potential in the management of diabetes mellitus. *Diabetologia* 1999; 42:1151–1167.
16. Becker RHA. Insulin glulisine complementing basal insulins: a review of structure and activity. *Diab Technol and Ther* 2007; 9:109–121.
17. Torlone E, Pampanelli S, Lalli C *et al.* Effects of the short-acting insulin analog [LYS(B28),PRO(B29)] on postprandial blood glucose control in IDDM. *Diabetes Care* 1996; 19:945–952.
18. Siebenhofer A, Plank J, Berghold A *et al.* Meta-analysis of short-acting insulin analogues in adult patients with type 1 diabetes: continuous subcutaneous insulin infusion versus injection therapy. *Diabetologia* 2004; 47:1895–1905.
19. Plank J, Siebenhofer A, Berghold A *et al.* Systematic review and meta-analysis of short-acting insulin analogues in patients with diabetes mellitus. *Arch Intern Med* 2005; 165:1337–1344.
20. Siebenhofer A, Plank J, Berghold A *et al.* Short-acting insulin analogues versus regular human insulin in patients with diabetes mellitus (Review). *The Cochrane Database of Systematic Reviews* 2006, Issue 2. Art.No.: CD003287.pub4. DOI: 10.1002/14651858.CD003287.pub4. (update of the version first published in 2004).
21. Zinman B, Tildesley H, Chiasson JL, Tsui E, Strack T. Insulin lispro in CSII: results of a double-blind crossover study. *Diabetes* 1997; 46:440–443.
22. Del Sindaco P, Ciofetta M, Lalli C *et al.* Use of the short-acting insulin analogue lispro in intensive treatment of IDDM: importance of appropriate replacement of basal insulin and time-interval injection-meal. *Diabet Med* 1998; 15:592–600.
23. Lalli C, Ciofetta M, Del Sindaco P *et al.* Long-term intensive treatment of type 1 diabetes with the short-acting insulin analogue lispro in variable combination with NPH insulin at mealtime. *Diabetes Care* 1999; 22:468–477.

24. Ashwell SG, Amiel SA, Bilous RW *et al*. Improved glycaemic control with insulin glargine plus insulin lispro: a multicentre, randomized, cross-over trial in people with type 1 diabetes. *Diabet Med* 2006; 23:285–292.

25. Porcellati F, Rossetti P, Pampanelli S *et al*. Better long-term glycaemic control with the basal insulin glargine as compared with NPH in patients with type 1 diabetes mellitus given meal-time lispro insulin. *Diabet Med* 2004; 21:1213–1220.

26. Hagedorn HC, Norman Jensen B, Krarup NB, Wodstrup I. Protamine insulinate. *JAMA* 1936; 106:177–180.

27. Lepore M, Pampanelli S, Fanelli C *et al*. Pharmacokinetics and pharmacodynamics of the long-acting human insulin analog glargine, NPH insulin, and ultralente human insulin injected subcutaneously, and continuous subcutaneous infusion of insulin lispro. *Diabetes* 2000; 49:2142–2148.

28. Porcellati F, Rossetti P, Busciantella Ricci N *et al*. Pharmacokinetics and pharmacodynamics of the long-acting insulin analog glargine after one week of use as compared to its first administration in subjects with type 1 diabetes mellitus. *Diabetes Care* 2007; 30:1261–1263.

29. Heise T, Nosek L, Ronn BB *et al*. Lower within-subject variability of insulin detemir in comparison to NPH insulin and insulin glargine in people with type 1 diabetes. *Diabetes* 2004; 53:1614–1620.

30. Porcellati F, Rossetti P, Fanelli CG, Bolli GB. Optimized use of glargine in intensive treatment of type 1 diabetes mellitus: benefits and a new question. (Abstract) *Diabetes* 2005; 54(Suppl 1):A129.

31. Porcellati F, Rossetti P, Busciantella S *et al*. Pharmacokinetics and –dynamics of therapeutic doses of the "long-acting" insulin analogs glargine and detemir at steady-state in type 1 diabetes mellitus. *Diabetes Care* 2007; 30:2447–2452.

32. Rossetti P, Porcellati F, Fanelli CG, Bolli GB. Mechanisms and Treatment of the 'Afternoon Phenomenon' in Patients with type 1 Diabetes Mellitus Using Glargine as Basal Insulin. (abstract) *Diabetes* 2005; 54(Suppl 1):A68.

33. Pieber TR, Treichel HC, Hompesch B *et al*. Comparison of insulin detemir and insulin glargine in subjects with type 1 diabetes using intensive insulin therapy. *Diabet Med* 2007; 24:635–642.

34. Hermansen K, Davies M. Does insulin detemir have a role in reducing risk of insulin-associated weight gain? *Diabetes Obes Metab* 2007; 9:209–217.

35. Pickup J, Mattock M, Kerry S. Glycaemic control with continuous subcutaneous insulin infusion compared with intensive insulin injections in patients with type 1 diabetes: meta-analysis of randomised controlled trials. *Br Med J* 2002; 324:1–6.

36. Bolli GB, Kerr D, Reena T *et al*. Comparison of a multiple daily insulin injection regime (basal once-daily glargine plus mealtime lispro) and CSII (lispro) in type 1 diabetes: a randomized open parallel multicenter study. *Diabetes Care* 2009; 32:1170–1176.

37. Bruttomesso D, Crazzolara D, Maran A *et al*. In type 1 diabetic patients with good glycaemic control, blood glucose variability is lower during continuous subcutaneous insulin infusion than during multiple daily injections with insulin glargine. *Diabet Med* 2008; 25:326–332.

38. Nathan DM, Buse JB, Davidson MB *et al*. Management of hyperglycemia in type 2 diabetes: a consensus algorithm for the initiation and adjustment of therapy. *Diabetes Care* 2006; 29:1963–1972.

39. Riddle MC, Rosenstock J, Gerich J. The treat-to-target trial: randomized addition of glargine or human NPH insulin to oral therapy of type 2 diabetic patients. *Diabetes Care* 2003; 26:3080–3086.

40. Hermansen K, Davies M, Derezinski T *et al*. A 26-week, randomized, parallel, treat-to-target trial comparing insulin detemir with NPH insulin as add-on therapy to oral glucose-lowering drugs in insulin-naïve people with type 2 diabetes. *Diabetes Care* 2006; 29:1269–1274.

41. Holman RR, Thorne KI, Farmer AJ *et al*. Addition of biphasic, prandial, or basal insulin to oral therapy in type 2 diabetes. *N Engl J Med* 2007; 357:1716–1730.

3

New developments in insulin administration

E. Renard

INTRODUCTION

From its discovery in 1922, insulin has been considered as a crucial therapeutic agent for blood glucose control. Insulin administration is vital in all situations of near-absolute insulin deficiency, such as type 1 diabetes mellitus or pancreatectomy. In partial insulin secretion defects, such as type 2 diabetes mellitus or chronic pancreatitis, insulin administration becomes necessary when oral antidiabetic drugs fail to achieve acceptable glucose control; contraindications to use these agents require earlier insulin administration, e.g. diabetic pregnancy. Stressful conditions that impair glucose control, such as in critically ill patients, have been more recently underscored as requiring insulin to restore near-normoglycaemia that improves patient outcomes [1].

Because of hormone proteolysis by gut enzymes, parenteral administration of insulin is mandatory. Insulin injections using the subcutaneous (SC) route have represented the usual means to deliver insulin until now. Because of the characteristics of time and duration of action after SC regular insulin injection, additives to insulin solution such as protamine or zinc have been used to prolong insulin action, especially for the night coverage. Over the past ten years or so, the development of bioengineering has allowed the synthesis of insulin analogues characterised by modifications of insulin primary sequence. These analogues keep the biological action of insulin while they either accelerate or slowdown its absorption after SC injection. The combination of a slow-acting analogue for basal coverage of insulin needs and a fast-acting analogue at mealtimes presently allows a better mimicry of physiological insulin secretion than previously used combinations of regular and Neutral Protamine Hagedorn (NPH) or lente insulin solutions [2].

However, the quest for tight and sustained blood glucose control cannot be fully satisfied by multiple daily SC insulin injections, even with the availability of effective insulin analogues.

The need for tight glucose control in the long term, aiming at sustained near-normoglycaemia, has been clearly demonstrated by the Diabetes Control and Complications Trial (DCCT) performed in type 1 diabetic patients [3] and the United Kingdom Prospective Diabetes Study (UKPDS) performed in type 2 diabetic patients [4]. In both trials, the lower the average HbA1c level for several years, the better were the outcomes in terms of diabetic complications. However, only limited subsets of patients are able to reach and maintain tight control, close to defined ideal goals, using daily SC insulin injections [3]. Besides defec-

Eric Renard, MD, PhD, Professor of Endocrinology, Diabetes and Metabolic Diseases, Senior Medical Practitioner in Endocrinology, Diabetes and Metabolic Diseases, Department of Endocrinology, Montpellier University Hospital; UMR CNRS 5232, University of Montpellier, Montpellier, France.

tive efficacy, the limitations of SC insulin injections include the risk excess of overshooting (resulting in hypoglycaemia) and cumbersome daily burden. Hence, improvements in insulin delivery are needed to overcome these limitations [5].

A first option, developed since the 1970s, is to consider continuous insulin infusion (CII) from portable pumps [6]. The initially investigated intravenous (IV) route for CII, although very effective in blood glucose control when insulin flow was modulated according to frequent blood glucose measurements [7], was revealed to be poorly feasible in ambulatory use, and the SC route (continuous subcutaneous insulin infusion, CSII) has been rapidly adopted in preference. However, intravenous insulin infusion remains a currently used means of insulin therapy for hospitalised patients. It is sometimes the only reliable mode of insulin administration to cover the widely fluctuating insulin needs of critically ill patients, in whom SC absorption of insulin can be poorly predictable. In ambulatory patients or in hospitalised patients with less erratic insulin needs, CSII has gradually improved over recent years. Progress in electronics and miniaturisation has led to reliable, user-friendly, programmable insulin infusion systems [8]. Improvements in catheter components and design have resulted in improved compatibility with insulin solutions and biocompatibility at infusion sites [8]. The availability of fast-acting insulin analogues increased the effectiveness of CSII on glucose control [9]. Presently, investigation of combinations of CSII with devices allowing continuous glucose monitoring should further optimise the effectiveness of this constantly innovating mode of insulin administration [10].

A second option is to deliver insulin continuously, but using the more physiological intraperitoneal (IP) route. From initial IP catheters implanted through the abdominal wall and connected to external insulin pumps, significant technical advances have resulted in the availability of implantable, programmable insulin pumps equipped with an IP catheter [11]. Although still in part under investigation, these delivery systems using the IP route have shown clear benefits on the stability of glucose control with a dramatic reduction of the incidence of severe hypoglycaemic events. In addition, the quality of life of patients has been significantly improved by the use of these implanted systems.

In order to overcome the limitations of SC insulin administration, various alternative routes of insulin delivery have been tested: per-oral (entericgastrointestinal), oral–buccal and sublingual, rectal, ocular, intravaginal, transdermal, intranasal, but none of them showed enough safety, reliability and effectiveness to allow fruitful clinical development [12]. More recently, the pulmonary route has been intensively investigated [12]. Absorption of inhaled insulin is helped by the large surface area of the lungs (similar to that of a tennis court), a highly permeable membrane, a rich blood perfusion and a lack of mucociliary clearance at the alveolar level. Moreover, painless, needle-free insulin administration is very attractive. Effectiveness of inhaled insulin is close to that of SC regular insulin at mealtimes, although requested doses for a similarly hypoglycaemic effect are much higher. Approval by the US Food and Drug Administration (FDA) of a model for insulin inhalation was expected to allow the clinical development of this new mode of insulin administration. Various persistent concerns about this mode of insulin delivery recently led most manufacturers to withdraw their projects in this field.

In this chapter, a current picture of recent innovations in and developments of insulin administration is presented. 'Biological insulin therapy' by allogenic islet transplantation is not addressed here.

CONTINUOUS SUBCUTANEOUS INSULIN INFUSION (CSII)

CSII from portable pumps is increasingly used for the treatment of type 1 diabetic patients and tends to become a more frequently considered option for insulin therapy in type 2 diabetic patients. More than 250 000 (25%) type 1 diabetic patients now use CSII in the USA, while this mode of insulin therapy is used in about 30 000 patients in Germany and 10 000 subjects in France, both being among the leading European countries for the utilisation of CSII.

This expansion of CSII use is relatively recent and has been mainly promoted by the results of the DCCT, during which CSII was used by almost one-half of the patients treated intensively [13]. It should be noted, though, that the initial steps in the use of CSII were taken in the 1970s. At that time, the efficacy of CSII appeared to be at least as effective as SC insulin injections, which included, in most cases, one or two daily injections of SC regular and NPH insulin [14]. After an enthusiastic period, during which insulin pumps were increasingly prescribed, the occurrence of severe acute complications such as fatal ketoacidosis, slowed their development [15]. Meanwhile, the availability of insulin pens, which helped the use of multiple daily insulin injections (MDI), also challenged the effectiveness of CSII. The combination of technical improvements, which produced safer delivery systems, and the persistent success of the technique in well-selected and better-trained patients, generated a renewed interest in CSII during the 1990s. Fast-acting analogues further improved the effectiveness of CSII by allowing a better glucose control after meals and a reduced occurrence of hypoglycaemia in the late post-absorptive period [9]. Wider and easier coverage of costs related to CSII use by health insurance companies finally helped the recent expansion of CSII in some countries. At the present time, CSII is considered as the gold standard of insulin therapy in type 1 diabetic patients [6, 16].

TECHNICAL ASPECTS OF CSII

Three main elements are involved in the performance of CSII: the pump itself, the catheter through which insulin is infused from the pump to the body and the insulin formulation itself.

All currently available pumps use pulsatile delivery, since peristaltic mechanisms of infusion have been shown to promote alterations of the insulin solution and required larger power supplies. They are about the size of small pagers ($100 \times 50 \times 20$ mm), with an average weight of 100 g. All offer programmable basal rates and some of them allow various bolus profiles. The insulin reservoir should be changed every 2–4 days, while the power supply comes from a battery that needs to be changed every month or two. Most devices record programmed orders in an incorporated memory. Specificities of the main models from the four major manufacturers are presented in Table 3.1. Pumps available today are safe and reliable thanks to improvements in microelectronics and built-in alarms. Most pumps can be continuously used for the expected operating time with a very low risk of failure [8].

Considerable improvements have also been achieved in the design of catheters [8]. All are internally covered with polyethylene, which is impermeable to carbon dioxide, thus avoiding impairments of the insulin's physical stability. Subcutaneous infusing cannulae are either made of stainless steel or Teflon™, with a better tolerance and a longer possibility of use for the latter (3–4 days versus 2), due to lesser trauma to the subcutaneous tissue. Their user-friendliness has also been enhanced by the availability of inserters to implant the soft cannula with the help of a removable needle in SC tissue on the one hand, and by the possibility of transitory disconnection of the infusing line from the cannula in most commonly used models. However, the catheter remains the weak link of the infusing system. The two main issues that may stop insulin delivery or impair insulin diffusion unexpectedly are:

1. A tip obstruction or a soft catheter bending.
2. Any subcutaneous reaction, e.g. haematoma, at insertion site.

Although built-in alarms in most pump models should warn the patient of any resistance to normal flow rate, common clinical experience indicates that cannula bending or minor reactions at the insertion site that impair insulin absorption are not usually detected by the

Table 3.1 Main characteristics of currently used insulin pumps for subcutaneous infusion

Models	H-TRON PLUS	D-TRON PLUS	ACCUCHEK SPIRIT	IR 1200	COZMO	PARADIGM 512	PARADIGM 712
Manufacturer	Roche Diagnostics	Roche Diagnostics	Roche Diagnostics	Animas	Smiths Medical	Medtronic-MiniMed	Medtronic-MiniMed
Length × width (mm)	97 × 55	117.6 × 48.1	81 × 55	90 × 51	88.9 × 50	83 × 50.5	95 × 52
Thickness (mm)	18.9	22.25	20	21.5	19	22	22
Weight (g)	105	124	110	98	93	103	108
Insulin reservoir	Specific reservoir or pre-filled cartridge	Pre-filled cartridge	Specific reservoir or pre-filled cartridge	Plastic syringe	Plastic syringe	Plastic syringe	Plastic syringe
Insulin units per reservoir	300	300	300	200	300	180	300
Type of insulin	Regular or fast-acting analogue or Insuman Infusat®	Humalog®	Regular or fast-acting analogue or Insuman Infusat®	Regular or fast-acting analogue	Regular or fast-acting analogue	Regular or fast-acting analogue	Regular or fast-acting analogue
Catheter connection	Luer-lock	Luer-lock	Luer-lock	Luer-lock	Luer-lock	Specific	Specific
Battery type	Specific (n = 2)	Specific (n = 1)	Standard AA	Lithium AA	Standard AAA	Standard AAA	Standard AAA
Battery life	1 month	2 months	1 month	8 weeks	1 month	4 weeks	4 weeks
Basal rates	24	24	24	12	48	48	48
Bolus profiles	1	3	4	3	3	3	3
Memory	no	yes	yes	yes	yes	yes	yes

alarm system. Education of the patient on how to behave in the case of persistent hyperglycaemia despite the addition of a corrective bolus is crucial: catheter replacement in such a case is mandatory, even in the absence of any evidence of catheter failure. Leakages at the connections between pump reservoir and catheter, or between infusion line and cannula, are also usually undetected by the warning system and the patient should be taught to consider this eventuality in the case of hyperglycaemia.

The insulin formulations used in pumps are dominated by fast-acting analogues [17]. No clear superiority of any of the available analogues is evident: lispro, aspart or glulisine can be considered equally effective. Only one pump model can host pre-filled lispro cartridges for insulin pens, whereas all of the other ones use reservoirs to be filled by the patients from 10 ml vials or pen cartridges, or pre-filled insulin pens. Although regular insulin can also be used in pumps, several studies have shown the metabolic benefits obtained with fast-acting analogues: lower average HbA1c, improved blood glucose stability, reduced occurrence of hypos [9, 18–20]. Only two pump models can use pre-filled cartridges of regular insulin specifically designed for pumps (Insuman Infusat®; Sanofi-Aventis, Paris, France). Due to technical improvements in the pumping mechanism and catheter components, both the physical and chemical stability of insulin solutions is now maintained for the average duration of use of the reservoir, namely 2–4 days.

METABOLIC RESULTS WITH CSII

The evidence of the benefits of pump use versus insulin injections has been debated for many years until published meta-analyses indicated a better average blood glucose control obtained with CSII.

Pickup and Keen in 2002 reported the first meta-analysis based upon a series of twelve randomised studies comparing CSII with MDI, all using no insulin analogue [6]. Mean benefits in favour of CSII included a weighted mean difference in blood glucose level of 0.9 mmol/l (95% confidence interval [CI] 0.5–1.2), and an HbA1c difference of 0.5% (0.2–0.7). Moreover, a 14% average reduction in daily insulin dose was associated with CSII superiority for blood glucose control. In contrast with the DCCT report, the frequency of severe hypoglycaemic episodes was reported to be 33–84% less with CSII from several studies. Diabetic ketoacidosis appeared to be similar with both modes of treatment after proper education and pump practice. Pickup and Sutton [22] further confirmed in a recent meta-analysis the benefit of CSII vs. multiple-daily insulin injections in terms of HbA1c with a mean difference of 0.62% (0.47–0.78) in favour of CSII, and by a rate ratio for severe hypoglycaemia of 4.19 (2.86–6.13) also in favour of CSII [21]. A meta-analysis of 52 studies with parallel or paired designs comparing CSII to MDI or conventional insulin therapy performed by Weissberg-Benchell and colleagues also reported a significantly higher effectiveness of CSII and a decreased frequency of hypoglycaemic episodes while using CSII [16].

Studies that compared CSII using regular insulin versus fast-acting insulin analogues further pointed to an improved glucose control with the latter [9, 18–20] (Table 3.2). An early comparison between CSII using lispro insulin and MDI combining lispro and NPH confirmed CSII using lispro as a better performing treatment [22]. However, a recently reported pooled analysis of three randomised controlled trials assessing this question, which included the aforementioned study, showed that higher baseline HbA1c increased the relative benefit of CSII over MDI [23]. No benefit could be expected if baseline HbA1c were 6.5%. Moreover, no significant difference in the rate of hypoglycaemic events was found.

Several recently reported studies investigated whether glargine, the first available long-acting analogue, as basal insulin and a fast-acting analogue at mealtimes could perform as well as CSII using fast-acting analogues [24]. Among six identified studies on this topic (Table 3.3), only three were randomised prospective trials [25–27]. Whereas one study per-

Table 3.2 Studies comparing lispro (LP) versus regular (R) insulin used for continuous subcutaneous insulin infusion in type 1 diabetic patients

Reference	Number of cases	Trial design (duration)	HbA1c (%)	SD blood glucose (mmol/l)	Hypoglycaemia/month (definition)
Zinman et al. [9]	30	Double-blind, crossover (2 × 3 months)	LP: 7.66 ± 0.13 R: 8.00 ± 0.16 (P = 0.0041)	NA	(<3 mmol/l) LP: 6.0 ± 0.9 R: 7.6 ± 1.0 (NS)
Melki et al. [18]	39	Opened, crossover (2 × 3 months)	(ΔHbA1c) LP: −0.62 ± 0.13 R: −0.09 ± 0.15 (P = 0.01)	LP: 3.44 ± 0.10 R: 3.80 ± 0.10 (P <0.0001)	(<2 mmol/l) LP: 0.05 ± 0.05 R: 0.47 ± 0.19 (P <0.05)
Renner et al. [19]	113	Opened, crossover (2 × 4 months)	LP: 6.8 ± 0.9 R: 6.9 ± 1.0 (P <0.02)	NA	(< 3.5 mmol/l) LP: 12.4 ± 13.9 R: 11.0 ± 11.2 (NS)
Johansson et al. [20]	41	Opened, crossover (2 × 2 months)	LP: 7.4 R: 7.6 (P = 0.047)	LP: 3.6 R: 3.9 (P = 0.012)	(< 3 mmol/l) LP: 9.7 R: 8.0 (NS)

NA = not available; NS = no significant difference.

Table 3.3 Studies comparing continuous subcutaneous insulin infusion (CSII) using a fast-acting insulin analogue versus multiple daily insulin injections (MDI) using fast-acting and long-acting analogues in type 1 diabetic patients

Reference	Number of cases (types) Study duration Trial design	Insulin used by multiple daily injections	Insulin analogues used in pumps	HbA1c (%) at end of trial CSII MDI	Other results
Bolli et al. [25]	57 (A) 6 months Randomised	Glargine + lispro	Lispro	CSII: 7.0 MDI: 7.2 (NS)	No difference: mean blood glucose, MAGE index, hypoglycaemia
Lepore et al. [30]	48 (A) 1 year Non-randomised	Glargine + lispro	Lispro	CSII: 8.0 MDI: 7.8 (NS)	No difference: hypoglycaemia CSII: lower MAGE index
Hirsch et al. [27]	100 (A) 10 weeks Randomised (crossover)	Glargine + lispro	Aspart	CSII: 7.1 MDI: 7.3 (NS)	No difference: hypoglycaemia CSII: lower fructosamine and 24-h blood glucose
Doyle et al. [26]	32 (C) 16 weeks Randomised	Glargine + aspart	Aspart	CSII: 7.2 MDI: 8.1 ($P < 0.05$)	CSII: lower blood glucose profile, insulin dose No difference: hypoglycaemia, quality of life
Schiaffini et al. [29]	36 (C) 6–12 months Retrospective	Glargine + regular	Lispro or Aspart	CSII: 8.5 → 7.6 ($P < 0.05$) MDI: 8.9 → 8.3 (NS)	
Alemzadeh et al. [28]	40 (C) 1 year Case-control matched on age and sex	Glargine + lispro	Lispro	CSII: 8.4 → 7.8 ($P < 0.002$) MDI: 8.5 → 8.2 (NS)	No difference: hypoglycaemia

Types of patients: A = adults, C = children and adolescents; h = hours; MAGE = mean amplitude of glycaemic excursions; NS = no significant difference.

formed in adults showed similarity of glucose control with the two options [25], one in children showed the superiority of CSII on HbA1c levels reached after 16 weeks with a significantly lower average insulin use [26]. The better basal coverage by using CSII in the latter study was apparent from lunch and dinner pre-meal and bedtime blood glucose values that were lower, whereas pre-breakfast values were similar [26]. The most recently published short-term crossover study comparing CSII and MDI including glargine reported lower fructosamine levels and reduced daily glycaemic exposure assessed by continuous glucose monitoring with CSII [26]. Among the other three studies [28–30], two of them showed an improvement of glucose control only with CSII in comparison with previous therapy using NPH or ultralente [28, 29], while a third reported significantly fewer glucose excursions with CSII only [30].

From currently available data, CSII allows the best blood glucose control in type 1 diabetic patients. Very recently published data further support the clear efficacy of CSII in patients who are poorly controlled by MDI and are showing wide blood glucose variability [31]. These observations are, however, valid for patients who were able to manage CSII and accepted the constraints of pump treatment. In common practice, these two prerequisites should be considered carefully if metabolic improvements are to be expected from CSII [24].

RISKS RELATED TO CSII

The main risk associated with CSII is under-delivery, which may result in ketoacidosis if undetected and not corrected by the patient [32]. This risk is inherent to the method because of a small insulin depot at the infusion site. In any case of significant under-delivery, insulin action will dramatically decrease after two hours. This phenomenon has been shown to occur even more quickly with the use of fast-acting analogues [33]. A similar metabolic impairment may occur when insulin requirements rapidly increase with no adaptation of the flow rate by the patient, in the case of infection for example [32]. Impairment of insulin absorption due to subcutaneous tissue alterations (e.g. lipodystrophy or skin infection at infusion site) can also result in a dangerous hyperglycaemic drift [32]. Whereas such events may occur easily in the case of patient unawareness of this risk, thorough selection and education of patients can prevent ketoacidosis by improving their knowledge and skill in correcting the delivery issue or increasing the insulin flow rate to correct the defect in insulin administration [6]. Although it remains a true risk of CSII, the current incidence of ketoacidosis in patients being treated by CSII is similar to that observed with MDI when patients have been well educated in the corrective measures to take in the case of a persistent hyperglycaemic drift [6].

Severe hypoglycaemic events can also be considered as a potential risk of CSII. The increased incidence of severe hypoglycaemia associated with the decrease of HbA1c level has been well recognised since the report of the DCCT results [3]. DCCT data even showed that CSII was associated with a significantly higher incidence of hypoglycaemic coma when compared with multiple daily insulin injections [13]. However, a more detailed analysis showed that these events dramatically decreased as the investigating centres acquired more experience in the management of CSII [3, 13]. A later study clearly demonstrated that the incidence of severe hypoglycaemia was, on the contrary, reduced by CSII [34]. A determining factor is, in fact, how much the patients using CSII are trained in tight control [6]. Pump over-delivery or runaway is well prevented by the safety mechanisms built into currently available devices. Fast-acting insulin analogues have reduced the variability of insulin absorption and action observed with regular insulin. Besides dosage errors of administered insulin due to the patient, the remaining reasons for the occurrence of severe hypoglycaemia when treated by CSII are hypoglycaemia unawareness and unreliable absorption of subcutaneous insulin in some patients.

INDICATIONS AND CONTRAINDICATIONS OF CSII

When taking into consideration the effectiveness of CSII on blood glucose control in terms of HbA1c levels, reduced blood glucose variability and decreased risk of hypoglycaemia, CSII can be considered as the reference therapy for all type 1 diabetic patients who are well-motivated to maintain tight glycaemic control [6]. More specifically, patients who are limited to reaching HbA1c levels close to 7% because of severe or recurrent mild hypoglycaemia when treated by multiple daily injections appear to be the best candidates for CSII. Since CSII allows a larger flexibility in terms of food intakes and scheduling of labour or leisure activities, it may also be a preferred mode of insulin therapy for socially active patients, for patients keen on frequent or intense sporting activity or for night-shift workers. Type 1 diabetic patients who are motivated for good diabetes control and are seeking an improved freedom and quality of life are currently an increasing source of CSII demand. The non-validated safety of long-acting insulin analogues during pregnancy remains a specific reason for promoting CSII use for women planning pregnancy. Present data allow the use of fast-acting analogues in pumps during pregnancy [35]. Finally, neonatal diabetes and type 1 diabetes in young children of pre-school age are good indications for CSII because they allow fine-tuning of insulin delivery in patients who require small doses of insulin with very fluctuating insulin needs and who are prone to frequent food intakes [36].

In fact, contraindications of CSII use are mainly those conditions in which intensive insulin therapy is not feasible, including:

- Severe psychological disorders affecting the reliability of adjustment of insulin dose and the self-monitoring of blood glucose (SMBG).
- Severe eating disorders that prevent any effective insulin therapy.
- Poor acceptance of diabetes mellitus and poor compliance with SMBG, which increases the risk of severe metabolic events by a lack of vigilance.
- A combination of diabetes with a severe disease that interferes in the accurate management of insulin therapy (e.g. Alzheimer's disease).

However, CSII may be helpful in preventing hypo- and hyperglycaemic deviations in patients affected by other pathological states that result in frequent fluctuations of insulin needs. When these patients are well trained, the reactivity of CSII in the modulation of insulin delivery may represent a valuable advantage.

The key contraindication of CSII remains the lack of acceptance of this mode of therapy, mostly for psychological reasons. For instance, patients who dislike depending on a device or showing their disease condition publicly, or for whom wearing a pump is an unwelcome reminder of their diabetes, are not good candidates for CSII. Even if their blood glucose profile while treated with insulin injections seems improvable by CSII, the caregiver must refrain from imposing on them CSII that they will never manage effectively.

Non-controlled ischaemic or pre-proliferative retinopathy represents a temporary contraindication of CSII until laser treatment has been completed. Lowering of blood glucose levels would increase the risk of microvascular retinal proliferation in such situations [37].

Blindness and deafness should no longer represent contraindications of CSII when the patients are motivated and able to learn, and well supported by helpful relatives. Patients living alone should also not be prevented from using pumps if they are able to organise safety measures to 'work around' this lack of assistance when needed.

The benefit of using CSII in insulin-requiring type 2 patients still lacks strong scientific evidence. However, recent studies showed a similar effectiveness as multiple daily injections in this population with no additional weight gain, but with an improvement in quality of life [38–40]. Further clinical studies are expected to better document these benefits, especially in obese patients who remain poorly controlled in spite of massive insulin doses.

Finally, a lack of finances or shortcomings in medical resources can also negatively influence the move to CSII. CSII has been shown to be cost-effective in type 1 diabetic patients who present at least two severe hypoglycaemic events per year, including one requiring hospitalisation [41]. Health insurance systems in Europe generally agree to pay for CSII when diabetes is shown to be poorly controllable by multiple daily insulin injections in spite of good compliance with recommended practice and medical follow-up. Significant differences remain, however, between countries or between regions in the same country. CSII training and medical follow-up also require a certain level of expertise, so even when no financial shortfall is present, limited medical expertise in CSII use may prevent access to CSII in some countries or regions.

EXPECTED DEVELOPMENTS OF CSII IN THE NEAR FUTURE

Besides financial and medical resources, the two main limiting factors of CSII use are the poor acceptance of current infusing systems as detailed above and the suboptimal blood glucose control obtained by this mode of therapy in a significant subset of patients.

The latter can be related to the limited information on blood glucose variations provided by SMBG while treated by CSII [42]. One may expect that continuous blood glucose monitoring (CBGM) could provide helpful data in order to better modulate insulin delivery according to actual needs. Warning alarms of hypoglycaemic trends would allow quicker flow rate reduction and could reduce the risk of severe hypoglycaemia. In addition, disclosure of hyperglycaemic peaks should induce immediate corrective actions and result in better control. The upcoming availability of glucose sensors, which continuously measure subcutaneous interstitial glucose and can provide accurate estimations of blood glucose after a delay of a few minutes, makes feasible this innovative approach of CSII. Moreover, a direct connection between a glucose sensor and an insulin pump is now under investigation [10]. In this configuration, the subcutaneous implanted sensor is linked to a transmitter that sends the glucose signal by telemetry to a receiver that is integrated in the infusion system. Blood glucose level is displayed on the pump screen, with associated information on the current trend of blood glucose variation. Whether this information on blood glucose at all times will allow improved control by CSII remains to be demonstrated, however. How patients will have to deal with these data still needs to be defined from the results of ongoing and future studies. The first closed-loop attempts have recently been reported in a hospital setting by linking the glucose sensor signal to the infusing system itself via algorithms [43]. Between-meals control appeared quite satisfactory, but meal excursions remained difficult to control.

Another promising development of CSII is the evolution of miniaturised pre-filled infusing devices with no catheter, thanks to a direct diffusion of insulin from the reservoir through the skin by transcutaneous puncture [44]. Once these devices have been demonstrated to be safe and effective, such disposable 'patch-pumps' could help in the further acceptance of CSII.

CONTINUOUS INTRAPERITONEAL INSULIN INFUSION (CIPII)

Intraperitoneal (IP) insulin delivery was initially used in diabetic patients with renal failure treated by peritoneal dialysis and has been shown to be effective and convenient in these subjects [45]. Several studies have since been performed in animal models to assess the characteristics of peritoneal insulin absorption. Insulin absorption from the peritoneal space was shown to be volume-, concentration- and time-dependent [46]. More interestingly, insulin was first distributed to the portal vein before entering the systemic circulation [47]. A positive gradient between portal and systemic blood insulin was further demonstrated by IP insulin administration that differed from intramuscular insulin injection but mimicked endogenous insulin secretion [47]. In humans, IP insulin delivery was shown to allow quicker insulin peaks than the subcutaneous (SC) route (70 vs. 120 minutes) and plasma insulin levels returned to baseline after 165 minutes, as in normal subjects [48]. While the rate of systemic appearance of IP infused insulin was lower than SC infused insulin at a steady state, the percentage increase in the rate of systemic appearance after an increase of infusion rate was higher with the IP route [49]. These data showed a quicker absorption of insulin from the peritoneum, which prefigured a higher reactivity in clinical use and suggested the likely role of the liver in modulating peripheral insulin delivery. As a result, a lower peripheral insulinaemia, close to physiological levels, was obtained in steady-state conditions with the IP route than with SC insulin delivery [49]. The answer to the question whether hepatic insulinisation secondary to IP insulin delivery better controls hepatic glucose output than systemic insulin delivery remains unclear, however. Studies in animals and in humans, comparing the effects of IP and IV insulin infusions showed similar reductions of hepatic glucose output [50].

First case-reports of IP insulin delivery from portable pumps via an indwelling in the peritoneal cavity through the abdominal wall indicated the effectiveness of this therapeutic mode in brittle diabetes after failures to achieve glucose control with SC, intramuscular (IM) and sometimes IV insulin [51–53]. Selam and colleagues reported considerable experience with this technique, accumulating 472 patient-months in 40 type 1 diabetic patients [54]. Metabolic control was significantly improved with reduced insulin doses. The technique was, however, associated with frequent local infectious complications around the implantation site of the catheter. Under-deliveries related to pump failures or catheter obstructions were also reported, so that 1-year survival rates of the pump and catheter were 46% and 70 %, respectively. Two technical variants of peritoneal insulin infusion from external pumps have been assessed to overcome these problems. The first consisted of the implantation of the catheter in the umbilical vein by reopening this physiologically occluded vein soon after birth [55]. The second variant has been the development of specific ports implanted in the abdominal wall through which the peritoneal catheter accessed the peritoneal space [56]. A new device (DiaPort®; Roche Diagnostics-Disetronic AG, Burgdorf, Switzerland) is currently under investigation in Europe. In spite of the drawbacks of these externally worn devices, dominated by skin infections and frequent catheter obstructions, IP insulin infusion has been shown to provide a tighter glucose control than SC infusion or injections over the time of use. A crucial benefit was the combination of a lower HbA1c or mean blood glucose and a very low incidence of severe hypoglycaemia.

In order to overcome the problems of CIPII from external pumps connected to catheters or ports that were implanted through the abdominal wall, fully implantable pumps using the IP route have been developed from the initial experience gained with implanted pumps using the IV route. Constant-flow implantable systems using IV delivery had been shown to be effective in improving blood glucose control and stability with a limited risk of infection and catheter occlusion in the long term [57]. However, the development of pumps using a pulsatile method of infusion has been associated with an increased incidence of catheter obstructions that has favoured the IP route since 1985.

TECHNICAL ASPECTS OF IMPLANTABLE INSULIN PUMPS

Essential requirements for implantable insulin pumps include:

- Physically and chemically stable insulin preparations.
- Miniaturised and telemetry-controlled safe and reliable infusion systems.
- Biocompatible materials for pump and catheter.
- A sustained power source for long-term infusion from the implanted pump.
- Easy access to the pump reservoir for insulin refills and to the peritoneal catheter in case of under-delivery.

The trend for insulin aggregation (i.e. physical instability) is a crucial phenomenon to overcome in the development of safe and reliable implanted insulin delivery devices. The two main mechanisms involved in insulin aggregation are iso-electric precipitation and non-covalent polymerization (or fibrillation) [58]. The elaboration of Genapol® (Hoechst AG, Frankfurt, Germany), a surface-active agent able to prevent hydrophobic interactions of insulin with the surface materials of pump reservoirs and tubing by providing hydrophilicity, has allowed considerable improvements in the physical stability of insulin preparation for implantable systems [59]. The resulting insulin solution presently available for implanted pumps, Hoe 21PH, is a pH-neutral buffered insulin formulation containing 400 IU/ml semi-synthetic human insulin, 111 µg/ml zinc ions with 2 mg/ml phenol as preservative, 16 mg/ml glycerol as an isotonicity agent, 50 mM of Tris buffer and 10 µg/ml polyethylene-polypropylene glycol (Genapol®). The stability of Hoe 21PH has been confirmed primarily in PIMS, an experimental model of pulsatile implantable insulin pump designed by MiniMed Inc. for IP infusion and has allowed clinical studies to be performed in subsequent years [59, 60].

Required components of an implantable insulin pump include:

■ An insulin reservoir.
■ A pump and valves.
■ A motor and a battery to supply power for the pump, a clock, a computer and a radio transmitter and receiver.

All of these elements are enclosed in a titanium case that comprises a connecting outlet for catheter attachment (Figure 3.1). An external programmer is used to modulate insulin delivery according to the patient's needs. The only currently available implantable insulin pump, MiniMed Implantable Pump (MIP) model 2007 (Medtronic-MiniMed, Northridge, CA, USA), is implanted in a subcutaneous 'pocket' created in a lower quadrant of the abdomen to allow easy access to the pump reservoir for insulin refills, which are performed every 6–8 weeks. The reservoir is under negative pressure according to the pulsatile pumping principle. The advantage of negative pressure is the prevention of insulin refills outside the reservoir since insulin passively enters the reservoir. The main advantages of a pulsatile pump are the reduction in energy demand and the minimised stress to the infused insulin [32]. The basal and bolus flow rates are determined by the frequency of pump strokes. Pump strokes are programmed by the use of an external telemetry programmer that orders pump cycles according to desired insulin delivery. All active pump procedures must be ordered by the computer in the system, following the programming performed by the patient using the external programmer. The clock allows programming of several basal rates over the day.

Safety mechanisms are needed to avoid over-delivery or runaway in case of computer error or in case of erroneous programming. Thus, MIP 2007 has been designed to stop insulin delivery and provide a corresponding warning sign to the patient on the programmer screen in a case of suspected electronic or mechanic malfunction of the device. Moreover, the physician can set a maximum limit of insulin dose per hour that can be programmed to prevent excessive insulin delivery following an erroneous order. On the other hand, under-delivery can be detected at each pump refill by comparing the volume of insulin expected to be remaining in the pump reservoir with the actual residual volume measured after insulin removal from the reservoir before a fresh insulin refill [61]. The expected residual volume is calculated by the pump programmer, which retains in its memory all programmed deliveries since the last pump refill. When actual residual volume exceeds the expected volume by more than 15%, under-delivery is considered significant and requires investigation [61, 62].

The power supply for the motor and the computer are provided by an internal battery that needs to have a lifespan of several years. The battery of the MIP 2007 may provide energy for 7–10 years.

In order to prevent CO_2 diffusion inside the catheter, which would promote insulin precipitation, polyethylene has been chosen as the interior component of the catheter. To avoid visceral or peritoneal trauma, a silicone coating is used on the external side of the catheter

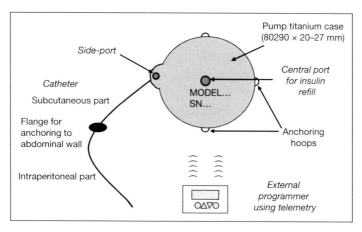

Figure 3.1 Scheme of an implantable insulin pump for intraperitoneal insulin delivery.

and the catheter tip is exclusively composed of silicone. The catheter is left free in the peritoneal cavity and made visible on X-ray by a specific index along its entire length. Various catheter lengths have been used in previous experiences of IP insulin delivery. Short catheters with their tip lying in the upper or middle part of the peritoneal cavity allow quicker insulin peaks but do not significantly influence average metabolic control [48]. The availability of a side-port at the proximal part of the catheter is a very useful tool to manage under-delivery events [50, 62]. This port is accessible by percutaneous puncture for diagnostic or therapeutic procedures.

METABOLIC RESULTS WITH IMPLANTABLE PUMPS

From the availability of Hoe 21PH, three manufacturer-sponsored pilot studies have been performed with three different pump models (Promedos ID1, PIMS and Infusaid model 1000) to assess the feasibility of CIPII using implantable programmable systems [60, 62, 63]. The metabolic results of these studies are presented in Table 3.4. Of note, some Promedos ID1 and Infusaid model 1000 pumps were tested for IV insulin delivery.

Selam and colleagues published a further randomised comparison of metabolic control achieved by the Infusaid model 1000 pump versus CSII [64]. Only the percentage of blood glucose values above 11 mmol/l and the standard deviation of blood glucose values happened to be significantly reduced by IP infusion.

The largest experience with the three available pump models at the beginning of 1990s was reported by the Evaluation dans le Diabète du Traitement par Implants Actifs (EVADIAC) study group, which collected in a central registry all data generated by seven French centres [65]. The whole experience represented 224 type 1 diabetic patients in whom 260 pumps were implanted (205 MIP 2001, a pump model derived from PIMS, 48 Infusaid model 1000 and 7 Promedos ID3) followed up for 353 patient-years. The EVADIAC experience highlighted the metabolic benefits of implantable pumps using the IP route. While HbA1c fell from 7.4 ± 1.8 to $6.8 \pm 1.0\%$, with a sustained improvement over 30 months, the incidence of severe hypoglycaemic events dramatically decreased from 15.2 to 2.5 per 100 patient-years ($P < 0.001$). Interestingly, severe hypoglycaemias were reported to recur in a subset of patients who went back to multiple daily injections or CSII after leaving the implantable pump trial, while HbA1c also went back to higher levels [66].

Table 3.4 Key studies for the assessment of feasibility and effectiveness of implantable insulin pumps for the treatment of type 1 diabetes mellitus

Authors [Ref No.] (Pump model, manufacturer)	Cumulated experience (patient-years)	HbA1c (%)		Severe hypoglycemia (n/p-y)	Local events (n/p-y)	Catheter obstructions (n/p-y)
		Initial	Final			
POINT STUDY GROUP* [63] (Promedos ID 1, Siemens AG)	18.2	7.6 (5.9–9.1)	7.0 (5.7–8.3) (P <0.05)	0.22	0.55	0.27
Saudek et al. [60] (PIMS, MiniMed Inc.)	28	9.2 ± 0.4	8.2 ± 0.4	0.00	0.04	0.14
Selam et al.* [64] (Model 1000, Infusaid)	73	7.4 ± 1.2	7.1 ± 1.0	0.05	0.03	0.29
Hanaire-Broutin et al. for EVADIAC [78] (MIP 2001, MiniMed Inc., Model 1000, Infusaid, Promedos ID 3, Siemens Elema)	353	7.4 ± 1.8	6.8 ± 1.0 (P <0.001)	0.025	0.08	0.13

*Intravenous and intraperitoneal catheters; n/p-y: number of events/patient-year.

Nathan and co-workers addressed the question of the mechanism of this reduction of severe hypoglycaemic events [67]. Attempts to induce hypoglycaemia were performed in eight patients using SC or IP/IV insulin administration at two different doses, the higher one being 1.75-fold, a dose normally used to cover a meal intake. The explanation for the higher occurrence of hypoglycaemia with SC insulin came from the measurements of plasma insulin levels, which were significantly higher at 180 and 240 minutes after SC insulin administration for both doses. Besides, Oskarsson and colleagues demonstrated that the glucagon response to a hypoglycaemia induced by IV insulin was improved after a prolonged IP insulin infusion from implantable pumps when compared with that obtained while the same patients were treated by CSII [68]. Glucagon response to exercise was similarly improved after prolonged IP insulin treatment using implantable pumps [69].

To address the potential usefulness of implantable pumps in type 2 diabetes mellitus, seven Veterans Affairs medical centres in the USA performed a randomised clinical trial to determine the effectiveness and the acceptability of this therapy in insulin-treated type 2 diabetic patients [70]. Mean blood glucose levels and HbA1c were improved in both groups, with no significant difference. However, blood glucose fluctuations, the incidence of mild clinical hypoglycaemia and weight gain were significantly lower with implantable pumps.

In recent years, the EVADIAC group further assessed the effectiveness of IP insulin delivery by implantable pumps in patients previously treated by CSII using lispro insulin. Reported data show that IP insulin treatment led to significantly lower blood glucose levels, noticeably concerning pre-meal values. HbA1c and blood glucose stability were also significantly improved by implantable pumps [71]. Another interesting experience was recently published by Dutch investigators looking at the use implantable insulin pumps in patients with brittle diabetes. A significant sustained reduction of HbA1c was obtained from 10.0 ± 2.3 to 9.0 ± 1.6% ($P = 0.023$) and average yearly hospital stay dramatically reduced from 45 to 13 days ($P = 0.005$) [72].

RISKS RELATED TO IMPLANTABLE INSULIN PUMPS

Although the studies reported above supported the long-term feasibility of implantable pump therapy in type 1 diabetic patients and suggested specific benefits for blood glucose control, most of them also reported adverse events that raised questions about the risk–benefit ratio of this technique.

Renard and colleagues first reported a significant incidence of 'pump-pocket' complications that were responsible for pump explantations in a series of 40 type 1 diabetic patients treated by MiniMed model 2001 pumps [73]. The Infusaid Multicenter Implantable Insulin Pump Study Group mentioned 23 complications at the implantation site occurring in 19 patients during a cumulated experience of 435 patient-years, resulting from 117 model 1000 pumps implanted at 16 centres [74]. The EVADIAC Study Group reported in the largest cumulative multicentre experience ever published (1180 patient-years) that 84 out of 352 patients (24%) were affected by complications at the implantation site [75]. Sixty-four per cent of these patients required pump explantations. Lesions included local inflammatory reactions, skin atrophy or erosion, chronic seromas or infections. No risk factor could be identified, but complications seemed to occur more frequently in centres with a limited number of implants, suggesting that a lack of experience in dealing with the occurrence of these events may be an issue. The cases that did not recover within a few days or weeks seemed unlikely to resolve even after surgical re-intervention, except in cases related to pump migration and/or with preserved skin integrity. Bacterial investigation of pump-pocket fluid accumulations can identify cases with a poor prognosis when microbial colonisation is present [76]. A consensus about preventive procedures includes the limitation of physical activity during the first month following implantation to allow the correct settlement of the pump and antibiotic coverage of implantation and surgical procedures. By following these consensual guidelines, a recent report of the EVADIAC group showed a dramatic reduction of 'pump-pocket' complications [77].

Insulin under-delivery is the major cause of adverse events that may occur when using implantable pumps. Acute under-deliveries related to pump electronic or mechanical failures are very uncommon events [78]. Premature battery depletions also remain anecdotal events only and do not seem widespread in their occurrence [60, 78]. The two main causes of insulin under-deliveries are catheter occlusions and insulin precipitates in pumps. Most incidents develop progressively and are suggested by a necessary increase of insulin dose programming to maintain glucose control. Because of the frequent time delay between gradual under-delivery and adaptation of insulin dose by the patients, impaired glucose control for an unknown reason is the common indicator of delivery problems [61]. The incidence of insulin under-deliveries with implantable pumps has been reported at very variable rates. If one considers reported gross incidences of IP catheter obstructions, they ranged from 7.8 to 57.3 per 100 patient-years [60, 62, 63, 78–81]. The Montpellier group pointed out that patients with previous use of IP insulin delivery using portable pumps accounted for the high incidence of IP catheter obstructions they reported, while patients with more than 21 years of diabetes duration also experienced more frequent catheter obstructions [81]. In a further report, these authors showed that, according to used insulin batches that differed in their preparation process, the incidence of catheter obstructions could vary from 9 to 79 per 100 patient-years [61]. More consensual are the reports on the nature of the obstruction materials. Two types of obstructions have been described:

1. Tip obstructions by fibrin clots.
2. Encapsulations forming a more or less extended 'sock' around the peritoneal catheter [60, 62, 79, 81].

Renard and colleagues first reported that amyloid deposits showing a positive staining by anti-insulin antibodies were present in encapsulation tissue and surrounded by a granulomatous inflammatory reaction involving giant cells and fibrous tissue [81]. Recurrent cases of catheter encapsulations have recently been related to an aseptic peritonitis characterised by similar histological features [82]. Besides these considerations about insulin involvement in catheter obstructions, the role of insulin in under-deliveries related to insulin aggregation is more clearly established. Flow slowdowns related to insulin aggregates in the accumulation chamber of Infusaid pump models 1000 affected 86% of investigated pumps after an average post-implantation time of 10 months in initial feasibility trial [62] and 100% of 48 pumps in the experience of the EVADIAC investigators after a similar post-implantation period [78]. All of these events were solved by rinsing of the pumps with NaOH. Both the design of the accumulation chamber and the lower concentration of used insulin (U-100 vs. U-400 in MiniMed pumps) that reduces the physical stability of the insulin solution have been suspected as promoters of this frequent insulin aggregation. Such incidents were uncommon with MIP 2001 until 1992 when a modification in the preparation procedure of Hoe 21PH insulin batches aimed at increasing its chemical stability resulted in high rates of under-deliveries related to insulin aggregation in pumps [61]. According to used insulin batches, incidence of these events ranged from 27.1 to 121 per 100 patient-years [61]. Udelsman and co-workers reported a similar incidence of 43.8 per 100 patient-years [80]. Investigations showed that insulin aggregation occurred on the titanium ferrule of the ejection chamber, which was in contact with the silicon rubber part of the pump piston, resulting in a backflow of insulin towards the reservoir, which is under negative pressure in MiniMed pumps. Clinical trials showed that a new insulin preparation (Hoe 21PH ETP) could decrease the incidence of backflows from 113 to 6 per 100 patient-years [83] and reduced pump flow impairments at a similar rate whether pump reservoirs were refilled every 45 or 90 days, indicating improved insulin–pump compatibility [84]. Meanwhile, the compliance of the catheter side-port was also improved to allow a better outflow of insulin. An EVADIAC trial reported a dramatic reduction of under-deliveries in 40 MIP 2001 devices that were equipped with this modified side-port and infused stabilised Hoe 21PH ETP insulin: a cumulative follow-up of 106 patient-years showed a stable incidence of four catheter obstructions per 100 patient-years but backflows still occurred with an incidence of 33.7 per 100 patient-years [77].

Whether the increased production of anti-insulin antibodies should be considered an adverse event of implantable insulin pump therapy is still controversial. The immunogenicity of peritoneal insulin delivery has been shown in animal studies as well as in humans treated by intraperitoneal insulin from external pumps. The Montpellier Group mentioned an average two- to three-fold increase of circulating anti-insulin antibodies detected by a radio-immunoelectrophoretic method after 6–84 months of IP insulin delivery from external pumps using U-40 acidic porcine insulin or U-100 neutral porcine insulin respectively [85]. A first report on anti-insulin antibodies in patients treated by implantable insulin pumps using the IP route was published by the Irvine Group [86]. Using a radio-immuno-assay (RIA) technique, they identified two groups of patients among a series of 25 type 1 diabetic subjects treated for 3–6 years – responders and non-responders, the former representing eleven of the total. The increase of antibodies in responders was slow over an average duration of 22 months, and was followed by a spontaneous decrease of titres regardless of whether or not IP therapy continued. Among the eleven responders, four subjects had clinical syndromes that consisted of increasing daily insulin requirements contrasting with nocturnal hypoglycaemia despite minimal basal infusion rates. Although these patients associated the clinical syndromes with high antibody titres, other patients with similarly high titres had no clinical symptoms. The causal relationship was thus not fully established, although altered pharmacokinetics of insulin had been previously described in patients treated by the SC route with high anti-insulin antibody levels [87]. Shortly afterwards, the Strasbourg Group similarly reported an increase of anti-insulin antibodies in about one-half of cases of a series of 62 type 1 diabetic patients treated by IP insulin from several pump models [88]. The Marseilles Group also reported increased anti-insulin antibody levels, detected by both RIA and enzyme-linked immunosorbent assay (ELISA) methods, in a series of 17 type 1 diabetic patients treated by implantable pumps using the IP route [89]. A recent EVADIAC study reported that a large series of 154 patients treated by implantable pumps did not show increased prevalence and incidence over one year of various anti-organ antibodies when matched with patients of similar sex, age and diabetes duration treated by CSII [90].

INDICATIONS AND CONTRAINDICATIONS OF IMPLANTABLE INSULIN PUMPS

Only about 450 diabetic patients worldwide are using such devices for insulin administration at the present time. Only one model of implantable insulin pump is commercially available in the European Union, but it is still under investigation in the USA. Insulin for these pumps is produced in limited volumes and its medical use is restricted to patients involved in research studies or to compassionate cases. Although insulin therapy using implantable pumps remains under investigation, both the results of the feasibility studies detailed above and data provided by recent clinical reports allow some proposals of indications for implantable pumps in type 1 diabetes mellitus [91].

The first proposal is that implantable pumps should be used only in 'last resort' conditions, when diabetic patients absolutely fail to achieve blood glucose control with any other means of insulin therapy, but may be reasonably improved by implantable pump therapy. These relatively uncommon situations include cases of alterations of subcutaneous absorption of insulin, which arise from rare cases of subcutaneous insulin resistance to local skin reactions to insulin injections (e.g. lipodystrophies), or to CSII catheters, or brittle diabetes of unknown origin [92, 93].

The second proposal, supported by the EVADIAC studies reported above, takes into account the documented improvements that IP insulin infusion may provide when compared with CSII using regular insulin or fast-acting analogues, i.e. better blood glucose stability, reduction of severe hypoglycaemia and lowered HbA1c in some studies. According to these data, any type 1 diabetic patient who cannot achieve tight metabolic control with optimised SC insulin therapy could be eligible for an implantable pump if no contraindication is present [89]. Patients who experience recurrent severe hypoglycaemia under intensive SC insulin therapy, in most cases because of hypoglycaemia unawareness, would represent first rank indications for implantable pumps. A non-exhaustive list of contraindications may include:

- Conditions in which the patient is unable to safely manage intensive insulin therapy.
- Situations in which pump use may be hazardous or prone to complications (e.g. work involving exposure to strong magnetic fields or the risk of repeated trauma to the pump-pocket).
- Repeated abdominal surgery that may alter peritoneal insulin infusion.
- Patients with serious associated disease, severe debilitating diabetic complications or an expected short life expectancy.
- High levels of anti-insulin antibodies [82].

It may, however, be argued that against this more liberal attitude, randomised controlled trials comparing implantable pumps with alternative modes of intensive insulin therapy have been very limited. Backing up these arguments is the poorly investigated cost-effectiveness of this technique, but opposing these objections is the better quality of life commonly reported by patients using implantable pumps for diabetes treatment.

EXPECTED DEVELOPMENTS OF IMPLANTABLE INSULIN PUMPS IN THE NEAR FUTURE

Several perspectives could hopefully influence this debate in favour of implantable pumps. Firstly, the expected improvements in pump technology and the insulin-manufacturing process should enable a reduction in the incidence of adverse events that still mar the metabolic effectiveness of this therapy [77]. Secondly, and related to the preceding expectations, the clinical use of implantable pumps is likely to be approved by healthcare authorities outside the European Union. These approvals should spur further clinical studies to assess many aspects of this therapeutic mode that remain unanswered or debated, e.g. cost-effectiveness [94]. It is important to remind ourselves that CSII only emerged as a therapy for diabetes almost 30 years after its initial trials and following many years of similar controversies.

Finally, the ultimate goal of implantable pump therapy is the availability of an artificial beta cell [95]. The first human implantations of a long-term sensor system (LTSS), designed by Medtronic-MiniMed, which connects an IV glucose sensor to an implantable insulin pump, have been performed from 2000 (Figure 3.2) [96]. Data from this trial reported by the Montpellier Group are very encouraging [97–99]. Alternative methods of continuous glucose monitoring using portable or subcutaneous implanted sensor models, currently under investigation, may also assist in the management of insulin delivery more closely matched to actual needs in the near future [11]. Whether used in open- or closed-loop conditions, the reliability and the reactivity of insulin delivery will be crucial to prevent blood glucose excursions. Intraperitoneal insulin infusion from implantable pumps may well take the lead to fulfil these requirements.

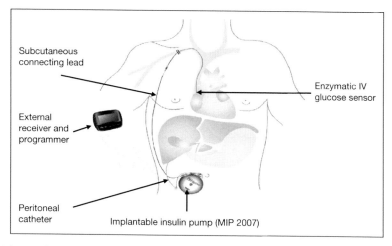

Subcutaneous
connecting lead

Enzymatic IV
glucose sensor

External
receiver and
programmer

Peritoneal
catheter

Implantable insulin pump (MIP 2007)

Figure 3.2 Scheme of human implantation of the Long-Term Sensor System (LTSS, Medtronic-MiniMed), a prototype of an artificial β-cell.
IV = intravenous.

INHALED INSULIN ADMINISTRATION

Pulmonary insulin administration has been considered as far back as the 1920s, but it only recently became feasible as a therapy as a result of an improved understanding of aerosol dynamics [12]. Efficient absorption of inhaled insulin at an alveolar level certainly depends on many factors, such as:

- Morphology and status of respiratory track.
- Smoking.
- Exercise.
- Patient skill in inhaler use.
- Breathing pattern.
- Size, surface morphology, charge, solubility and hygroscopicity of inhaled insulin particles [100].

Inhalation at the beginning of a slow and deep inspiration improves alveolar deposition; therefore, breath-activated inhalers improve the bioavailability of inhaled insulin and lower the doses necessary for effective action [101]. Dry powder and liquid aerosol are the two presently available formulations of insulin. The ideal particle size of insulin aerosol should be 1.5–2.5 μm, larger particles being blocked prior to reaching the alveolar surface and smaller ones being exhaled [12]. However, specifically designed insulin particles may offer original characteristics that improve diffusion at the alveolar surface. Thus, large, porous insulin particles of 10–20 μm size and low mass density obtained by using a biodegradable polymer matrix composed of phospholipids in Alkermes/Eli Lilly system have a reduced tendency to aggregate, disperse easily and may be less susceptible to phagocytosis [102]. Trapped insulin in self-assembled microspheres formed by a diketo-piperazine derivative at low pH is quickly released at neutral pH in the Technosphere™/Medtone™ system [103]. Presently, various combinations of insulin formulations or preparations and inhalers are used for clinical investigations (Table 3.5).

Table 3.5 Different systems for insulin inhalation

Device	Nektar/Exubera	AER$_X$ IDMS	Aerodose Inhaler	Advanced Inhalation Research	Medtone/Technosphere
Type of device	Dry powder inhaler	Aqueous mist inhaler	Liquid insulin inhaler	Dry powder inhaler	Dry powder high impedance inhaler
Manufacturer	Nektar Therapeutics, Pfizer Inc, Aventis Pharma	Aradigm Corp, Novo Nordisk A/S	Aerogen Inc	Alkermes, Eli-Lilly	Mannkind Biopharmaceuticals
Type of insulin	Insulin powder	Liquid insulin	Liquid insulin (Humalin I®)	Insulin powder	Insulin powder
Insulin presentation	Blisters of 1 or 3 mg (28 or 84 IU)	Strips (equivalent to 1 IU SC insulin)	500 IU/ml	Capsules of 0.9 or 2.6 mg (equivalent to 2 or 6 IU SC insulin)	Capsules of 6, 12 or 24 IU (equivalent to 2, 4 or 8 IU SC insulin)
MMAD (μm)	3	2	3.3	1–3	3.3
Breath-activation	No	Yes	Yes	Yes	No

MMAD = mass median aerodynamic diameter (of insulin particles); SC = subcutaneous.

PHARMACOLOGICAL CHARACTERISTICS OF INHALED INSULIN

A persistent limitation of the current options for inhaled insulin delivery comes from bio-availability and biopotency between 10 and 15%, resulting in the necessary use of large amounts of insulin to obtain insulin action. The Mannkind Biopharmaceuticals option is somewhat different in that bioavailability and biopotency of 26 and 19% relative to SC insulin have been reported, respectively [12].

Average time to plasma insulin peak is shorter after insulin inhalation than after SC injection of regular insulin with the Nektar/Exubera system: 55 vs. 148 minutes [104], AERx® iDMS: 7–20 vs. 100–120 minutes [98] and Aerodose™ Inhaler: 50 vs. 85 minutes [12], and close to that after SC lispro insulin injection with the Alkermes/Eli Lilly system: 45 minutes for both [105]. The Technosphere™/Medtone™ system allows a very short time to plasma insulin peak of 13 minutes [106]. Thus, insulin action is quicker with inhaled insulin with an earlier average time of maximal insulin effect of 143 minutes (versus 193 minutes after SC regular insulin), which is similar to SC lispro insulin (137 minutes) with the Nektar/Exubera system [104]. The duration of insulin action after inhalation is close to that after SC delivery of regular insulin: 392 ± 95 vs. 413 ± 108 minutes, but longer than that after SC lispro insulin: 309 ± 45 minutes [101]. The average time to maximal activity is shorter with the Technosphere™/Medtone™ system: 39 minutes, but the duration of action does not exceed 2–3 hours [106].

Onset and duration of inhaled insulin action are not modified according to insulin dose, while maximal effect follows insulin dose. Intra-subject variability of action is similar to that of SC regular or lispro insulin: 14–25 versus 11–27% [107]. Of note, smokers or recent past smokers show a higher insulin absorption rate whereas asthmatics absorb less inhaled insulin [108, 109]. Mild upper respiratory tract infections are associated with a slightly shorter time to peak plasma insulin. Age does not seem to influence absorption rate and action profile of inhaled insulin [12].

METABOLIC RESULTS WITH INHALED INSULIN

In type 1 diabetes mellitus, two randomised studies have been recently published comparing inhaled insulin at mealtime versus SC regular or lispro insulin, in combination with twice daily NPH insulin or glargine as basal insulin. The Nektar/Exubera system was used in the comparison with SC regular insulin, and in association with NPH [110]. The Alkermes/Eli Lilly system was tested in the other study versus SC regular or lispro insulin, and in association with glargine [111]. Both studies showed no difference in terms of HbA1c levels and post-meal blood glucose levels. Fasting blood glucose was significantly lower in both studies where inhaled insulin was used. In the study with NPH as basal insulin, the incidence of hypoglycaemia was similar with SC or inhaled insulin, but severe hypoglycaemic episodes occurred more frequently with inhaled insulin (6.5 vs. 3.3 events per 100 patient-months). In the study using glargine as basal insulin, the incidence of hypoglycaemic episodes was also similar with inhaled or SC regular or lispro insulin, but nocturnal hypoglycaemic episodes were more frequent with inhaled insulin (4.2 vs. 2.7 events per 30 days). So, no metabolic advantage was found in favour of inhaled insulin in type 1 diabetic patients; the increased rate of severe or nocturnal hypoglycaemic episodes may even be worrisome.

Five randomised studies have been reported with inhaled insulin in type 2 diabetic patients at various stages of evolution. In patients experiencing failure of glucose control with diet and exercise [112], 82.7% of patients who used the Nektar/Exubera system once or twice daily reached an HbA1c level below 8% versus 58.2% of patients to whom 8 mg daily rosiglitazone was allocated. Weight gain and hypoglycaemic events were, however, higher with inhaled insulin. In patients with failure while using oral drugs, HbA1c was dramatically improved after 12 weeks by a mean difference of 2.2% in the patients who added inhaled insulin to their oral drugs [113]. A recent study in a similar population of patients showed a mean decrease of HbA1c by 1.67% when pre-meal inhaled insulin (Nektar/Exubera) was added to oral drugs, and by 1.44% with pre-meal inhaled insulin alone, versus –1.18% in the control group who continued taking oral drugs only [114]. Hypoglycaemia rate and mild weight gain were, however, higher with inhaled insulin. When compared to pre-meal SC regular insulin and associated with NPH twice daily, HbA1c decreased by 0.69% with inhaled insulin ($AER_X^®$ / IDMS) versus 0.77% with SC regular insulin [115]. With ultralente as basal insulin, inhaled insulin (Nektar/Exubera) also showed no significant difference versus 2–3 regular daily SC insulin injections (-0.71%) [116]. In summary, inhaled insulin in type 2 diabetic patients is very effective when these patients experience failure of oral drugs. Inhaled insulin can also be a good substitute for mealtime SC injections in patients who require multiple injections. Since inhaled insulin may be easier to accept by these patients, it could prevent the usual delay of treatment adaptation when insulin is needed or more frequent insulin injections become necessary to improve glucose control. Indeed, patient satisfaction was highly rated after trials of inhaled insulin, and most of them agreed to continue with it after studies [117, 118].

RISKS RELATED TO INHALED INSULIN

The main question raised by inhaled insulin is whether it may induce pulmonary adverse events. Until now, the only reported symptom in around 10% of patients who used inhaled insulin was a throat-clearing cough, which tended to decrease with time. Data obtained from reported studies show no significant difference on forced expiratory volume (FEV_1) or diffusing capacity (DLCO), although some studies found a fall in DLCO that vanished after interruption of insulin inhalation [12]. In these reports, use of inhaled insulin was limited to a few months and clearer information is needed on longer-term usage. Specific data in limited groups of patients will have to be collected by alveolar lavage or high resolution computed tomography. Moreover, analyses of pulmonary function versus well-matched control patients will have to be gathered, based upon precise criteria. Theoretical risk includes asthma, lung fibrosis, impairments of pressure in pulmonary artery and lung cancer, but no data recorded until now confirmed these hypotheses.

The second question is about the potential consequences of anti-insulin antibodies whose plasma levels have been reported to increase with inhaled insulin [115, 119]. Until now, no relationship has been found between anti-insulin antibody titres and metabolic parameters [12]. However, keeping in mind the phenomena observed with IP insulin, a careful survey of antibody levels and their potential consequences will be needed.

INDICATIONS AND CONTRAINDICATIONS OF INHALED INSULIN

Presently, no specific indication for inhaled insulin has been validated. Contraindications should reasonably include any respiratory tract disease and all serious cardiac diseases. Patients with high anti-insulin antibody titres should also be considered as relative contraindications, because they are potential further 'responders' with inhaled insulin. At least until more safety data have been collected, young patients mostly affected by type 1 diabetes with a long-term potential use of inhaled insulin should be excluded.

The best initial indication would likely be meal insulin coverage of type 2 diabetic patients who are poorly controlled with oral drugs or with basal insulin only.

EXPECTED FUTURE DEVELOPMENTS OF INHALED INSULIN

Development of insulin inhalation has, for some time, remained highly dependent on the answers to a number of safety issues [5, 12]. If reassuring initial data had been confirmed, inhaled insulin could likely become the most widely used method of 'non- invasive' insulin therapy.

As a matter of fact, almost two years after initial approval of the Nektar/Exubera system for clinical use by the US FDA in January 2006, this tool for inhaled insulin administration was withdrawn from the market by the manufacturer in October 2007. The other companies that were developing systems for insulin inhalation stopped their development programmes shortly afterwards, except Mannkind Biopharmaceuticals. Beside sales below expectations and limited acceptance of the Nektar/Exubera system, several concerns including cost, efficacy, safety, patient eligibility and convenience have contributed to the failure of inhaled insulin to be embraced by patients and healthcare providers [120]. The amount of cumulated clinical data with inhaled insulin will remain a valuable source from technological, scientific and medical points of view.

SUMMARY

The development of new methods of insulin administration is motivated by a desire to increase insulin's effectiveness, safety and ease of use. 'Patch' micro-pumps connected to discrete and reliable continuous glucose monitoring systems, which will likely represent the next generation of devices for CSII, could take the lead in the near future as the reference method of insulin therapy. However, these systems will require education that not all patients will be able to follow. Patients with frequent hypoglycaemic events and erratic blood glucose swings will be good candidates for IP insulin delivery; others will apply for implanted devices because this treatment minimises the visible manifestation of their disease and for quality of life reasons. The real challenge will occur when comparing these insulin delivery methods with the development of cell therapy of diabetes, provided it restores insulin secretion on a sustained duration with limited adverse outcomes in relation to tolerance. Insulin delivery by inhalation – or buccal or transdermal administration, if they become feasible – could at least reduce the burden of currently used insulin therapy for a while until more sophisticated means of treatment become widely available. When facing the expected worldwide diabetes epidemic, the question of cost will, however, play a key role in these developments.

REFERENCES

1. Van den Berghe G, Wouters P, Weekers F et al. Intensive insulin therapy in critically ill patients. N Engl J Med 2001; 345:1359–1367.
2. Bolli GB. Physiological insulin replacement in type 1 diabetes mellitus. Exp Clin Endocrinol Diabetes 2001; 109(suppl 2):S317–S332.
3. The Diabetes Control and Complications Trial Research Group. The effect of intensive treatment of diabetes on the development and progression of long-term complications in insulin-dependent diabetes mellitus. N Engl J Med 1993; 329:977–986.
4. UK Prospective Diabetes Study Group. Intensive blood-glucose control with sulfonylureas or insulin compared with conventional treatment and risk of complications in patients with type 2 diabetes (UKPDS 33). Lancet 1998; 352:837–853.
5. Gomez-Perez FJ, Rull JA. Insulin therapy: current alternatives. Arch Med Res 2005; 36:258–272.
6. Pickup J, Keen H. Continuous subcutaneous insulin infusion at 25 years: evidence base for the expanding use of insulin pump therapy in type 1 diabetes. Diabetes Care 2002; 25:593–598.
7. Slama G, Hautecouverture M, Assan R, Tchobroutsky G. One to five days of continuous intravenous insulin infusion on seven diabetic patients. Diabetes 1974; 23:732–738.
8. Plodkowski RA, Edelman SV. The state of insulin pump therapy: 2002. Curr Opin Endocrinol Diabetes 2002; 9:329–337.
9. Zinman B, Tildesley H, Chiasson JL, Tsui E, Strack T. Insulin lispro in CSII: results of double-blind crossover study. Diabetes 1997; 46:440–443.

10. Fisher LK, Halvorson M. Future developments in insulin pump therapy: progression from continuous subcutaneous insulin infusion to a sensor-pump system. *Diabetes Educ* 2006; 32(suppl 1):47S–52S.
11. Renard E. Implantable closed loop glucose-sensing and insulin delivery: the future for insulin pump therapy. *Curr Opin Pharmacol* 2002; 2:708–716.
12. Owens DR, Zinman B, Bolli G. Alternative routes of insulin delivery. *Diabet Med* 2003; 20:886–898.
13. The Diabetes Control and Complications Trial Research Group. Implementation of treatment protocols in the Diabetes Control and Complications Trial. *Diabetes Care* 1995; 18:361–376.
14. Mecklenburg RS, Benson JW Jr, Becker NM *et al*. Clinical use of the insulin infusion pump in 100 patients with type 1 diabetes. *N Engl J Med* 1982; 307:513–718.
15. Mecklenburg RS, Benson EA, Benson JW Jr *et al*. Acute complications associated with insulin infusion therapy. Report of experience with 181 patients. *JAMA* 1984; 252:3265–3269.
16. Weissberg-Benchell J, Antisdel-Lomaglio J, Seshadri R. Insulin pump therapy: a meta-analysis. *Diabetes Care* 2003; 26:1079–1087.
17. Radermecker RP, Scheen AJ. Continuous subcutaneous insulin infusion with short-acting insulin analogues or human regular insulin: efficacy, safety, quality of life, and cost-effectiveness. *Diabetes Metab Res Rev* 2004; 20:178–188.
18. Melki V, Renard E, Lassmann-Vague V *et al*. Improvement of HbA1c and blood glucose stability in IDDM patients treated with lispro insulin analog in external pumps. *Diabetes Care* 1998; 21:977–982.
19. Renner R, Pfützner A, Trautmann M *et al*. Use of insulin lispro in continuous subcutaneous insulin infusion treatment. Results of a multicenter trial. *Diabetes Care* 1999; 22:784–788.
20. Johansson UB, Adamson UCK, Lins PES, Wredling RAM. The Swedish Multicenter Lispro Insulin Study. Improved blood glucose variability, HbA1c and less insulin requirement in IDDM patients using lispro in CSII. *Diabetes Metab* 2000; 26:192–196.
21. Hanaire-Broutin H, Melki V, Bessieres-Lacombe S, Tauber JP. The Study Group for the Development of Pump Therapy in Diabetes. Comparison of continuous subcutaneous insulin infusion and multiple daily injection regimens using insulin lispro in type 1 diabetic patients on intensified treatment. *Diabetes Care* 2000; 23:1232–1235.
22. Pickup JC, Sutton AJ. Severe hypoglycaemia and glycaemic control in Type 1 diabetes: meta-analysis of multiple daily insulin injections compared with continuous subcutaneous insulin infusion. *Diabet Med* 2008; 25:765–774
23. Retnakaran R, Hochman J, DeVries JH *et al*. Continuous subcutaneous insulin infusion versus multiple daily injections. The impact of baseline A1c. *Diabetes Care* 2004; 27:2590–2596.
24. Renard E. Intensive insulin therapy today: 'basal-bolus' using multiple daily injections or CSII? *Diabetes Metab* 2005; 31:4S40–4S44.
25. Bolli GB, Capani F, Home PD *et al*. Comparison of a multiple daily injection daily with once-daily insulin glargine basal insulin and mealtime lispro, to continuous subcutaneous insulin infusion: a randomised, open, parallel study. *Diabetes* 2004; 53(suppl 2):A107–A108.
26. Doyle (Boland) EA, Weinzimer SA, Steffen AT, Ahern JAH, Vincent M, Tamborlane WV. A randomized, prospective trial comparing the efficacy of continuous subcutaneous insulin infusion with multiple daily injections using insulin glargine. *Diabetes Care* 2004; 27:1554–1558.
27. Hirsch IB, Bode BW, Garg S *et al*. Continuous subcutaneous insulin infusion (CSII) of insulin aspart versus multiple daily injection of insulin aspart/insulin glargine in type 1 diabetic patients previously treated with CSII. *Diabetes Care* 2005; 28:533–538.
28. Alemzadeh R, Ellis JN, Holzum MK, Parton EA, Wyatt DT. Beneficial effects of continuous subcutaneous insulin infusion and flexible multiple daily insulin regimen using insulin glargine in type 1 diabetes. *Pediatrics* 2004; 114:91–95.
29. Schiaffini R, Ciampalini P, Spera S, Cappa M, Crino A. An observational study comparing continuous subcutaneous insulin infusion (CSII) and insulin glargine in children with type 1 diabetes. *Diabetes Metab Res Rev* 2005; 21:347–352.
30. Lepore G, Dodesini AR, Nosari I, Trevisan R. Effect of continuous subcutaneous insulin infusion vs multiple daily injection with glargine as basal insulin; an open parallel long-term study. *Diabetes Nutr Metab* 2004; 17:84–89.
31. Pickup JC, Kidd J, Burmiston S, Yemane N. Determinants of glycaemic control in type 1 diabetes during intensified therapy with multiple daily injections or continuous subcutaneous insulin infusion: importance of blood glucose variability. *Diabetes Metab Res Rev* 2006; 22:232–237.
32. Selam JL, Charles MA. Devices for insulin administration. *Diabetes Care* 1990; 13:955–979.

33. Guerci B, Meyer L, Salle A et al. Comparison of metabolic deterioration between insulin analog and regular insulin after a 5-hour interruption of a continuous subcutaneous insulin infusion in type 1 diabetic patients. *J Clin Endocrinol Metab* 1999; 84:2673–2678.
34. Bode BW, Steed RD, Davidson PC. Reduction in severe hypoglycaemia with long-term subcutaneous insulin infusion in type 1 diabetes. *Diabetes Care* 1996; 19:324–327.
35. Garg SK, Frias JP, Anil S, Gottlieb PA, MacKenzie T, Jackson WE. Insulin lispro therapy in pregnancies complicated by type 1 diabetes: glycemic control and maternal and fetal outcomes. *Endoc Pract* 2003; 9:187–193.
36. Fox LA, Buckloh LM, Smith SD, Wysocki T, Mauras N. A randomized controlled trial of insulin pump therapy in young children with type 1 diabetes. *Diabetes Care* 2005; 28:1277–1281.
37. Dahl-Jorgensen K, Brinchmann-Hansen O, Hanssen KF, Sandvik L, Aegenes O, Aker Diabetes Group. Rapid tightening of blood glucose control leads to transient deterioration of retinopathy in insulin dependent diabetes mellitus: the Oslo Study. *Br Med J* 1985; 290:811–815.
38. Raskin P, Bode BW, Marck JB et al. Continuous subcutaneous insulin infusion and multiple daily injection therapy are equally effective in type 2 diabetes: a randomized, parallel-group, 24-week study. *Diabetes Care* 2003; 26:2598–2603.
39. Wainstein J, Metzger M, Boaz M et al. Insulin pump therapy vs multiple daily injections in obese type 2 diabetic patients. *Diabet Med* 2005; 22:1037–1046.
40. Herman WH, Ilag LL, Johnson SL et al. A clinical trial of continuous subcutaneous insulin infusion versus multiple daily injections in older adults with type 2 diabetes. *Diabetes Care* 2005; 28:1568–1573.
41. Scuffham P, Carr L. The cost-effectiveness of continuous subcutaneous insulin infusion compared with multiple daily injections for the management of diabetes. *Diabet Med* 2003; 20:586–593.
42. Renard E. Insulin therapy by insulin pump: continuous or conventional self-blood glucose monitoring? *Diabetes Metab* 2003; 29:2S54–2S62.
43. Steil GM, Saad MF. Automated insulin delivery for type 1 diabetes. *Curr Opin Endocrinol Diabetes* 2006; 13:205–211.
44. Wang PM, Cornwell M, Hill J, Prausnitz MR. Precise microinjection into skin using hollow microneedles. *J Invest Dermatol* 2006; 126:1080–1087.
45. Diagnostic and therapeutic technology assessment. Continuous peritoneal insulin infusion and implantable insulin infusion pumps for diabetic control. *JAMA* 1989; 262:3195–3198.
46. Schade DS, Eaton RP, Davis T et al. The kinetics of peritoneal insulin absorption. *Metabolism* 1981; 30:149–155.
47. Nelson JA, Stephen R, Landau ST, Wilson DE, Tyler FH. Intraperitoneal insulin administration produces a positive portal-systemic blood insulin gradient in unanesthetized, unrestrained swine. *Metabolism* 1982; 31:969–972.
48. Selam JL, Raymond M, Jacquemin JL, Orsetti A, Richard JL, Mirouze J. Pharmacokinetics of insulin infused intra-peritoneally via portable pumps. *Diabetes Metab* 1985; 11:170–173.
49. Giacca A, Caumo A, Galimberti G et al. Peritoneal and subcutaneous absorption of insulin in type 1 diabetic subjects. *J Clin Endocrinol Metab* 1993; 77:738–742.
50. Olsen CL, Liu G, Charles MA. Novel Routes of insulin delivery. In: Marshall SM, Home PD (eds). *The Diabetes Annual/8.* Elsevier Science BV, New York, 1994, pp 243–276.
51. Irsigler K, Kritz H. Alternate routes of insulin delivery. *Diabetes Care* 1980; 3:219–228.
52. Pozza G, Spotti D, Micossi P et al. Long-term continuous intraperitoneal insulin treatment in brittle diabetes. *Diabetes* 1983; 286:255–256.
53. Selam JL, Slingeneyer A, Hedon B, Mares P, Beraud JJ, Mirouze J. Long-term ambulatory peritoneal insulin infusion of brittle diabetes with portable pumps: comparison with intravenous and subcutaneous routes. *Diabetes Care* 1983; 6:105–111.
54. Selam JL, Slingeneyer A, Saeidi S, Mirouze J. Experience with long-term peritoneal insulin infusion with portable pumps. *Diabetic Med* 1985; 2:41–44.
55. Shishko PI, Kovalev PA, Goncharov VG, Zajarny IU. Comparison of peripheral and portal (via the umbilical vein) routes of insulin infusion in IDDM patients. *Diabetes* 1982; 41:1042–1049.
56. Wredling R, Adamson U, Lins PE, Backman L, Lundgren D. Experience of a long-term intraperitoneal insulin treatment using a new percutaneous access device. *Diabet Med* 1991; 8:597–600.
57. Blackshear PJ, Shulman GI, Roussell AM et al. Metabolic response to three years of continuous, basal rate intravenous insulin infusion in type II diabetic patients. *J Clin Endocrinol Metab* 1985; 61:753–760.
58. Brange J, Havelund S. Insulin pumps and insulin quality. Requirements and problems. *Acta Med Scand* 1983; (suppl 671):135–138.

59. Grau U, Saudek CD. Stable insulin preparation for implanted insulin pumps. Laboratory and animal trials. *Diabetes* 1987; 36:1453–1459.

60. Saudek CD, Selam JL, Pitt HA *et al.* A preliminary trial of the programmable implantable medication system for insulin delivery. *N Engl J Med* 1989; 321:574–579.

61. Renard E, Bouteleau S, Jacques-Apostol D *et al.* Insulin underdelivery from implanted pumps using peritoneal route: determinant role of insulin-pump compatibility. *Diabetes Care* 1996; 19:812–817.

62. Selam JL, Micossi P, Dunn FL, Nathan DM. Clinical trial of programmable implantable insulin pumps for type 1 diabetes. *Diabetes Care* 1992; 15:877–885.

63. Point Study Group. One-year trial of a remote-controlled implantable insulin infusion system in type I diabetic patients. *Lancet* 1988; i:864–869.

64. Selam JL, Raccah D, Jeandidier N, Lozano JL, Waxman K, Charles MA. Randomized comparison of metabolic control achieved by intraperitoneal insulin infusion with implantable pumps versus intensive subcutaneous insulin therapy in type I diabetic patients. *Diabetes Care* 1992; 15:53–58.

65. Broussolle C, Jeandidier N, Hanaire-Broutin H, for The Evadiac Study Group. French multicentre experience with implantable insulin pumps. *Lancet* 1994; 343:514–515.

66. Jeandidier N, Selam JL, Renard E *et al*, for The Evadiac Study Group. Decreased severe hypoglycaemia frequency during intraperitoneal insulin infusion using programmable implantable pumps. *Diabetes Care* 1996; 19:780.

67. Nathan DM, Dunn FL, Bruch J *et al.* Postprandial insulin profiles with implantable pump therapy may explain decreased frequency of severe hypoglycemia, compared with intensive subcutaneous regimens, in insulin-dependent diabetes mellitus patients. *Am J Med* 1996; 100:412–417.

68. Oskarsson PR, Lins PE, Backman L, Adamson UC. Continuous intraperitoneal insulin infusion partly restores the glucagon response to hypoglycemia in type 1 diabetic patients. *Diabetes Metab* 2000; 26:118–124.

69. Oskarsson PR, Lins PE, Wallberg-Henriksson H, Adamson UC. Metabolic and hormonal responses to exercise in type 1 diabetic patients during continuous subcutaneous, as compared to continuous intraperitoneal, insulin infusion. *Diabetes Metab* 1999; 25:491–497.

70. Saudek CD, Duckworth WC, Giobbie-Hurder A *et al*, for the Department of Veterans Affairs Implantable Insulin Pump Study Group. Implantable insulin pumps vs. multiple dose insulin for non-insulin-dependent diabetes mellitus: a randomized clinical trial. *JAMA* 1996; 276:1322–1327.

71. Catargi B, Meyer L, Melki V, Renard E, Jeandidier N, for the EVADIAC Study Group. Comparison of blood glucose stability and HbA1c between implantable insulin pumps using U400 HOE 21Ph insulin and external pumps using lispro in type 1 diabetic patients: a pilot study. *Diabetes Metab* 2002; 28:133–137.

72. De Vries JH, Eskes SA, Snoek FJ *et al.* Continuous intraperitoneal insulin infusion in patients with 'brittle' diabetes: favourable effects on glycaemic control and hospital stay. *Diabet Med* 2002; 19:496–501.

73. Renard E, Bringer J, Jacques-Apostol D *et al.* Complications of the pump-pocket may represent a significant cause of incidents with implanted systems for intraperitoneal insulin delivery. *Diabetes Care* 1994; 17:1064–1066.

74. Scavini M, Cristallo M, Sarmiento M, Dunn FL, The Infusaid Multicenter Implantable Insulin Pump Study Group. Pump-pocket complications during long-term insulin delivery using an implanted programmable pump. *Diabetes Care* 1996; 19:384–385.

75. Belicar P, Lassmann-Vague V, The EVADIAC Study Group. Local adverse events associated with long-term treatment by implantable insulin pumps. *Diabetes Care* 1998; 21:325–326.

76. Renard E, Rostane T, Carriere C *et al.* Implantable insulin pumps: infections most likely due to seeding from skin flora determine severe outcomes of pump-pocket seromas. *Diabetes Metab* 2001; 27:62–65.

77. Gin H, Renard E, Melki V *et al*, and the EVADIAC Study Group. Combined improvements in implantable pump technology and insulin stability allow safe and effective long term intraperitoneal insulin delivery in type 1 diabetic patients: the EVADIAC experience. *Diabetes Metab* 2003; 29:602–607.

78. Hanaire-Broutin H, Broussolle C, Jeandidier N *et al*, the EVADIAC Study Group. Feasibility of intraperitoneal insulin therapy with programmable implantable pumps in IDDM: a multicenter study. *Diabetes Care* 1995; 18:388–392.

79. Scavini M, Galli L, Reich S, Eaton RP, Charles MA, Dunn FL, the Implantable Insulin Pump Trial Study. Catheter survival during long-term insulin therapy with an implanted programmable pump. *Diabetes Care* 1997; 20:610–613.

80. Udelsman R, Chen H, Loman K, Pitt HA, Saudek CD. Implanted programmable insulin pumps: one hundred fifty-three patient years of surgical experience. *Surgery* 1997; 122:1005–1011.

81. Renard E, Baldet P, Picot MC *et al*. Catheter complications with implantable systems for peritoneal insulin delivery. An analysis of frequency, predisposing factors and obstructing materials. *Diabetes Care* 1995; 18:300–306.

82. Renard E, Raingeard I, Costalat G *et al*. Aseptic peritonitis revealed through recurrent catheter obstructions in type 1 diabetic patients treated with continuous peritoneal insulin infusion. *Diabetes Care* 2004; 27:276–277.

83. Renard E, Souche C, Jacques-Apostol D *et al*. Improved stability of insulin delivery from implanted pumps using a new preparation process for infused insulin. *Diabetes Care* 1999; 22:1371–1372.

84. Boivin S, Belicar P, Melki V, EVADIAC Group. Assessment of *in vivo* stability of a new insulin preparation for implantable insulin pumps. *Diabetes Care* 1999; 22:2089–2090.

85. Bousquet-Rouaud R, Chante MA, Orsetti A, Mirouze J. Increase of antiinsulin antibody titer during continuous peritoneal insulin infusion. *Artif Organs* 1990; 14(suppl 3):241–243.

86. Olsen CL, Chan E, Turner DS *et al*. Insulin antibody responses after long-term intraperitoneal insulin administration via implantable programmable insulin delivery systems. *Diabetes Care* 1994; 17:169–176.

87. Sodoyez JC, Koch M, Sodoyez-Goffaux F. Anticorps anti-insuline: méthodologie et implications cliniques. *Diabetes Metab* 1991; 17:255–269.

88. Jeandidier N, Boivin S, Sapin R *et al*. Immunogenicity of intraperitoneal insulin infusion using programmable implantable devices. *Diabetologia* 1995; 38:577–584.

89. Lassmann-Vague V, Belicar P, Raccah D, Vialettes B, Sodoyez JC, Vague P. Immunogenicity of long-term intraperitoneal insulin administration with implantable programmable pumps. *Diabetes Care* 1995; 18:498–503.

90. Dufaitre-Patouraux L, Riveline JP, Renard E *et al*. Continuous intraperitoneal insulin infusion does not increase the risk of organ-specific autoimmune disease in type 1 diabetic patients: results of a multicentric, comparative study. *Diabetes Metab* 2006; 32(5 Pt 1):427–432.

91. Renard E, Schaepelynck-Bélicar P, EVADIAC Group. Implantable insulin pumps. A position statement about their clinical use. *Diabetes Metab* 2007; 33:158–166.

92. Riveline JP, Vantyghem MC, Fermon C *et al*. Subcutaneous insulin resistance successfully circumvented on long term by peritoneal insulin delivery from an implantable pump in four diabetic patients. *Diabetes Metab* 2005; 31:496–498.

93. Baillot-Rudoni S, Apostol D, Vaillant G, Brun JM, Renard E, on behalf of the EVADIAC study group. Implantable pump therapy restores metabolic control and quality of life in type 1 diabetic patients with Buschke's non systemic scleroderma. *Diabetes Care* 2006; in press.

94. Haardt MJ, Selam JL, Slama G *et al*. A cost-benefit comparison of intensive diabetes management with implantable pumps versus multiple subcutaneous injections in patients with type 1 diabetes. *Diabetes Care* 1994; 17:847–851.

95. Jaremko J, Rorstad O. Advances toward the implantable artificial pancreas for treatment of diabetes. *Diabetes Care* 1998; 21:444–450.

96. Renard E, Costalat G, Moran B, Kolopp M, Lebel R, Bringer J. First combined implantations of a long-term IV glucose sensor and an intra-peritoneal insulin pump in diabetic patients. *Diabetes* 2001; 50(suppl 2):A3.

97. Renard E, Shah R, Miller M *et al*. Accuracy of real-time blood glucose measurement by long-term sensor system allows automated insulin delivery in diabetic patients. *Diabetes* 2002; 51(suppl 2):A126.

98. Renard E, Shah R, Miller M, Kolopp M, Costalat G, Bringer J. Sustained safety and accuracy of central IV glucose sensors connected to implanted insulin pumps and short-term closed-loop trials in diabetic patients. *Diabetes* 2003; 52(suppl 2):A36.

99. Renard E, Costalat G, Chevassus H, Bringer J. Artificial beta-cell: clinical experience toward an implantable closed-loop insulin delivery system. *Diabetes Metab* 2006; 32(5 Pt 2):497–502.

100. Patton JS, Bukar J, Nagarajan S. Inhaled insulin. *Advanced Drug Delivery Rev* 1992; 8:179–196.

101. Farr SJ, McElduff A, Mather LE *et al*. Pulmonary insulin administration using the AER$_X$™ system: physiological and physiochemical factors influencing insulin effectiveness in healthy fasting subjects. *Diabetes Technol Therapeutics* 2000; 2:185–197.

102. Edwards DA, Ben-Jerbria A, Eskew ML, Langer R. Recent advances in pulmonary drug delivery using large, porous inhaled particles. *J Appl Physiol* 1998; 85:379–385.

103. Pfutzner A, Mann A, Steiner S. Technosphere™/insulin-a new approach for effective delivery of human insulin via the pulmonary route. *Diabetes Technol Therapeutics* 2002; 4:589–593.

104. Rave K, Bott S, Heinemann L *et al*. Time-action profile of inhaled insulin in comparison with subcutaneously injected insulin lispro and regular human insulin. *Diabetes Care* 2005; 28:1077–1082.

105. Rave KM, Nosek L, De La Pena A *et al*. Dose response of inhaled dry-powder insulin and dose equivalence to subcutaneous insulin lispro. *Diabetes Care* 2005; 28:2400–2405.
106. Rave KM, Heise T, Pfutzner A, Steiner S, Heinemann L. Results of a dose-response study with a new pulmonary insulin formulation and inhaler. *Diabetes* 2000; 49(suppl 1):A7.
107. Heinemann L, Klappoth W, Rave K *et al*. Intra-individual variability of the metabolic effect of inhaled insulin together with an absorption enhancer. *Diabetes Care* 2000; 23:1343–1347.
108. Himmelmann A, Jendle J, Mellen A *et al*. The impact of smoking on inhaled insulin. *Diabetes Care* 2003; 26:677–682.
109. Henry RR, Mudaliar SR, Howland WC III *et al*. Inhaled insulin using the AERx Insulin Diabetes Management System in healthy and asthmatic subjects. *Diabetes Care* 2003; 26:764–769.
110. Skyler JS, Weinstock RS, Raskin P *et al*, The Inhaled Insulin Phase III Type 1 Diabetes Study Group. Use of inhaled insulin in a basal/bolus insulin regimen in type 1 diabetic subjects. *Diabetes Care* 2005; 28:1630–1635.
111. Garg S, Rosenstock J, Silverman BL *et al*. Efficacy and safety of preprandial human insulin inhalation powder versus injectable insulin in patients with type 1 diabetes. *Diabetologia* 2006; 49:891–899.
112. DeFronzo R, Bergenstal RM, Cefalu WT *et al*, for the Exubera Phase III Study Group. Efficacy of inhaled insulin in patients with type 2 diabetes not controlled with diet and exercise. *Diabetes Care* 2005; 28:1922–1928.
113. Weiss SR, Cheng SL, Kourides IA *et al*. Inhaled insulin provides improved glycemic control in patients with type 2 diabetes mellitus inadequately controlled with oral agents: a randomized controlled trial. *Arch Intern Med* 2003; 163:2277–2282.
114. Rosenstock J, Zinman B, Murphy LJ *et al*. Inhaled insulin improves glycaemic control when substituted for or added to oral combination therapy in type 2 diabetes. *Ann Intern Med* 2005; 143:549–558.
115. Hermansen K, Ronnemaa T, Petersen AH *et al*. Intensive therapy with inhaled insulin via the AERx insulin diabetes management system: a 12-week proof-of-concept trial in patients with type 2 diabetes. *Diabetes Care* 2004; 27:162–167.
116. Cefalu WT, Skyler JS, Kourides IA *et al*. Inhaled human insulin treatment in patients with type 2 diabetes mellitus. *Ann Intern Med* 2001; 134:203–207.
117. Cappelleri JC, Cefalu WT, Rosenstock J *et al*. Treatment satisfaction in type 2 diabetes: a comparison between an inhaled insulin regimen and a subcutaneous insulin regimen. *Clin Ther* 2002; 24:552–564.
118. Gerber RA, Cappelleri JC, Kourides IA, Gelfand RA. Treatment satisfaction with inhaled insulin in patients with type 1 diabetes: a randomized controlled trial. *Diabetes Care* 2001; 24:1556–1559.
119. Finberg SE, Schatz D, Krasner A. Results of insulin antibody monitoring during phase II and phase III clinical studies of inhaled insulin (Exubera®) in patients with type 1 or type 2 diabetes. *Diabetologia* 2002; 45(suppl 2):A17.
120. Mitri J, Pittas AG. Inhaled insulin–what went wrong. *Nat Clin Pract Endocrinol Metab* 2009; 5:24–25.

4

Metformin: new understanding and uses for an old drug

A. A. Vaag, S. S. Lund

INTRODUCTION

Metformin is a chemical derivative of the compound guanidine extracted from the plant *Galega officinalis*. *Galega officinalis* was used several hundred years ago for the treatment of polyuria, and to treat plague as well as other medical conditions. Metformin was introduced for the treatment of patients with type 2 diabetes more than 50 years ago. Together with phenformin, metformin belongs to the class of biguanides. Phenformin was, like metformin, initially used for the treatment of patients with type 2 diabetes. However, due to substantial increased risk of lactate acidosis with phenformin treatment, it has not been used for the treatment of patients with type 2 diabetes since the late 1970s. In contrast, metformin has become the oral antidiabetic drug (OAD) of first choice for the treatment of patients with type 2 diabetes including both obese and non-obese phenotypes, either as monotherapy or in combination with other antidiabetic treatment modalities. The are many reasons why metformin plays such an important role in the treatment of patients with type 2 diabetes including its mode of action to improve insulin action, side-effects and the costs of newer 'insulin sensitisers', its documented role in the prevention of type 2 diabetes and not least its putative role in the prevention of cardiovascular disease (CVD) in patients with type 2 diabetes. The focus of this chapter is to provide an updated critical review of recent advances in our knowledge of metformin's mode of action on glucose and fat metabolism, as well as on the cardiovascular system and to review the current 'state-of-the-art' of the clinical use of metformin in mono- or combination therapies in patients with type 2 diabetes, as well as in other states of insulin resistance including polycystic ovary syndrome (PCOS), and even type 1 diabetes. Finally, the potential future role of pharmacogenetics in metformin treatment will be addressed.

MONOTHERAPY, PHARMACOKINETICS AND PHARMACODYNAMICS

The decision on which drug to give a patient is made from a number of different perspectives including efficacy, safety, cost, availability, tolerability and convenience. Based on these criteria, metformin was recommend as the OAD of first choice to treat drug-naïve patients with type 2 diabetes including both obese and non-obese patients in a recent joint consensus statement of the European Association for the Study of Diabetes (EASD) and American

Allan Arthur Vaag, MD, PhD, DMSc, Endocrinologist, Steno Diabetes Center, Gentofte, Denmark; Chief Physician and Adjunct Professor of Metabolism and Clinical Diabetes Research, Lund University, Sweden.

Søren Søgaard Lund, MD, Steno Diabetes Center, Gentofte, Denmark.

Diabetes Association (ADA) [1]. The potency of metformin to reduce glycaemia is (surprisingly) similar to most other oral OADs including insulin secretagogues (sulphonylureas [SU] and glinides) and glitazones, all of which reduce glycosylated haemoglobin (HbA1c) levels between 0.6 and 2.4% in patients with type 2 diabetes when given either as mono- or combination therapy [2–5]. Metformin reduces blood glucose levels in type 2 diabetes regardless of age, gender, ethnicity, duration of diabetes or residual β-cell function [2, 3]. Although metformin, due to its effects on body weight and insulin resistance, may have advantages in obese patients, recent studies have shown that metformin is non-inferior to insulin secretagogues according to efficacy even in non-obese patients with type 2 diabetes, a topic which will be addressed in more detail later in this review.

The weight-reducing effect of metformin compared with other OADs involves both a reduction of total fat mass as well as abdominal obesity and visceral fat content [5]. Although it has been speculated that the weight-reducing effect of metformin may be due to its well-established gastrointestinal side-effects, this important effect of metformin is more likely to be mediated via an improvement of insulin action and the concomitant compensatory reduction of endogenous insulin secretion, subsequently diminishing appetite at the level of the hypothalamus [5, 6].

To reduce or prevent the gastrointestinal side-effects, it is recommended to initiate metformin treatment with a low dose of 500 mg with a meal. If additional glucose lowering is required, after one week, metformin doses may be increased gradually over a period of 1–4 weeks to the maximal recommended daily dose of 2000 mg (with the option of up to 3000 mg). Only marginal additional hypoglycaemic effects of metformin can be achieved with total daily doses exceeding 2000 mg [7].

After absorption, metformin circulates in plasma in its native and unmodified form with no protein binding, and it is ultimatively cleared by the kidneys [5,8]. The bioavailability of metformin is around 50% after oral ingestion. Accordingly, metformin has a relatively large distribution volume with the highest tissue accumulation in the wall of the small intestine [5, 8].

COMBINATION THERAPY: METABOLIC ASPECTS

A major pathophysiological feature of type 2 diabetes is the progressive loss of β-cell function with time, which eventually leads to a need to intensify antidiabetic therapy with OAD combinations and ultimately to insulin treatment in most patients with type 2 diabetes. In the United Kingdom Prospective Diabetes Study (UKPDS), after 3 years, half of the patients who received only one glucose-lowering drug achieved an HbA1c <7%, and after 9 years, this was achieved by only one quarter of the patients [9]. Metformin has been shown to be effective in reducing HbA1c in combination with all currently available antidiabetic therapies [2, 4, 5]. When used in combination with SU, metformin reduces average HbA1c by around 0.5% more than when used in monotherapy, as illustrated for instance in the UKPDS trial [10].

In patients with type 2 diabetes insulin treatment may be initiated with any of the current available insulin preparations, with or without combination with metformin or other OADs. It has been reported that bedtime long- or intermediate-acting (basal) insulin administration in combination with metformin is superior to insulin alone — or other insulin OAD combination therapies — with respect to the reduction of HbA1c and the risk of hypoglycaemia as well as minimising weight gain [11]. However, with a longer duration of diabetes, only a minority of patients can obtain a target HbA1c below 6.5 or 7.0% with basal insulin administration alone. These patients need additional insulin injections of rapid-acting or mixed insulin preparations. Combination therapy of metformin with other insulin treatment regimens (for example, premixed or basal bolus insulin therapies) has demonstrated at least similar beneficial results to basal insulin treatment with respect to HbA1c, insulin dose and risk of weight gain, whereas the effect on hypoglycaemia has been conflicting [12–14]. The 'Treating to Target in Type 2 Diabetes' study in 708 patients with type 2 diabetes followed for one year suggested combination therapy of metformin (plus SU) together with basal insulin therapy was less efficient than combination therapy of metformin (plus SU) together with either premixed or basal bolus insulin therapies with respect to HbA1c. In contrast, basal insulin therapy resulted in less weight gain and less hypoglycaemia than premixed or basal bolus insulin therapies [15]. Recently, the Hyperinsulinaemia: the Outcome of its Metabolic Effects (HOME) trial suggested combination therapy with insulin plus metformin versus insulin alone to reduce the risk of cardiovascular outcomes (see further details below).

In conclusion, there are many data to suggest that combination treatment with metformin and insulin is beneficial in patients with type 2 diabetes, but more knowledge is needed regarding the combination with different insulin treatment regimens including insulin analogues, and the combination of insulin treatment with both metformin and insulin secretagogues. Future investigations of metformin in combination with other glucose-lowering treatments should focus on relevant endpoints including glycaemic control, and on the risk of micro- and macrovascular complications.

PREVENTION OF DIABETES

In the Diabetes Prevention Program (DPP) study, metformin reduced the risk of developing type 2 diabetes in pre-diabetic subjects with impaired glucose tolerance (IGT) by 31% over a mean intervention period of 2.8 years [16]. The preventive effect of metformin persisted at least 2 weeks after withdrawal of metformin, indicating that metformin prevents type 2 diabetes beyond its acute blood glucose lowering effects [17]. Although metformin treatment prevented type 2 diabetes in the DPP study, this effect was significantly lower than lifestyle intervention. Therefore, metformin is not to be recommended for the treatment of pre-diabetic subjects with IGT. It is not known whether metformin treatment may prevent or postpone development of overt type 2 diabetes in pre-diabetic subjects with isolated impaired fasting glucose (IFG). In particular, pre-diabetic subjects with IFG are predominantly characterised by reduced pancreatic insulin secretion and less peripheral insulin resistance and it is therefore uncertain if treatment with metformin targeting insulin resistance may prevent overt type 2 diabetes in IFG subjects. Metformin works equally effectively in preventing type 2 diabetes in young and elderly subjects, but is less effective in preventing type 2 diabetes in non-obese compared with obese subjects [16, 17].

PREVENTION OF MICRO- AND MACROVASCULAR COMPLICATIONS

Regardless of treatment modality, improvement of glycaemic regulation and reduction of HbA1c appears to reduce the risk and prevalence of microvascular complications including diabetic retinopathy, nephropathy and neuropathy in both patients with type 1 and type 2 diabetes [18, 19]. Although, in the landmark metformin trials, convincing statistical trends have suggested that metformin treatment also improves microvascular risk, a statistically significant reduction of microvascular complications by metformin therapy has in fact not yet been demonstrated — probably due to a lack of statistical power [13, 20, 21]. Patients with type 2 diabetes have a two-fold elevated risk of macrovascular disease and a risk of myocardial infarction and mortality similar to non-diabetic subjects with a previous myocardial infarction [22, 23], which needs to be addressed and/or prevented as far as possible. This explains why there is general agreement to treat type 2 diabetes patients as a 'CVD equivalent' with aggressive blood pressure lowering therapy, cholesterol lowering therapy, smoking cessation etc.

Epidemiological data from the UKPDS showed that a 1% reduction in the HbA1c value during treatment was associated with a 21% reduction in diabetes-related deaths, a 16% reduction in heart failure, a 14% reduction in myocardial infarctions and a 12% reduction in strokes [24]. Despite this, the extent to which extensive glucose lowering using other antidiabetic drugs including SUs, glitazones as well as insulin may reduce the risk of CVD in

Table 4.1 Impact of metformin (n = 342) versus conventional treatment policy (n = 411) in overweight and obese patients with type 2 diabetes in the UKPDS

- 32% reduction in any diabetes-related endpoints
- 42% reduction in diabetes-related death
- 36% reduction in all cause mortality
- 39% reduction in myocardial infarction

patients with type 2 diabetes remains highly controversial. Recently, large-scale clinical trials investigating intensive versus conventional glucose control on the risk of major cardiovascular outcomes have underscored that a major challenge in the treatment of patients with type 2 diabetes are the absence of any conclusive data showing that pharmacological treatment of hyperglycaemia *per se* prevents CVD [25–27]. In fact, in terms of mortality, such treatment could be harmful [25]. In contrast, subsequent meta-analyses of these trials have suggested a pharmacological reduction of blood glucose to result in a lowering of the cardiovascular risk, without adversely affecting mortality [28, 29].

In the UKPDS, overweight patients with newly diagnosed type 2 diabetes were randomised to metformin versus either chlorpropamide, glibenclamide or insulin treatment [20]. The control group of overweight type 2 diabetes patients were treated with conventional diet therapy. Both drug-treated groups achieved equal degrees of glycaemic control with a median HbA1c of 7.4% after 10 years. The conventionally treated group obtained a median HbA1c value of 8.0% [20]. Metformin treatment was associated with a significant risk reduction of 30–40% in any diabetes-related endpoints, myocardial infarction and mortality as compared with conventional diet treatment (Table 4.1) [20]. When analysing these data in the context of the impact of glycaemic control on complications, the impact of metformin seems to be almost fully explained by the degree of glycaemic control between the metformin and diet groups. However, compared with the (combined) group of SU- or insulin-treated patients, despite equal effects on HbA1c levels, metformin was superior in preventing any diabetes-related endpoints and reducing both total mortality and stroke [20], supporting the idea that metformin might possess cardiovascular protective effects independent of its blood glucose reducing effects.

Notably, compared with the conventionally (diet-only) treated group, and despite the achievement of similar post-study levels of glycaemic control, the recent 10-year follow-up of the UKPDS, confirmed the lower risk of CVD in the group of overweight patients with type 2 diabetes with prior allocation to metformin monotherapy. Also, as a new finding, a decreased risk of CVD and mortality was shown in the group of (obese and non-obese) patients with prior allocation to SU or insulin [21]. From the original or the 10-year follow-up UKPDS investigation, data have not been published comparing the metformin versus the SU or insulin groups separately with respect to clinical outcomes. However, as outlined, the 10-year follow-up of the UKPDS suggests that besides metformin therapy, insulin-providing therapies (that is, insulin or insulin secretagogues) might also have long-term beneficial effects on cardiovascular outcomes.

The HOME trial randomly allocated 390 patients with type 2 diabetes to either placebo or metformin in addition to ongoing insulin therapy [13]. Patients were overweight/obese (mean BMI at enrolment of 30 kg/m^2) and after a follow-up of 4.3 years there was no significant decrease in the risk of the primary outcome (an aggregate of microvascular disease, CVD and mortality). However, metformin treatment significantly reduced the risk of (secondary) CVD outcomes (e.g. myocardial infarction, stroke and peripheral arterial reconstruction) by 39% (P = 0.02). The reduction in microvascular outcomes was non-significant (P = 0.43). Compared with insulin plus placebo, the combination of insulin and metformin reduced body weight, insulin requirements and HbA1c (0.4% difference in HbA1c). The changes in body weight partly explained the difference in CVD [13]. Hence, the HOME study represents a much-needed reinforcement of the findings from the UKPDS of potential beneficial CVD effects of metformin therapy.

Besides the HOME trial, with respect to the potential favourable effects of metformin treatment on CVD, the UKPDS results have been supported by at least two subsequent retrospective studies comparing mortality in type 2 diabetes patients treated with metformin versus SU as well as by the DIGAMI-2 trial comparing metformin, SU or insulin treatment in patients with type 2 diabetes having a myocardial infarction [30–32].

In contrast, the UKPDS results have recently been challenged in a retrospective study of a total of 39 721 type 2 diabetes patients from the Veterans Health Administration (VHA) Diabetes Epidemiology Cohort [33]. In this study, metformin compared with SU treatment was neither associated with any beneficial — nor adverse — outcome according to all-cause mortality when data were adjusted for many (or most) confounding factors including comorbidity and comedication, age, duration of diabetes, HbA1c, low-density lipoprotein (LDL)-cholesterol etc. using the elegant propensity score methodology [33]. Therefore, the UKPDS metformin mortality data urgently needs to be confirmed in other prospective studies.

A somewhat surprising outcome of the UKPDS was that metformin, when added to SU treatment (due to failure of SU monotherapy) was associated with a significant increase in diabetes-related death in patients with type 2 diabetes [20]. The finding of an excess mortality in type 2 diabetes patients treated with a combination of metformin and SU was subsequently reported in three other independent retrospective studies [34–36]. In contrast, in other subsequent retrospective studies of larger samples of type 2 diabetes patients identified as 'new users' of OAD [31] or with heart failure [32], the combination of metformin with SU was associated with lower mortality compared with SU monotherapy after correction for age, gender, nitrate use and a modified chronic disease score [31, 32]. However, a recently published meta-analysis of such observational studies indicated an increased frequency of CVD by combined intervention with metformin and insulin secretagogues compared with diet or monotherapy [37].

The different and sometimes opposite outcomes seen with metformin as monotherapy versus metformin as an 'add on' in SU failure in the UKPDS was explained by its authors to be due to differences in the patients studied, including relatively few patients in the SU plus metformin combination arm. Indeed, these SU-failure patients were on average 5 years older, more hyperglycaemic (baseline median fasting plasma glucose = 9.1 vs. 8.1 mmol/l), less overweight and followed up for, on average, 5 years less as the entire UKPDS cohort [20]. Also, as suggested by the UKPDS authors, a lower than expected diabetes-related mortality in the SU monotherapy group could have contributed to the adverse finding of increased mortality with combined metformin and SU treatment versus SU monotherapy (14 diabetes-related deaths occurred in the SU monotherapy group and 35 such deaths were expected) [38]. Moreover, the retrospective studies reporting either increased or decreased mortality in patients treated with metformin and SU combination therapy may all, to various unknown extents, be influenced by confounding by indication and therefore flawed in one or other direction. Indeed, in the recent VHA study using the propensity score method to correct for confounding clinical variables, metformin plus SU combination treatment was associated with the same mortality rate as both metformin and SU monotherapies [33].

There are data to suggest that newer generations of SUs including glimepiride and gliclazide are safer drugs in relation to the risk of CVD [39]. In support of this, the recently published A Diabetes Outcome Progression Trial (ADOPT) study somewhat surprisingly suggested that the third generation SU glimepiride was associated with a reduced incidence of cardiovascular events compared with both metformin and glitazone over a 4-year period in patients with type 2 diabetes [40].

In conclusion, the current state-of-the-art opinion is that the combination of metformin and insulin secretagogues — and in particular the novel generation of SUs — remains an attractive therapeutic option when metformin in monotherapy has failed. Nevertheless, there is an urgent need for more knowledge about the extent to which metformin, and in fact all currently available glucose lowering therapies, protect against CVD in patients with type 2 diabetes. Hence, as outlined, with respect to metformin treatment, the beneficial findings from the UKPDS need to be confirmed.

MECHANISM OF ACTION ON GLUCOSE AND FAT METABOLISM

Metformin may indirectly improve pancreatic insulin secretion by reducing free fatty acids (FFA) (lipotoxicity) or hyperglycaemia (glucose toxicity). However, metformin does not increase pancreatic insulin secretion in itself [41]. The glucose-lowering effect of metformin is due to an improvement of insulin action in the liver and possibly, to a minor extent, to an improvement of insulin action in skeletal muscle and adipose tissue. The presence of insulin is required for metformin to exert its full action to enhance peripheral glucose transport and glycogen and lipid synthesis in subjects with pre-existing insulin resistance [42]. However, metformin increases cellular glucose transport in cultured skeletal muscle cells even in the absence of insulin [43, 44].

The increased hepatic glucose production in patients with type 2 diabetes is primarily caused by an increased rate of gluconeogenesis (formation of glucose from non-carbohydrate substrates) and probably to a lesser extent by affecting glycogenolysis (breakdown of glycogen). Indeed, metformin reduces hepatic glucose production primarily by reducing gluconeogenesis, and only to a minor extent by inhibition of glycogenolysis [45] (Figure 4.1).

The precise molecular mechanism by which metformin reduces hepatic gluconeogenesis and stimulates glucose uptake and non-oxidative glucose metabolism in different tissues including liver, muscle and adipose tissue remains unclear, but inhibition of mitochondrial respiratory chain oxidation of complex I substrates may play a role [5, 46]. Inhibition of cellular respiration leads to a decrease in adenosine triphosphate (ATP) levels and to increased cellular adenosine monophosphate (AMP) and adenosine diphosphate (ADP) levels, subsequently activating the AMP-activated protein kinase (AMPK) in many different tissues including the liver, skeletal muscle and possibly adipose tissue [46]. AMPK acts as an intracellular energy regulator and is activated by a decline of the ATP–ADP ratio and/or in the phosphocreatinine–creatinine ratio. Increased AMPK activity is associated with increased translocation of GLUT4 glucose transporters to the plasma membrane in skeletal muscle as well as GLUT1 in liver cells [47], which subsequently increases glucose transport into the cell and causes an inhibition of gluconeogenesis and hepatic glucose production [47]. Thus, activation of AMPK seems to be central for metformin both to inhibit the hepatic glucose production and to increase glucose uptake into skeletal muscle and adipose tissue, as well as the effect to increase fat oxidation in liver cells.

In the adipose tissue, metformin inhibits the release of FFA by inhibition of lypolysis and by increasing re-esterification of FFA. This subsequently leads to a reduced lipid oxidation and moreover facilitates the effect of metformin in reducing gluconeogenesis and increasing tissue glucose uptake.

The uptake of metformin in the liver is regulated and controlled by the organic cation transporter (OCT) and possibly also to some extent by passive diffusion. In support of a role of OCT, metformin levels were reduced in the liver and intestine of Oct1–/– mice [48], while kidney and circulating metformin levels were comparable in Oct1–/– and control mice. The Oct2 is expressed in the kidneys regulating renal transport and secretion of metformin [49]. The effect of metformin in regulating cellular glucose and fat metabolism is reproduced in Figure 4.2 and involves additional cellular signalling molecules and transcription factors including LKB, alias of serine-threonine kinase 11 (STK11), peroxisome proliferator activated receptor γ– coactivator 1 α (PGC-1α), target of rapamycin complex 2 (TORC2) and sterol regulatory element binding protein (SREBP)-1.

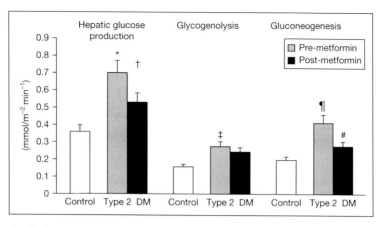

Figure 4.1 Metformin decreases hepatic glucose production in patients with type 2 diabetes by inhibition of hepatic gluconeogenesis (with permission from [28]).
DM = diabetes mellitus.

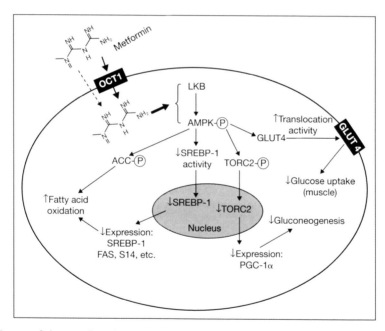

Figure 4.2 Impact of the organic cation transporter 1 (OCT1) on the cellular mechanism of action of metformin. OCT1 plays a central role in the cellular uptake of metformin in the liver cell, thereby influencing the pharmacological effects in the liver (bold arrow). In addition to the role of OCT1, passive diffusion and other transporters may account for small portion of hepatic uptake of metformin (dashed arrow). Other transporters may control metformin uptake into other tissues, such as skeletal muscle. Factors such as genetic variation in transporter genes may alter transporter activity and thus metformin response (with permission from [73]).
ACC = acetyl-CoA carboxylase; AMPK = AMP-dependent protein kinase; FAS = fatty acid synthetase; GLUT4 = glucose transporter 4; LKB = alias of serine-threonine kinase 11 (STK11); OCT1 = organic cation transporter 1; PGC-1α = peroxisome proliferator activated receptor γ coactivator 1 α; SREBP-1 = sterol regulatory element binding protein-1; TORC2 = target of rapamycin complex 2.

MECHANISM OF ACTION ON THE CARDIOVASCULAR SYSTEM

As mentioned above, perhaps the most important effect of metformin in patients with type 2 diabetes is its putative effect in protecting against CVD. Although incompletely understood, several direct or indirect effects of metformin on both conventional and non-conventional CVD risk factors may contribute to this. Firstly, there is no doubt that metformin treatment causes less weight gain when compared with most other drugs used to lower plasma glucose in patients with diabetes. Besides reducing or maintaining total weight, the weight effects of metformin include a reduction of the degree of abdominal obesity and probably also the accumulation of fat in the liver [50, 51]. Although previous studies reported an antihypertensive effect of metformin in animals [52], most studies in patients with diabetes have failed to document any clinically significant reduction of the blood pressure [2, 3, 5, 53–55].

It has been indicated from some studies that metformin has a beneficial effect on a number of well-established biochemical cardiovascular and arteriosclerotic risk markers related to inflammation, endothelial dysfunction, coagulation and the formation of advanced glycolysation end-products. These biomarkers include high-sensitivity C-reactive protein, tumour necrosis factor-α, soluble intercellular adhesion molecule-1, soluble vascular cell adhesion molecule-1, von Willebrand factor, sE-selectin, tissue-type plasminogen activator antigen, plasminogen activator inhibitor antigen type 1 and methylglyoxal (i.e. a major precursor in the formation of advanced glycosylated end-products) [55–64]. Furthermore, studies in animals have shown that metformin has a beneficial effect on a number of molecular mechanisms involved in the development of the arteriosclerotic vascular lesion including fat accumulation in the vessel wall, attraction of leukocytes to the endothelial cells, formation of so-called vascular foam cells, proliferation of smooth muscle cells, attraction and aggregation of thombocytes and finally, beneficial effects on the degree of oxidative stress in the cell (reviewed in [65]). In addition, in patients with type 1 or type 2 diabetes, metformin treatment has been shown to have a potential beneficial effect on lipid levels by reducing levels of triglycerides and/or levels of pro-atherogenic cholesterol (total, low-density lipoprotein and non-high-density lipoprotein cholesterol) [66–68]. Thus, there are indeed many pathways and molecular mechanisms by which metformin may prevent the development and progression of atherosclerosis, which may or may not be interrelated and/or associated with insulin resistance, obesity or glycaemic regulation (Table 4.2). However, the extent to which most of these effects are due to reduction of glucose *per se*, is restricted to some type 2 diabetes sub-phenotypes such as obese patients, and is present with or without combination with other glucose lowering therapy including insulin, and whether these effects may play a role in clinical practice, remains to be established. Finally, it has for many years been speculated that hyperinsulinaemia *per se* may, to some extent, be involved in the development of atherosclerosis, and the possibility remains that the putative beneficial effects on the risk of CVD of reducing hyperglycaemia with insulin in patients with type 2 diabetes may be counteracted by the concomitant elevations of plasma insulin levels. A key conclusion of the UKPDS was that the absence of an excess risk of CVD in the insulin treated patients provided near conclusive evidence for the rejection of the hypothesis that insulin treatment in type 2 diabetes increases the risk of atherosclerosis [19]. Another key conclusion of the UKPDS was that the supposed excess risk of CVD and cardiac arrest associated with the earliest generations of SUs was not supported by the UKPDS data [19]. However, assuming that both the excess CVD risk of insulin and the earliest generations of SU is correct, then these effects might have masked or counteracted the beneficial effects of improved glycaemia in the UKPDS. The logical subsequent question to ask would then be whether the supposedly beneficial non-glycaemic effects of metformin on CVD and mortality in the UKPDS were explained by an excess risk of CVD with insulin and SUs, and that the non-glycaemic CVD effect of metformin may therefore be explained entirely by its insulin lowering and sparing effects.

Table 4.2 Beneficial 'non-glycaemic' effects of metformin on CVD risk factors.

Conventional
- Obesity (visceral) ↓
- Plasma lipoprotein-lipids (TC, LDL, TG) ↓
- Blood pressure (- ?)

Non-conventional
- Inflammation (hsCRP↓)
- Endothelial Function (VCAM↓, forearm blood flow↑)
- Coagulation (PAI-1↓, tPA(↓), Fibrinogen(↓), FactorVII↓, Factor XIII(↓))
- Advanced glycation products (Methylglyoxal↓)
- Microcirculation (arteriolar vasomotion↑capillary density and flow↑, capillary permeability↓) (rats and hamsters))
- Foam cell formation (LDL uptake in vitro in monocytes↓)
- Oxidative stress? (reactive oxygen species↓?)
- Plasma insulin ↓

hsCRP = high-sensitivity C-reactive protein; LDL = low-density lipoprotein; PAI-I = type I plasminogen activator inhibitor; TC = total cholesterol; TG = triglycerides; tPA = tissue-type plasminogen activator; VCAM = vascular cell adhesion molecule.

SIDE-EFFECTS AND CONTRAINDICATIONS

The most important side-effects of metformin treatment include gastrointestinal discomfort, diarrhoea and flatulence [5]. These symptoms are dose-dependent and, usually, they can be ameliorated or completely avoided by slow titration and/or reduction of the dose [5]. Around 5% of patients cannot tolerate treatment because of gastrointestinal side-effects [3, 5, 7]. After long-term metformin therapy, around 10–30% of patients develop decreased levels of total Vitamin B_{12} potentially because of Vitamin B_{12} malabsorption [3, 5]. In the ileum, by influencing the intracellular mucosa cell handling of calcium, metformin disrupts the calcium-dependent absorption of Vitamin B_{12}. Fortunately, the reduced levels of Vitamin B_{12} are most often without clinical significance [3, 5] and may be prevented by increased calcium intake [69].

Metformin treatment is contraindicated in patients with cardiac congestion, kidney or liver failure, severe hypoxia due to chronic obstructive pulmonary disease, and in patients with severe infections [5]. These conditions may increase the production or decrease the utilisation of lactic acid thereby increasing the risk of lactic acidosis [5]. Also, by causing hypotension with peripheral tissue hypoxia and reduced renal perfusion, general anaesthesia might lead to lactate accumulation [5, 70, 71]. Moreover, the use of radiocontrast could impair kidney function thereby potentially decreasing the clearance of metformin and resulting in toxic levels of the drug. Therefore, in urgent surgery or when using radiocontrast, metformin should be withheld and hydration maintained until preserved kidney function has been ensured, usually one or two days after such procedures [5, 70, 71]. Similarly, in elderly patients, metformin treatment should be used with some caution, but not necessarily avoided [5, 70, 71].

Compared to treatment with insulin secretagogues and insulin, hypoglycaemia occurs less frequently during metformin treatment. The reason for this is unknown, but may be due to the effect of metformin on the liver (reduces gluconeogenesis) with no enhancement of pancreatic insulin secretion.

Lactic acidosis is a very rare but potentially fatal complication of biguanide therapy. Mortality rates of up to 50% has been reported in previous studies [70, 71]. The estimated incidence of lactate acidosis during metformin therapy is around one case per 3000 patient-years [3, 70, 71]. Metformin increases plasma lactate levels by interfering with mitochondrial oxidative phosphorylation. Interestingly, the development of lactic acidosis seems not to depend on plasma metformin concentrations [70, 71] and even markedly elevated metformin levels in some patients with chronic renal insufficiency may not necessarily cause lactic acidosis [72]. In contrast, development of lactic acidosis is mostly seen in patients with renal insufficiency or coexistent hypoxia including pulmonary diseases or cardiac congestion. Thus, overt lactic acidosis may in most cases be precipitated by the underlying metabolic and hypoxic condition, rather than by lactate accumulation *per se*, providing an explanation for the increased mortality rate. Thus, metformin treatment should be avoided in patients with markedly compromised renal function or co-existing hypoxic conditions [5].

OBESE VERSUS NON-OBESE PATIENTS WITH TYPE 2 DIABETES

At least 20% of Caucasian patients with type 2 diabetes are not obese [73–76], and some ethnic groups with a high prevalence of type 2 diabetes, including Asians, develop type 2 diabetes at markedly lower levels of body mass index (BMI) compared with Europeans. In the UKPDS, non-obese patients with type 2 diabetes did not receive treatment with metformin in monotherapy or in combination with insulin [20]. Moreover, the excess diabetes-related deaths in patients receiving combined SU and metformin treatment in the UKPDS were suggested to be partly due to the fact that these patients were leaner (17% had a BMI $<25 \text{ kg/m}^2$) than the patients receiving metformin monotherapy [20]. This indirectly implied that non-obese patients with type 2 diabetes may not benefit from metformin treatment to the same extent as obese patients. The reason for not initially randomising non-obese type 2 diabetes patients to receive metformin monotherapy in the UKPDS was that, due to a more deficient insulin-secretion and less insulin-resistance compared with obese patients with type 2 diabetes [76], they have, for many years, been treated predominantly with insulin-secretagogues and/or insulin instead of metformin therapy. However, since obese and non-obese patients with type 2 diabetes carry a similar cardiovascular risk [77, 78], the use of metformin even in non-obese patients with type 2 diabetes might theoretically be beneficial to protect against CVD. As outlined, the 10-year UKPDS follow-up, confirmed the beneficial effects of metformin therapy on CVD outcomes in overweight type 2 diabetes patients, but also demonstrated reduced CVD risk in the group of patients treated with SU or insulin. This latter group included obese and non-obese patients with type 2 diabetes (mean BMI at enrolment was 27.5 kg/m^2 in this group) [19, 21]. Hence, based on these findings, there is no clear evidence to suggest that either of metformin, SU or insulin should necessarily be superior as the treatment(s) of first choice for non-obese patients with type 2 diabetes. However, since 2006, the EASD/ADA have recommended the use of metformin therapy as the 'drug of first choice' in all patients with type-2 diabetes, regardless of BMI [1, 79]. Also, this EASD/ADA consensus statement provided no evidence from clinical trials to support such recommendation for the non-obese patient with type 2-diabetes [1, 79]. Previous studies investigating the use of metformin in non-obese type 2 diabetes patients were either small, open-labelled, without a matching control group or without data on HbA1c [80–87] (but suggested a glucose-lowering effect of metformin also in these patients). Moreover, data from two observational studies suggested a similar glycaemic response to metformin treatment in non-obese versus obese patients with type 2 diabetes [88, 89]. Recently, in a randomised, double-blind trial, our group demonstrated equal antihyperglycaemic effect (as measured by HbA1c) between metformin versus an insulin secretagogue (repaglinide), both as monotherapy, in about 100 non-obese Caucasian patients with type 2 diabetes [90]. Thus, the empirical argument that non-obese type 2 diabetes patients need an insulin secretagogue to restore insulin secretion and obtain the most significant glucose-lowering effect was refuted [90]. Also, in these patients, metformin treatment appeared to have improved effects compared with repaglinide on lipids and a number of other CVD biomarkers [55, 67]. Hence, in support of the EASD/ADA recommendations of 'metformin for all patients with type 2 diabetes', some evidence for the use of metformin treatment in the non-obese type 2 diabetes patients has become available. However, the decision as to whether the OAD of first-choice in non-obese patients is metformin or an insulin secretagogue should be based on potential differences in the efficacy to prevent complications including CVD, and of course on the important issues of safety, cost, availability, tolerability and convenience. However, as outlined, except for the UKPDS data showing increased mortality in the group of obese and non-obese patients treated with a combination of metformin and SU, no long-term data of metformin therapy with respect to CVD outcomes are available in non-obese patients with type 2 diabetes. Important issues to resolve in future studies are therefore the effects of metformin versus insulin secretagogues in mono- and/or in combination therapy regimens with or without, for example insulin and/or other OADs on the risk of CVD in non-obese patients with type 2 diabetes.

POSITIONING IN RELATION TO OTHER OADs

In addition to lifestyle interventions, type 2 diabetes can now be treated with seven classes of approved oral drugs including SUs, glinides, biguanides, α-glucosidase inhibitors, thiazolidinediones, amylin mimetics and dipeptidyl peptidase-4 inhibitors. Furthermore, insulin treatment plays a more central role than previously in the management and treatment of type 2 diabetes and the recently introduced glucagon-like peptide-1 (GLP-1) analogues and mimetics seem very promising as replacements and/or add-ons in the earliest phases of type 2 diabetes. As outlined, in a recent joint consensus statement of EASD and ADA, metformin was recommend as the OAD of first choice to treat drug-naïve patients with type 2 diabetes [1]. Although it was initially claimed that glitazones, due to their insulin-sensitizing effects, might be associated with reduced CVD in patients with type 2 diabetes, a recent meta-analysis indicated that rosiglitazone treatment is associated with an increased risk of myocardial infarction [91]. Obviously, an increased risk of myocardial infarction makes the finding from the ADOPT study of improved pancreatic β-cell conservation and prolonged durability of rosiglitazone compared with metformin and glimepiride monotherapy less clinically relevant [40]. With this report of increased risk of myocardial infarction the increased price of glitazones, combined with the additional side-effects of this class of drugs, including excess risk of bone fractures and an increase in body weight and fluid retention, the future role of glitazones in the treatment of patients with type 2 diabetes is uncertain. An interesting finding in the ADOPT study was that glimepiride treatment — despite its cardiovascular benefits, as outlined — was associated with a more rapid decline of β-cell function with time when compared with both metformin and rosiglitazone [40] (Figure 4.3). Thus, despite the expected initial increase of insulin secretion in patients treated with glimepiride, their absolute insulin secretion after 5 years was similar to that of patients treated with rosiglitazone and approaching the insulin secretion of patients treated with metformin (Figure 4.3, panel d). In patients with type 2 diabetes, an observational study of CVD events suggested the insulin secretagogue and the glinide, repaglinide, to have similar CVD protective effects as metformin, whereas most SUs could be less favourable [92].

Taken together, although the evidence is incomplete, metformin remains the OAD of first-choice to treat patients with type 2 diabetes. While glitazones seem not to threaten this leading position of metformin, the novel generations of SUs or glinides remain attractive alternatives, and if the novel GLP-1 mimetics and dipeptidyl peptidase-4 inhibitors prove their supposed long-term efficacy in maintaining β-cell function, reducing body weight and

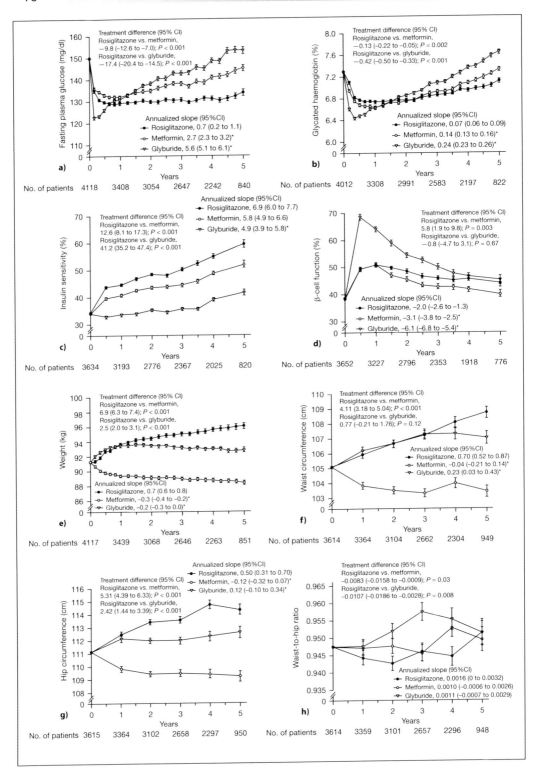

No. of patients   4118   3408   3054   2647   2242   840

No. of patients   4012   3308   2991   2583   2197   822

No. of patients   3634   3193   2776   2367   2025   820

No. of patients   3652   3227   2796   2353   1918   776

No. of patients   4117   3439   3068   2646   2263   851

No. of patients   3614   3364   3104   2662   2304   949

No. of patients   3615   3364   3102   2658   2297   950

No. of patients   3614   3359   3101   2657   2296   948 perhaps protecting against CVD, they may in the long run replace metformin as the OAD of first choice in type 2 diabetes patients.

TYPE 1 DIABETES AND POLYCYSTIC OVARY SYNDROME (PCOS)

Despite intensive insulin treatment and patient care, many patients with type 1 diabetes have long-standing suboptimal metabolic regulation with HbA1c levels much higher than the recommended goal of HbA1c <7.0%. Given that even patients with type 1 diabetes exhibit insulin resistance [93] and that, like patients with type 2 diabetes, they have a substantial increased risk of morbidity and mortality from CVD [22, 23, 94, 95], it has been suggested that they may also benefit from metformin treatment. Several small and short-term studies (typically including ≤60 patients or followed for ≤6 months) have investigated metformin treatment in patients with type 1 diabetes with conflicting results [96–107]. Some of these studies suggested metformin treatment to improve glycaemic control [96, 97, 100, 101, 103–106] as well as to lower insulin dose [96, 99, 100, 102, 104–107] and body weight [100, 107]. Recently, our group published data from a randomised, double-blind trial of one-year of treatment with metformin versus placebo in 100 patients with type 1 diabetes having persistent poor glycaemic control (HbA1c 9.3% at baseline) and preserved hypoglycaemic awareness. In this group of patients, which included non-obese as well as overweight and obese patients, we suggested that metformin treatment resulted in a transient lowering of HbA1c of 0.5% during the initial three months or so, but, with no significant difference in glycaemic control after one year of treatment ($P = 0.422$ for the 0.13% HbA1c difference at one year). In contrast, metformin treatment significantly lowered body weight and insulin doses by about two kilograms and six units, respectively [108]. Hence, the transient lowering of HbA1c during the first three months can potentially explain why previous, shorter-term trials suggested a lowering of glucose levels after metformin treatment in patients with type 1 diabetes. In our study, we did not observe any beneficial effect of metformin treatment on glycaemic control in subgroups of patients according to, for example, the degree of obesity or the magnitude of the insulin dose (as potential markers of insulin sensitivity) [108]. In contrast, metformin treatment resulted in a small but significant lowering of cholesterol levels, which appeared to be enhanced in those patients already receiving statin treatment (about 0.5 mmol/l lowering of LDL cholesterol) [68]. In general, metformin treatment was well-tolerated, with side-effects, including gastrointestinal, comparable to that of placebo. Overall, minor and major hypoglycaemia was similar between treatments. However, we noted some evidence for events of major hypoglycaemia being more severe with metformin treatment [108]. Also, metformin treatment decreased Vitamin B_{12} levels significantly by about 80 pmol/l and increased plasma potassium levels significantly by 0.2 mmol/l. Hence, the most consistent effect of metformin treatment in patients with type 1 diabetes is its insulin-sparring effect as well as some lowering of body weight [96–108]. Thus, at this stage, treating patients with type 1 diabetes with metformin seems to have some potential beneficial effects if, for example, a reduction in body weight, insulin dose or cholesterol is desired, but not as an option for improving long-term

Figure 4.3 Impact of metformin versus rosiglitazone versus glyburide as initial treatment for recently diagnosed type 2 diabetes on fasting plasma glucose (panel a), glycated haemoglobin (panel b), insulin sensitivity (panel c), β-cell function (panel d), weight (panel e), waist circumference (panel f), hip circumference (panel g), and waist-to-hip ratio (panel h). Results from the double-blind, randomised, controlled clinical ADOPT trial involving 4360 patients. The patients were treated for a median of 4.0 years. Data are presented as mean ± SE. Insulin sensitivity and β-cell function were determined by homeostasis model assessment (HOMA 2) and are expressed as a percentage of the value in a normal reference population. The treatment difference is expressed as the relative percent difference between the rosiglitazone group and each comparison group at 4 years; the slopes represent the annual percentage change. Asterisks denote significant differences between the rosiglitazone group and the other treatment groups with the Hochberg adjustment (with permission from [24]).

glycaemic control. If metformin treatment is initiated in patients with type 1 diabetes, attention should be paid to the risk of major hypoglycaemia as well as to the plasma Vitamin B_{12} and potassium levels. However, long-term trials with clinical outcomes (micro- and macrovascular) are still needed to give more definitive answers about the potential role of metformin therapy in patients with type 1 diabetes.

Insulin resistance and/or hyperinsulinaemia have been suggested to play a role in the development of PCOS in women [109–111]. Hyperinsulinaemia is a potent stimulus to enhance testosterone production by the ovaries [110] and to decrease the formation of sex hormone-binding globulin in the liver [109], which subsequently increases levels of total and free testosterone. Metformin treatment causes an improvement of insulin action as well as a reduction of hyperinsulinaemia in women with PCOS, which in turn is associated with decreased levels of testosterone and increased levels of oestradiol [109, 112]. Importantly, in many women with PCOS, metformin treatment improves hirsutism and normalises menstrual cycles, which subsequently leads to ovulation [109, 111, 113]. Metformin is now indicated, therefore, to treat these symptoms in women with PCOS.

PHARMACOGENETICS

The term 'pharmacogenetics' defines the enabling of more rational decisions of pharmacological strategies based on the individual's genetic constitution. Clinically relevant examples of pharmacogenetics in diabetes related to metformin therapy include the finding that patients with diabetes caused by mutations in the hepatocyte nuclear factor 1-α– gene (i.e. MODY3) exhibit a markedly better glucose lowering response to SU as compared with metformin treatment [86]. Most recently, Shu and colleagues reported that genetic variation in the OCT1 gene affects the response to metformin by regulating the uptake of metformin in hepatocytes [114] (Figure 4.4). However, data on the effect of OCT1 polymorphisms on the response to metformin treatment in humans have been conflicting, maybe due to the small number of patients studied [114, 115].

Recently, the transcription factor 7-like 2 (TCF7L2) gene was identified as a significant type 2 diabetes susceptibility gene, so far the most important risk gene [116]. The exact mechanism of action of TCF7L2 has not been identified, but has been linked to impaired insulin secretion. Surprisingly, the TCF7L2 risk-alleles are also associated with a lower BMI (that is, with a leaner phenotype) [117].

In subjects with impaired glucose tolerance, the Diabetes Prevention Program (DPP) study reported no significant difference between TCF7L2 genotypes on the progression to diabetes after interventions with placebo, life-style modification or metformin [117]. In contrast, an observational and retrospective study including predominantly overweight patients with type 2 diabetes, reported an increased glycaemic failure rate by treatment with insulin secretagogues compared to metformin in individuals being homozygotes for the risk-variants of TCF7L2 [118]. Thus, it is likely that these — and perhaps other unknown — type 2 diabetes susceptibility genes defines subgroups of patients with type 2 diabetes responding in different ways to any of the currently available antidiabetic treatments, including metformin.

SUMMARY

Metformin remains the OAD of first choice to treat both obese and non-obese patients with the common form of type 2 diabetes in monotherapy or in combination with other OADs or insulin due to its glucose-lowering effect as well as its putative effect in protecting against CVD. Furthermore, metformin treatment now has an established role in the treatment of PCOS. In contrast, patients with type 1 diabetes should not routinely receive metformin treatment. Although our understanding of the molecular mechanisms of action of metformin has increased substantially during recent years, including the identification of a central role

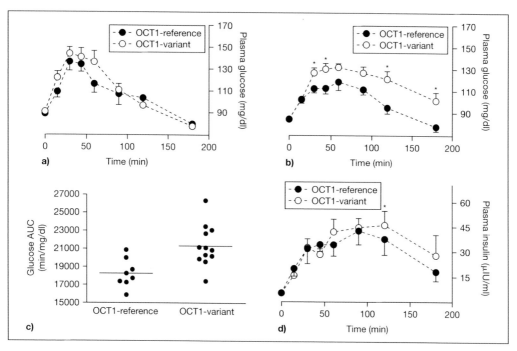

Figure 4.4 OCT1 genetic variants may be associated with different responses to metformin in healthy human volunteers. Panel a: The time course of plasma glucose concentrations for a baseline OGTT without metformin treatment in healthy subjects having only reference OCT1 alleles ($n = 8$) and those having at least one reduced-function OCT1 allele ($n = 12$). The data are expressed as mean ± SEM. Panel b: The time course of plasma glucose concentrations for OGTT after metformin treatment in the same healthy subjects represented in A. The data are expressed as mean ± SEM; *P <0.05 compared with volunteers with only reference OCT1 alleles. (unpaired Student's t test). Panel c: The glucose exposure with OGTT (area under curve; AUC) after metformin treatment for healthy subjects represented in B. The horizontal lines represent mean values for the two groups. The mean value for volunteers with only reference OCT1 alleles is significantly lower than that for the variant group. $P = 0.004$ (unpaired Student's t test). Panel d: The time course of insulin levels during the OGTT after metformin administration in the same healthy individuals represented in A. The data are expressed as mean ± SEM; *P <0.05 compared with individuals with only OCT1-reference alleles (unpaired 1-tailed Student's t test) (with permission from [73]).
OCT1 = organic cation transporter 1; OGTT = oral glucose tolerance test; SEM = standard error of the mean.

for activation of AMPK and the role of OCT1 regulating the cellular uptake of metformin, much more knowledge of the actions of metformin is required to understand (and fully accept) its potential cardiovascular protective effects. Pharmacogenetics also needs to be used to identify responders and non-responders to metformin therapy.

REFERENCES

1. Nathan DM, Buse JB, Davidson MB *et al.* Management of hyperglycaemia in type 2 diabetes: a consensus algorithm for the initiation and adjustment of therapy: a consensus statement from the American Diabetes Association and the European Association for the Study of Diabetes. *Diabetologia* 2006; 49:1711–1721.
2. Hermann LS, Schersten B, Bitzen PO, Kjellstrom T, Lindgarde F, Melander A. Therapeutic comparison of metformin and sulfonylurea, alone and in various combinations. A double-blind controlled study. *Diabetes Care* 1994; 17:1100–1109.

3. DeFronzo RA, Goodman AM Efficacy of metformin in patients with non-insulin-dependent diabetes mellitus. The Multicenter Metformin Study Group. *N Engl J Med* 1995; 333:541–549.

4. Johansen K. Efficacy of metformin in the treatment of NIDDM: Meta- analysis. *Diabetes Care* 1999; 22:33–37.

5. Kirpichnikov D, McFarlane SI, Sowers JR. Metformin: An update. Ann Intern Med 2002; 137:25–33.

6. Yki-Jarvinen H, Nikkila K, Mäkimattila S. Metformin prevents weight gain by reducing dietary intake during insulin therapy in patients with type 2 diabetes mellitus. *Drugs* 1999; 58(suppl 1):53–54.

7. Garber AJ, Duncan TG, Goodman AM, Mills DJ, Rohlf JL. Efficacy of metformin in type II diabetes: results of a double-blind, placebo-controlled, dose-response trial. *Am J Med* 1997; 103:491–497.

8. Davidson MB, Peters AL. An overview of metformin in the treatment of type 2 diabetes mellitus. *Am J Med* 1997; 102:99–9110.

9. Turner RC, Cull CA, Frighi V, Holman RR, for the UK Prospective Diabetes Study Group Glycemic Control With Diet, Sulfonylurea, Metformin, or Insulin in Patients With Type 2 Diabetes Mellitus: Progressive Requirement for Multiple Therapies (UKPDS 49). *JAMA* 1999; 281:2005–2012.

10. UKPDS 28: a randomized trial of efficacy of early addition of metformin in sulfonylurea-treated type 2 diabetes. UK Prospective Diabetes Study Group. *Diabetes Care* 1998; 21:87–92.

11. Yki-Jarvinen H, Ryysy L, Nikkila K, Tulokas T, Vanamo R, Heikkila M. Comparison of bedtime insulin regimens in patients with type 2 diabetes mellitus. A randomized, controlled trial. *Ann Intern Med* 1999; 130:389–396.

12. Douek IF, Allen SE, Ewings P, Gale EAM, Bingley PJ. Continuing metformin when starting insulin in patients with Type 2 diabetes: A double-blind randomized placebo-controlled trial. *Diabet Med* 2005; 22:634–640.

13. Kooy A, de Jager J, Lehert P *et al*. Long-term Effects of Metformin on Metabolism and Microvascular and Macrovascular Disease in Patients With Type 2 Diabetes Mellitus. *Arch Intern Med* 2009; 169:616–625.

14. Kabadi UM, Kabadi M. Comparative efficacy of glimepiride and/or metformin with insulin in type 2 diabetes. *Diabetes Res Clin Pract* 2006; 72:265–270.

15. Holman RR, Thorne KI, Farmer AJ *et al*. Addition of biphasic, prandial, or basal insulin to oral therapy in type 2 diabetes. *N Engl J Med* 2007; 357:1716–1730.

16. Diabetes Prevention Program Research Group Reduction in the Incidence of Type 2 Diabetes with Lifestyle Intervention or Metformin. *N Engl J Med* 2002; 346:393–403.

17. Diabetes Prevention Program Research Group Effects of withdrawal from metformin on the development of diabetes in the diabetes prevention program. *Diabetes Care* 2003; 26:977–980.

18. The Diabetes Control and Complications Trial Research Group. The effect of intensive treatment of diabetes on the development and progression of long-term complications in insulin-dependent diabetes mellitus. *N Engl J Med* 1993; 329:977–986.

19. UK Prospective Diabetes Study (UKPDS) Group Intensive blood-glucose control with sulphonylureas or insulin compared with conventional treatment and risk of complications in patients with type 2 diabetes (UKPDS 33). *Lancet* 1998; 352:837–853.

20. UK Prospective Diabetes Study (UKPDS) Group Effect of intensive blood-glucose control with metformin on complications in overweight patients with type 2 diabetes (UKPDS 34). *Lancet* 1998; 352:854–865.

21. Holman RR, Paul SK, Bethel MA, Matthews DR, Neil HA. 10-Year Follow-up of Intensive Glucose Control in Type 2 Diabetes. *N Engl J Med* 2008; 359:1577–1589.

22. Schramm TK, Gislason GH, Kober L *et al*. Diabetes Patients Requiring Glucose-Lowering Therapy and Nondiabetics With a Prior Myocardial Infarction Carry the Same Cardiovascular Risk: A Population Study of 3.3 Million People. *Circulation* 2008; 117:1945–1954.

23. Haffner SM, Lehto S, Rönnemaa T, Pyörälä K, Laakso M. Mortality from coronary heart disease in subjects with type 2 diabetes and in nondiabetic subjects with and without prior myocardial infarction. *N Engl J Med* 1998; 339:229–234.

24. Stratton IM, Adler AI, Neil HA *et al*. Association of glycaemia with macrovascular and microvascular complications of type 2 diabetes (UKPDS 35): prospective observational study. *BMJ* 2000; 321:405–412.

25. The Action to Control Cardiovascular Risk in Diabetes Study Group Effects of Intensive Glucose Lowering in Type 2 Diabetes. *N Engl J Med* 2008; 358:2545–2559.

26. ADVANCE Collaborative Group, Patel A, MacMahon S *et al*. Intensive blood glucose control and vascular outcomes in patients with type 2 diabetes. *N Engl J Med* 2008; 358:2560–2572.

27. Duckworth W, Abraira C, Moritz T et al. Glucose Control and Vascular Complications in Veterans with Type 2 Diabetes. N Engl J Med 2008; 360:129–139.

28. Mannucci E, Monami M, Lamanna C, Gori F, Marchionni N. Prevention of cardiovascular disease through glycemic control in type 2 diabetes: A meta-analysis of randomized clinical trials. Nutr Metab Cardiovasc Dis 2009; In Press, Corrected Proof.

29. Ray KK, Seshasai SR, Wijesuriya S et al. Effect of intensive control of glucose on cardiovascular outcomes and death in patients with diabetes mellitus: a meta-analysis of randomised controlled trials. Lancet 2009; 373:1765–1772.

30. Mellbin LG, Malmberg K, Norhammar A, Wedel H, Ryden L, for the DIGAMI The impact of glucose lowering treatment on long-term prognosis in patients with type 2 diabetes and myocardial infarction: a report from the DIGAMI 2 trial. Eur Heart J 2008; 29:166–176.

31. Johnson JA, Majumdar SR, Simpson SH, Toth EL. Decreased mortality associated with the use of metformin compared with sulfonylurea monotherapy in type 2 diabetes. Diabetes Care 2002; 25:2244–2248.

32. Eurich DT, Majumdar SR, McAlister FA, Tsuyuki RT, Johnson JA. Improved clinical outcomes associated with metformin in patients with diabetes and heart failure. Diabetes Care 2005; 28:2345–2351.

33. Kahler KH, Rajan M, Rhoads GG et al. Impact of oral antihyperglycemic therapy on all-cause mortality among patients with diabetes in the Veterans Health Administration. Diabetes Care 2007; 30:1689–1693.

34. Olsson J, Lindberg G, Gottsäter M et al. Increased mortality in Type II diabetic patients using sulphonylurea and metformin in combination: a population-based observational study. Diabetologia 2000; 43:558–560.

35. Mannucci E, Monami M, Masotti G, Marchionni N. All-cause mortality in diabetic patients treated with combinations of sulfonylureas and biguanides. Diabetes Metab Res Rev 2004; 20:44–47.

36. Fisman EZ, Tenenbaum A, Boyko V et al. Oral antidiabetic treatment in patients with coronary disease: time-related increased mortality on combined glyburide/metformin therapy over a 7.7-year follow-up. Clin Cardiol 2001; 24:151–158.

37. Rao AD, Kuhadiya N, Reynolds K, Fonseca VA. Is the Combination of Sulfonylureas and Metformin Associated With an Increased Risk of Cardiovascular Disease or All-Cause Mortality?: A meta-analysis of observational studies. Diabetes Care 2008; 31:1672–1678.

38. Turner RC, Holman R, Stratton I. The UK Prospective Diabetes Study: Authors' reply. Lancet 1998; 352:1934.

39. Thisted H, Johnsen SP, Rungby J. Sulfonylureas and the risk of myocardial infarction. Metabolism 2006; 55:S16–S19.

40. Kahn SE, Haffner SM, Heise MA et al. Glycemic Durability of Rosiglitazone, Metformin, or Glyburide Monotherapy. N Engl J Med 2006; 355:2427–2443.

41. Wiernsperger NF, Bailey CJ. The antihyperglycaemic effect of metformin: therapeutic and cellular mechanisms. Drugs 1999; 58(suppl 1):31–39.

42. Klip A, Gumà A, Ramlal T, Bilan PJ, Lam L, Leiter LA. Stimulation of hexose transport by metformin in L6 muscle cells in culture. Endocrinology 1992; 130:2535–2544.

43. Hundal HS, Ramlal T, Reyes R, Leiter LA, Klip A. Cellular mechanism of metformin action involves glucose transporter translocation from an intracellular pool to the plasma membrane in L6 muscle cells. Endocrinology 1992; 131:1165–1173.

44. Hundal RS, Krssak M, Dufour S et al. Mechanism by which metformin reduces glucose production in type 2 diabetes. Diabetes 2000; 49:2063–2069.

45. Zhou G, Myers R, Li Y et al. Role of AMP-activated protein kinase in mechanism of metformin action. J Clin Invest 2001; 108:1167–1174.

46. Hardie DG. AMP-Activated Protein Kinase as a Drug Target. Annu Rev Pharmacol Toxicol 2007; 47:185–210.

47. Patanè G, Piro S, Rabuazzo AM, Anello M, Vigneri R, Purrello F. Metformin restores insulin secretion altered by chronic exposure to free fatty acids or high glucose: a direct metformin effect on pancreatic beta-cells. Diabetes 2000; 49:735–740.

48. Wang DS, Jonker JW, Kato Y, Kusuhara H, Schinkel AH, Sugiyama Y. Involvement of Organic Cation Transporter 1 in Hepatic and Intestinal Distribution of Metformin. J Pharmacol Exp Ther 2002; 302:510–515.

49. Kimura N, Masuda S, Tanihara Y et al. Metformin is a superior substrate for renal organic cation transporter OCT2 rather than hepatic OCT1. Drug Metab Pharmacokinet 2005; 20:379–386.

50. Angelico F, Burattin M, Alessandri C, Del-Ben M, Lirussi F. Drugs improving insulin resistance for non-alcoholic fatty liver disease and/or non-alcoholic steatohepatitis. *Cochrane Database Syst Rev* 2007;CD005166.
51. Vuppalanchi R, Chalasani N. Nonalcoholic fatty liver disease and nonalcoholic steatohepatitis: Selected practical issues in their evaluation and management. *Hepatology* 2009; 49:306–317.
52. Sowers JR, Epstein M, Frohlich ED. Diabetes, Hypertension, and Cardiovascular Disease: An Update. *Hypertension* 2001; 37:1053–1059.
53. Wulffele MG, Kooy A, de Zeeuw D, Stehouwer CD, Gansevoort RT. The effect of metformin on blood pressure, plasma cholesterol and triglycerides in type 2 diabetes mellitus: a systematic review. *J Intern Med* 2004; 256:1–14.
54. Wulffele MG, Kooy A, Lehert P, Betst D, Donker AJM, Stehouwer CDA. Does metformin decrease blood pressure in patients with Type 2 diabetes intensively treated with insulin? *Diabet Med* 2005; 22:907–913.
55. Lund SS, Tarnow L, Stehouwer CD *et al*. Impact of metformin versus repaglinide on non-glycaemic cardiovascular risk markers related to inflammation and endothelial dysfunction in non-obese patients with type 2 diabetes. *Eur J Endocrinol* 2008; 158:631–641.
56. Abbasi F, Chu JW, McLaughlin T, Lamendola C, Leary ET, Reaven GM. Effect of metformin treatment on multiple cardiovascular disease risk factors in patients with type 2 diabetes mellitus. *Metabolism* 2004; 53:159–164.
57. Chu NV, Kong AP, Kim DD *et al*. Differential effects of metformin and troglitazone on cardiovascular risk factors in patients with type 2 diabetes. *Diabetes Care* 2002; 25:542–549.
58. De Jager J, Kooy A, Lehert P *et al*. Effects of short-term treatment with metformin on markers of endothelial function and inflammatory activity in type 2 diabetes mellitus: a randomized, placebo-controlled trial. *J Intern Med* 2005; 257:100–109.
59. Asagami T, Abbasi F, Stuelinger M *et al*. Metformin treatment lowers asymmetric dimethylarginine concentrations in patients with type 2 diabetes. *Metabolism* 2002; 51:843–846.
60. Beisswenger PJ, Howell SK, Touchette AD, Lal S, Szwergold BS. Metformin reduces systemic methylglyoxal levels in type 2 diabetes. *Diabetes* 1999; 48:198–202.
61. Amador-Licona N, Guizar-Mendoza J, Vargas E, Sanchez-Camargo G, Zamora-Mata L. The short-term effect of a switch from glibenclamide to metformin on blood pressure and microalbuminuria in patients with type 2 diabetes mellitus. *Arch Med Res* 2000; 31:571–575.
62. Grant PJ. The effects of high- and medium-dose metformin therapy on cardiovascular risk factors in patients with type II diabetes. *Diabetes Care* 1996; 19:64–66.
63. Testa R, Bonfigli AR, Piantanelli L, Manfrini S, Testa I, Gregorio F. Relationship between plasminogen activator inhibitor type-1 plasma levels and the lipoprotein(a) concentrations in non-insulin-dependent diabetes mellitus. *Diabetes Res Clin Pract* 1996; 33:111–118.
64. Grant PJ, Stickland MH, Booth NA, Prentice CR. Metformin causes a reduction in basal and post-venous occlusion plasminogen activator inhibitor-1 in type 2 diabetic patients. *Diabet Med* 1991; 8:361–365.
65. Vague P. Cardiovascular benefits of metformin. *Diabetes & Metabolism* 2003; 29:6S1–6S122.
66. Bolen S, Feldman L, Vassy J *et al*. Systematic Review: Comparative Effectiveness and Safety of Oral Medications for Type 2 Diabetes Mellitus. *Ann Intern Med* 2007; 147:386–399.
67. Lund SS, Tarnow L, Frandsen M *et al*. Impact of metformin versus the prandial insulin secretagogue, repaglinide, on fasting and postprandial glucose and lipid responses in non-obese patients with type 2 diabetes. *Eur J Endocrinol* 2008; 158:443–445.
68. Lund SS, Tarnow L, Astrup AS *et al*. Effect of adjunct metformin treatment on levels of plasma lipids in patients with type 1 diabetes. *Diabetes Obes Metab* 2009;DOI: 10.1111/j.1463-1326.2009.01079.x.
69. Bauman WA, Shaw S, Jayatilleke E, Spungen AM, Herbert V. Increased intake of calcium reverses Vitamin B12 malabsorption induced by metformin. *Diabetes Care* 2000; 23:1227–1231.
70. Cusi K, DeFronzo RA. Metformin: a review of its metabolic effects. *Diabetes Review* 1998; 6:89–131.
71. Lalau JD, Race JM. Lactic acidosis in metformin therapy. *Drugs* 1999; 58(suppl 1):55–60.
72. Lalau JD, Andrejak M, Moriniere P *et al*. Hemodialysis in the treatment of lactic acidosis in diabetics treated by metformin: a study of metformin elimination. *Int J Clin Pharmacol Ther Toxicol* 1989; 27:285–288.
73. Skarfors ET, Selinus KI, Lithell HO. Risk factors for developing non-insulin dependent diabetes: a 10 year follow up of men in Uppsala. *BMJ* 1991; 303:755–760.
74. Dalton M, Cameron AJ, Zimmet PZ *et al*. Waist circumference, waist-hip ratio and body mass index and their correlation with cardiovascular disease risk factors in Australian adults. *J Intern Med* 2003; 254:555–563.

75. Garancini MP, Calori G, Ruotolo G et al. Prevalence of NIDDM and impaired glucose tolerance in Italy: an OGTT-based population study. *Diabetologia* 1995; 38:306–313.
76. Arner P, Pollare T, Lithell H. Different aetiologies of type 2 (non-insulin-dependent) diabetes mellitus in obese and non-obese subjects. *Diabetologia* 1991; 34:483–487.
77. Manson JE, Colditz GA, Stampfer MJ et al. A prospective study of maturity-onset diabetes mellitus and risk of coronary heart disease and stroke in women. *Arch Intern Med* 1991; 151:1141–1148.
78. Adlerberth AM, Rosengren A, Wilhelmsen L. Diabetes and long-term risk of mortality from coronary and other causes in middle-aged Swedish men. A general population study. *Diabetes Care* 1998; 21:539–545.
79. Nathan DM, Buse JB, Davidson MB et al. Medical management of hyperglycaemia in type 2 diabetes mellitus: a consensus algorithm for the initiation and adjustment of therapy: a consensus statement from the American Diabetes Association and the European Association for the Study of Diabetes. *Diabetologia* 2009; 52:17–30.
80. Collier A, Watson HHK, Patrick AW, Ludlam CA, Clarke BF. Effect of glycemic control metformin and gliclazide on platelet density and aggregability in recently diagnosed type 2 non-insulin-dependent diabetic patients. *Diabet Metab* 1989; 15:420–425.
81. Boyd K, Rogers C, Boreham C, Andrews WJ, Hadden DR. Insulin, glibenclamide or metformin treatment for non insulin dependent diabetes: heterogenous responses of standard measures of insulin action and insulin secretion before and after differing hypoglycaemic therapy. *Diabetes Res* 1992; 19:69–76.
82. DeFronzo RA, Barzilai N, Simonson DC. Mechanism of metformin action in obese and lean noninsulin-dependent diabetic subjects. *J Clin Endocrinol Metab* 1991; 73:1294–1301.
83. Clarke BF, Campbell IW. Comparison of metformin and chlorpropamide in non-obese, maturity-onset diabetics uncontrolled by diet. *BMJ* 1977; 2:1576–1578.
84. Derosa G, Mugellini A, Ciccarelli L, Crescenzi G, Fogari R. Comparison of glycaemic control and cardiovascular risk profile in patients with type 2 diabetes during treatment with either repaglinide or metformin. *Diabetes Res Clin Pract* 2003; 60:161–169.
85. Perriello G, Misericordia P, Volpi E et al. Acute antihyperglycemic mechanisms of metformin in NIDDM. Evidence for suppression of lipid oxidation and hepatic glucose production. *Diabetes* 1994; 43:920–928.
86. Pearson ER, Starkey BJ, Powell RJ, Gribble FM, Clark PM, Hattersley AT. Genetic cause of hyperglycaemia and response to treatment in diabetes. *Lancet* 2003; 362:1275–1281.
87. Josephkutty S, Potter JM. Comparison of tolbutamide and metformin in elderly diabetic patients. *Diabet Med* 1990; 7:510–514.
88. Donnelly LA, Doney AS, Hattersley AT, Morris AD, Pearson ER. The effect of obesity on glycaemic response to metformin or sulphonylureas in Type 2 diabetes. *Diabet Med* 2006; 23:128–133.
89. Ong CR, Molyneaux LM, Constantino MI, Twigg SM, Yue DK. Long-Term Efficacy of Metformin Therapy in Nonobese Individuals With Type 2 Diabetes. *Diabetes Care* 2006; 29:2361–2364.
90. Lund SS, Tarnow L, Stehouwer CD et al. Targeting hyperglycaemia with either metformin or repaglinide in non-obese patients with type 2 diabetes: results from a randomized crossover trial. *Diabetes Obes Metab* 2007; 9:394–407.
91. Nissen SE, Wolski K. Effect of rosiglitazone on the risk of myocardial infarction and death from cardiovascular causes. *N Engl J Med* 2007; 356:2457–2471.
92. Schramm TK, Gislason GH, Vaag A et al. Differences in Risk of Cardiovascular Death According to Type of Oral Glucose-Lowering Therapy in Patients with Diabetes: A Nationwide Study. *Diabetes* 2009; 58(suppl). Ref Type: Abstract.
93. DeFronzo RA. Hepatic and peripheral insulin resistance: a common feature of type 2 (non-insulin-dependent) and type 1 (insulin-dependent) diabetes mellitus. *Diabetologia* 1982; 23:313–319.
94. Laing SP, Swerdlow AJ, Slater SD et al. Mortality from heart disease in a cohort of 23,000 patients with insulin-treated diabetes. *Diabetologia* 2003; 46:760–765.
95. Nathan DM, Cleary PA, Backlund JY et al. Intensive diabetes treatment and cardiovascular disease in patients with type 1 diabetes. *N Engl J Med* 2005; 353:2643–2653.
96. Pagano G. Metformin reduces insulin requirement in Type 1 (insulin-dependent) diabetes. *Diabetologia* 1983; 24:351–354.
97. Coscelli C, Palmari V, Saccardi F, Alpi O, Bonora E. Evidence that metformin addition to insulin induces an amelioration of glycemic profile in type I (insulin-dependent) diabetes mellitus. *Curr Ther Res* 1984; 35:1058–1064.

98. Gin H. Metformin improved insulin resistance in type I, insulin-dependent, diabetic patients. *Metab Clin Exp* 1985; 34:923–925.

99. Janssen M, Rillaerts E, De Leeuw I. Effects of metformin on haemorheology, lipid parameters and insulin resistance in insulin-dependent diabetic patients (IDDM). *Biomed Pharmacother* 1991; 45:363–367.

100. Lacigova S, Rusavy Z, Jankovec Z, Kyselova P. Metformin in the treatment of type 1 diabetics–a placebo controlled study. *Cas Lek Cesk* 2001; 140:302–306.

101. Gomez R, Mokhashi MH, Rao J et al. Metformin adjunctive therapy with insulin improves glycemic control in patients with type 1 diabetes mellitus: a pilot study. *J Pediatr Endocrinol Metab* 2002; 15:1147–1151.

102. Meyer L, Bohme P, Delbachian I et al. The benefits of metformin therapy during continuous subcutaneous insulin infusion treatment of type 1 diabetic patients. *Diabetes Care* 2002; 25:2153–2158.

103. Särnblad S, Kroon M, Aman J. Metformin as additional therapy in adolescents with poorly controlled type 1 diabetes: randomised placebo-controlled trial with aspects on insulin sensitivity. *Eur J Endocrinol* 2003; 149:323–329.

104. Hamilton J, Cummings E, Zdravkovic V, Finegood D, Daneman D. Metformin as an adjunct therapy in adolescents with type 1 diabetes and insulin resistance: a randomized controlled trial. *Diabetes Care* 2003; 26:138–143.

105. Khan AS, McLoughney CR, Ahmed AB. The effect of metformin on blood glucose control in overweight patients with Type 1 diabetes. *Diabet Med* 2006; 23:1079–1084.

106. Moon RJ, Bascombe LA, Holt RI. The addition of metformin in type 1 diabetes improves insulin sensitivity, diabetic control, body composition and patient well-being. *Diabetes Obes Metab* 2007; 9:143–145.

107. Jacobsen IB, Henriksen JE, Beck-Nielsen H. The Effect of Metformin in Overweight Patients with Type 1 Diabetes and Poor Metabolic Control. *Basic Clin Pharmacol Toxicol* 2009;DOI: 10.1111/j.1742-7843.2009.00380.x.

108. Lund SS, Tarnow L, Astrup AS et al. Effect of Adjunct Metformin Treatment in Patients with Type-1 Diabetes and Persistent Inadequate Glycaemic Control. A Randomized Study. *PLoS ONE* 2008; 3:e3363.

109. Pasquali R, Gambineri A, Biscotti D et al. Effect of long-term treatment with metformin added to hypocaloric diet on body composition, fat distribution, and androgen and insulin levels in abdominally obese women with and without the polycystic ovary syndrome. *J Clin Endocrinol Metab* 2000; 85:2767–2774.

110. Pugeat M, Ducluzeau PH. Insulin resistance, polycystic ovary syndrome and metformin. *Drugs* 1999; 58(suppl 1):41–46.

111. Nestler JE, Powers LP, Matt DW et al. A direct effect of hyperinsulinemia on serum sex hormone-binding globulin levels in obese women with the polycystic ovary syndrome. *J Clin Endocrinol Metab* 1991; 72:83–89.

112. Glueck CJ, Wang P, Fontaine R, Tracy T, Sieve-Smith L. Metformin-induced resumption of normal menses in 39 of 43 (91%) previously amenorrheic women with the polycystic ovary syndrome. *Metabolism* 1999; 48:511–519.

113. Velazquez EM, Mendoza S, Hamer T, Sosa F, Glueck CJ. Metformin therapy in polycystic ovary syndrome reduces hyperinsulinemia, insulin resistance, hyperandrogenemia, and systolic blood pressure, while facilitating normal menses and pregnancy. *Metabolism* 1994; 43:647–654.

114. Shu Y, Sheardown SA, Brown C et al. Effect of genetic variation in the organic cation transporter 1 (OCT1) on metformin action. *J Clin Invest* 2007; 117:1422–1431.

115. Shikata E, Yamamoto R, Takane H et al. Human organic cation transporter (OCT1 and OCT2) gene polymorphisms and therapeutic effects of metformin. *J Hum Genet* 2006; 52:117–122.

116. Grant SFA, Thorleifsson G, Reynisdottir I et al. Variant of transcription factor 7-like 2 (TCF7L2) gene confers risk of type 2 diabetes. *Nat Genet* 2006; 38:320–323.

117. Florez JC, Jablonski KA, Bayley N et al. TCF7L2 Polymorphisms and Progression to Diabetes in the Diabetes Prevention Program. *N Engl J Med* 2006; 355:241–250.

118. Pearson ER, Donnelly LA, Kimber C et al. Variation in TCF7L2 influences therapeutic response to sulfonylureas: a GoDARTs study. *Diabetes* 2007; 56:2178–2182.

5

Glitazones and glitazars: targeting PPARγ and PPARα in diabetes

A. J. Gilde, B. Staels

INTRODUCTION

In 1990, Issemann and Green elucidated the mechanism by which hypolipidaemic fibrates induced peroxisome proliferation in the rodent liver [1, 2] and identified a member of the steroid hormone receptor superfamily, designated peroxisome proliferator-activated receptor (PPAR), to be the mediators of this response. The PPAR family belongs to the nuclear receptor superfamily [3] and consists of three isoforms, PPARα, PPARβ (also known as δ) and PPARγ, each with their own tissue distribution pattern [4–6].

The structure of these nuclear receptors is organised in a modular fashion (Figure 5.1) with an amino acid N-terminal A/B domain containing the activating function 1 (AF-1) that possesses ligand-independent transactivation properties; the C-domain, which is responsible for DNA-binding; and the D-, E- and F-domains comprising a hinge region for conformational flexibility, and the ligand binding domain containing the AF-2 activation domain. Like the other members of the nuclear receptor superfamily, PPARs are conserved in nature and are found in a variety of species [7] (*www.receptors.org/NR/*).

While PPARα is predominantly expressed in tissues with a high oxidative capacity such as the heart and liver, PPARγ is expressed most highly in adipose tissue, whereas PPARβ/δ, which is more ubiquitously expressed, is abundant in skeletal muscle and intestine. PPARs can be activated by an array of natural (endogenous) ligands, ranging from long chain fatty acids to eicosanoids, which all bind with different affinity [8–10], as well as by synthetic ligands. Upon ligand binding, PPARs transactivate gene expression by heterodimerization with another nuclear receptor, the retinoic X receptor (RXR), and this complex binds to a direct repeat sequence designated PPAR responsive element (PPRE) [11] (Figure 5.2). Alternatively, PPARs are able to down-regulate or transrepress gene expression via a signal transduction disrupting mechanism independent of deoxyribonucleic acid (DNA) binding (Figure 5.2) [12, 13].

Andries J. Gilde, PhD, Post-doctoral Fellow, INSERM U545, Department of Atherosclerosis, Institut Pasteur de Lille, Lille, France.

Bart Staels, PhD, Professor of Pharmacy and Group Leader, Department of Atherosclerosis, Unit 545 INSERM, Institut Pasteur, University of Lille 2, Lille, France.

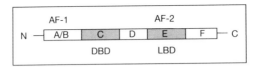

Figure 5.1 Schematic representation of the nuclear receptor structure. N is the amino terminus of the protein followed by the A/B domain containing the activating function-1 (AF-1) for ligand-independent transactivation, the C domain is responsible for DNA binding (DBD); and the D, E and F domains contain a hinge region for conformational flexibility and ligand binding domain (LBD) containing the AF-2 activation domain at the C-carboxyl terminus.

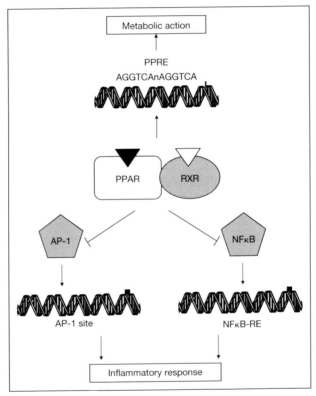

Figure 5.2 Schematic representation of ligand-mediated peroxisome proliferator activated-receptor (PPAR) activation and heterodimer formation with retinoic X receptor (RXR). Heterodimer formation results in binding to the consensus PPAR responsive element (PPRE) DNA-sequence mediating gene expression and inflammatory gene transrepression.

PPARγ ACTIVATION

PPARγ

In humans, PPARγ has been found to be predominantly expressed in white adipose tissue, although small amounts are also present in the heart, liver and skeletal muscle [14,

15]. Two isotypes were identified, designated PPARγ1 and PPARγ2, the expression of the latter being restricted mainly to adipose tissue as a mediator of adipocyte differentiation [16].

Genetic studies in humans revealed the PPARγ gene to influence body fat composition [17]. Loss-of-function mutations in humans result in partial lipodystrophy, which differs from other inherited forms of partial lipodystrophy such as the Lamin A/C mutation. These mutations are characterised by a loss of subcutaneous fat from the limbs and gluteal region and the relative preservation of abdominal subcutaneous and visceral depots. Subjects with mutations in the PPARγ gene have an increased risk of cardiovascular disease (CVD) [18, 19].

The creation of mice with a genetically altered PPARγ gene has proven to be useful in the study of PPARγ function in pathophysiology. Mice homozygous for PPARγ deficiency or in which the wild type gene is replaced by a dominant negative PPARγ mutation L466A die *in utero* at embryonic day 10.5–11.5 [20]. In addition to these whole body transgenic models, the tissue-specific knockout models for PPARγ have proven valuable in delineating the role of this receptor in specific tissues. Adipose tissue-specific ablation of PPARγ results in a decrease of white and brown adipose tissue mass [21, 22]. In contrast, the selective knockout of PPARγ2 in adipose tissue resulted in the reduction of white adipose tissue but not of brown adipose tissue [23]. Interestingly, introduction of the Pro12Ala mutation in exon B of the PPARγ gene resulted in a reduced expression of both PPARγ1 and PPARγ2 in white and PPARγ2 in brown adipose tissue [24]. Skeletal muscle-specific deletion of PPARγ resulted in glucose intolerance and insulin resistance [25, 26].

Taken together, the data obtained from tissue-selective PPARγ knockout models clearly confirm the role of this isoform in adipose tissue generation and function.

THIAZOLIDINEDIONES AND DIABETES

Thiazolidinediones (TZDs), also called glitazones, are a class of PPARγ agonists widely used in the treatment of type 2 diabetes since their discovery in the early 1980s [2, 27–29]. The principal mechanism by which TZDs exert their insulin sensitisation effect is via the activation of PPARγ in adipose tissue, inducing the differentiation of subcutaneous adipocytes and thus decreasing the visceral to subcutaneous adipose tissue ratio, resulting in the storage of free fatty acids in less harmful depots. Furthermore, PPARγ activation results in a reduced cell size of the adipocytes that coincides with an increased glucose transport [30]. In parallel, the expression of fatty acid transport proteins like CD36 and aP2 is increased in adipose tissue, increasing the uptake and storage of free fatty acids [31]. This results in improved insulin sensitivity of skeletal muscle and liver due to the decrease in free fatty acid load [32]. Moreover, TZDs increase the level of adiponectin in type 2 diabetic patients [33], an adipokine that was shown to be a diabetes susceptibility gene in humans [34]. Adiponectin levels correlate with liver fat content in type 2 diabetic patients and an increase of adiponectin improves insulin resistance [35]. In addition, adiponectin increases the activity of fatty acid oxidation enzymes in skeletal muscle and liver, probably via activation of the AMP-kinase (AMPK) pathway [36]. In addition, it was shown that macrophage accumulation in adipose tissue is correlated with obesity and insulin resistance [37]. In part, this is the result of macrophage excretory factors that reduce adipocyte differentiation and increase the expression of nuclear factor κB (NFκB) regulated inflammatory genes [38, 39]. The PPARγ agonist pioglitazone was shown to reduce macrophage infiltration in adipose tissue, improve insulin sensitivity and decrease plasma tumour necrosis factor-alpha (TNF-α) levels in human subjects [40].

The TZDs on the market today are rosiglitazone and pioglitazone, which each have different effects on blood lipid levels, whereas their effects on glucose homeostasis are comparable [2]. The recent GLAI study, which investigated differences between rosiglitazone and pioglitazone as monotherapy in type 2 diabetic patients, illustrated these differences (Table 5.1). Both drugs decreased fasting glucose and insulin levels, glycosylated haemoglobin A1c (HbA1c), plasminogen activator inhibitor-1 (PAI-1) and C-reactive protein (CRP), as well as free fatty acids, whereas pioglitazone but not rosiglitazone decreased plasma triglyceride levels. Both drugs increased high-density lipoprotein-cholesterol (HDL-C), low-density lipoprotein-cholesterol (LDL-C), and total cholesterol concentrations, but LDL particle concentrations decreased with pioglitazone and increased with rosiglitazone. Both TZDs increase LDL particle size, resulting in a decrease of atherogenic small dense low-density lipoprotein (sdLDL). The impact of these TZDs on CVD and the mechanisms behind these differences in lipid levels are not clear. Whereas pioglitazone may have limited PPARα activating properties, thus mimicking some of the effects of fibrates, such as the decrease of triglycerides [41] (Table 5.2), selective PPAR modulator (SPPARM) effects could also be involved.

In addition to their effects on glucose homeostasis, TZDs possess anti-inflammatory properties. PPARγ is expressed in cells of the vascular system such as endothelial cells, macrophages, vascular smooth muscle cells, lymphocytes and platelets. This raised the hypothesis that TZDs may also be useful to combat the development and progression of atherosclerotic plaque formation [42]. Different studies showed that PPARγ activation resulted in a decrease of plasma cytokines and other inflammatory mediators like MMP9 and soluble CD40-ligand expression as well as a reduction of TNF-α, interleukin (IL)-6, IL-8, the acute phase reactants fibrinogen and CRP, and the endothelial cell activation markers E-selectin and von Willebrand factor, not only in type 2 diabetics but also in non-diabetic patients [43–47]. These effects might contribute to the outcome of the recent PROspective pioglitAzone Clinical Trial In macroVascular Events (PROactive) study that investigated the effect of pioglitazone on macrovascular morbidity and mortality in type 2 diabetic patients over a 34.5-month period [48]. Although all-cause mortality (primary endpoint) was not significantly changed, the results showed a significant reduction of the principal secondary endpoint by pioglitazone, i.e. death from all causes, non-fatal myocardial infarction (MI) and stroke in type 2 diabetic patients (hazard ratio [HR] 0.84; 95% confidence interval [CI] 0.72–0.98; $P = 0.027$). Furthermore, pioglitazone decreased triglycerides, LDL/HDL ratio and HbA1c. Additionally, pioglitazone reduced the progression of diabetes as indicated by a lower initiation of insulin (2.7% vs. 12.4% in placebo; $P <0.0001$). These effects on CVD were observed in addition to the use of statins (55%) and angiotensin converting enzyme (ACE)-inhibitors (63%), drugs previously shown to be beneficial in attenuating cardiovascular disease [49, 50]. A first *post hoc* analysis of the PROactive trial, investigating the subgroup of patients with previous MI, showed that pioglitazone significantly reduced recurrent cardiovascular events (Late Breaking News, AHA 2005, E. Erdmann [*www.proactive-results.com*]).

Unfortunately, the use of TZDs is accompanied by certain adverse effects. Among these is the gain of body weight as a result of adipocyte differentiation and increased body fat. Contributing to this weight gain is TZD-induced fluid retention due partly to PPARγ-mediated fluid and salt retention in the collecting duct of the kidney [51, 52]. Fluid retention, together with increased vascular permeability, may result in oedema. In type 2 diabetics with diminished cardiac function, this could precipitate congestive heart failure [53, 54]. From this perspective, it is reassuring that the recent PROactive study showed that pioglitazone does not increase mortality due to heart failure [48]. Furthermore, the recent Rosiglitazone Early versus Sulphonylurea Titration (RESULT) study, investigating the addition of rosiglitazone to regular glipizide treatment, revealed no increase of heart failure due to rosiglitazone as compared to the glipizide control group [55]. Interestingly, this study showed a 50% reduction in hospitalisation upon use of rosiglitazone (0.4 events per 1000 patient-days) in a study population with 65% of the patients above 65 years.

Table 5.1 The effect of different PPAR agonists on plasma markers

Agonist	Study	Subjects	HbA1c	FPG	FPI	FFA	TG	Tchol	LDL	HDL	Ref.
Rosiglitazone	GLAI/RESULT	T2D	→	→			↑	↑	↑	↑	[55, 69]
Pioglitazone	PROactive/GLAI	T2D	→	→	→	→	↑	↑	↑	↑	[48, 69]
Fenofibrate	FIELD	T2D	-	→		→	↓	↓	→	↑	[58]
Muraglitazar		T2D-drug naïve	→	→	→	→	↓	↓	↓	↑	[63]
Ragaglitazar		T2D	→	→	→	→	↓	↓	→	↑	[64]
Tesaglitazar		IR	→	→	→	→	↓	→	→	↑	[70]
KRP297/MK-767		Healthy individuals				→	↓	↓	→	↓	[71]

FIELD = Fenofibrate Intervention and Event Lowering in Diabetes; GLAI = no abbreviation; IR = insulin resistance; PROactive = PROspectieve pioglitAzone Clinical Trial In macroVascular Events; RESULT = Rosiglitazone Early vs SULphonylurea Titration; T2D = type 2 diabetes; ↑ = increase; ↓ = decrease; - = no change.

Table 5.2 Summary of clinical and pre-clinical safety issues regarding PPAR agonsts

Agonist	Phase	Clinical safety issues	Ref. No.	Pre-clinical safety issues	EC50 PPARα (nM)	EC50 PPARγ (nM)	Status
Muraglitazar	III	Weight gain, oedema, MI, TIA, heart failure	[65]	No issues known	320 [72]	110 [72]	Stopped
Ragaglitazar	II	Weight gain, oedema, anaemia, Hb↓		Urothelial cancer [73, 74]	3000	93	Stopped
Tesaglitazar	III	Plasma creatinine↑, glomerular filtration rate↓		No issues known	3000	149	Stopped
KRP297/MK-767	III	Abnormal liver enzymes		Hemangiosarcoma	149	83	Stopped
TAK-559	III			No data	67 [75]	31 [75]	On-hold
Fenofibrate		Pancreatitis 0.8%, pulmonary embolism 1%, creatinine 2%	[58]	Hepatocarcinoma	30 000 (76)		On market (Tricor)
Rosiglitazone		Oedema, heart failure			n.a.[a]	22	On market (Avandia)
Pioglitazone		Oedema, heart failure	[48]		>10 000[a]	326	On market (Actos)

EC50 values were obtained using a chimeric human PPAR promoter/reporter assay in our lab[a], or [77] unless mentioned otherwise, n.a., not active. Hb = haemoglobin; MI = myocardial infarction; TIA = transient ischaemic attack.

DUAL PPAR ACTIVATORS

Recently, studies on the development of single drugs as dual PPAR activators have begun, combining the activation of two PPAR isoforms in a single drug. The focus of this field of research has initially been on dual PPARγ/PPARα activation since both isoforms are expressed in insulin sensitising tissues such as adipose tissue, liver and skeletal muscle. In addition, clinical efficacy of PPARβ/δ-activators remains to be demonstrated. To understand the beneficial effects of combined PPARγ and PPARα, certain biological effects mediated by PPARα will be discussed in the following section of this chapter.

PPARα

PPARα-activating fibrates have been used in the treatment of dyslipidaemia improving the plasma lipid profile by lowering triglyceride and, for certain fibrates, also LDL-cholesterol levels and increasing HDL-cholesterol [41]. These effects are achieved by a variety of mechanisms such as an increase in lipoprotein lipase (LPL) expression, reduction of apolipoprotein CIII (apoCIII) expression, inhibition of triglyceride synthesis and very low-density lipoprotein-cholesterol (VLDL) production. Furthermore, fibrates exert transrepression effects influencing the expression of pro-inflammatory genes such as TNF-α, IL1β, IL6, matrix metalloproteinase 9 (MMP9) and tissue factor [56].

Clinical studies show that PPARα-activating drugs effectively reduce CVD in pre-diabetic and diabetic patients without previous CVD [2, 57]. The recent Fenofibrate Intervention and Event Lowering in Diabetes (FIELD) study evaluated the effect of fenofibrate in 9795 type 2 diabetes patients over a 5-year period [58]. Although fenofibrate did not significantly reduce the primary outcome (coronary heart disease death or non-fatal MI), it significantly reduced the secondary outcome of total cardiovascular disease events by 11% (cardiovascular disease mortality, non-fatal MI, stroke, and coronary and carotid artery revascularisation), due to a significant reduction of non-fatal MI and coronary revascularisation. Furthermore, fenofibrate reduced plasma total- and LDL-cholesterol and triglyceride concentrations by 16%, 21% and 25% respectively, while HDL-cholesterol increased only by 3%. A major confounder of this study was the supplementation of other lipid-lowering drugs (mainly statins) during the trial, the placebo group receiving significantly more as compared to the fenofibrate treated group, which likely contributed to the lack of significance of the primary endpoint.

Combining the effect of both PPARγ and PPARα activation in one drug could have additional beneficial effects over the use of TZDs or fibrates in monotherapy, in part related to their different tissue distribution patterns (Figure 5.3). Moreover, pre-clinical studies show that fibrates and TZDs exert different effects in pancreatic islets [59] or cardiac myocytes [60]. Dual agonists could thus not only act on insulin sensitivity as well as lipid homeostasis but may also improve diabetes progression through complementary activities. In obese (ob/ob) mice, the adverse effects of rosiglitazone on adiposity were attenuated by concomitant fenofibrate treatment, suggesting potential additional benefits of a dual-agonist compared to single PPARγ activation [61]. Furthermore, the study of Wagner and colleagues [62] showed, in non-diabetic healthy individuals, that addition of fenofibrate to rosiglitazone treatment increased LPL activity, decreased triglyceride, free fatty acids, LDL-cholesterol and total cholesterol concentrations, and increased HDL cholesterol concentrations, proving the concept of dual activation to be relevant.

GLITAZARS

Consequently, a new class of PPAR activators, the glitazars, have been synthesised, which combine the properties of multiple PPAR isoforms in one drug thus yielding more global effects

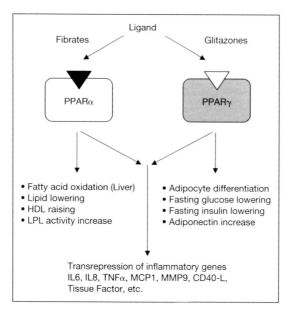

Figure 5.3 Schematic representation of the separate and combined actions of fibrates and glitazones in obesity and diabetes.

as compared to isoform-specific agonists. Clinical trials show favourable effects of glitazars on plasma lipids, insulin and glucose concentrations in type 2 diabetic and insulin-resistant patients, proving the concept of combined PPARα/γ activation in the clinic (Table 5.1).

In a multicentre, double-blind, placebo-controlled trial the effect of the dual PPARα/γ agonist muraglitazar was tested as monotherapy in drug-naïve type 2 diabetic patients for 24 weeks [63]. The results of this study showed a reduction in glycosylated haemoglobin, triglycerides, total- and LDL-cholesterol, and apoB. Furthermore, HDL-cholesterol was increased and fasting glucose, insulin and C-peptide levels were decreased, together showing results that are most favourable in reducing the risk of CVD. In parallel, a dose-finding study with ragaglitazar identified favourable effects of this drug in type 2 diabetic patients [64]. As shown in Table 5.1, several other glitazars improve insulin resistance as evidenced by the reduction in fasting glucose and insulin levels as well as the decrease in triglycerides, LDL- and total- cholesterol and the increase in HDL concentrations. Overall, the effects of glitazars on plasma glucose, insulin and lipids are a combination of the effects observed with fibrates and TZDs.

Unfortunately, several compounds were withdrawn from further development due to adverse effects (Table 5.2). Muraglitazar, approved by the US Food and Drug Administration (FDA), was withdrawn from the market due to hints of an excess incidence of death from adverse cardiovascular events, including MI and heart failure, as compared to placebo or pioglitazone [65]. Tesaglitazar was withdrawn, reportedly due to an increase in plasma creatinine levels and decrease in glomerular filtration rate (GFR), suggesting that the drug may lead to progression of renal failure in type 2 diabetes (AstraZeneca press release). Furthermore, the development of MK-767 was stopped due to an increased cancer incidence in pre-clinical animal models, mainly rodents, while the drug was tested in parallel to the phase III clinical trial [66] and TAK-559 is on hold for clinical use after the report of abnormal liver enzyme tests (Takeda press release).

These observations preclude the further development of these dual-agonists for clinical purposes and call for further attention to critical safety issues. The question remains whether the adverse effects observed in these studies are compound or target-related effects. Close observation of Table 5.2 reveals different toxicological effects, including urothelial cancer, plasma creatinine and liver enzyme elevation, suggesting compound rather than target-related effects. However, the withdrawn dual agonists display low EC_{50} values for PPARγ, suggesting that some of the adverse effects such as oedema, weight gain and heart failure may be target (PPARγ) related. Previous studies with the pan-agonist (PPARα, β/δ, and γ) bezafibrate, which activates multiple PPAR isoforms, have revealed it to be safe (Bezafibrate Infarction Prevention [BIP] study [67]; St Mary's, Ealing, Northwick Park Diabetes Cardiovascular Disease Prevention [SENDCAP] study [68]) substantiating the concept of multiple PPAR targets in a single drug.

Although the development of new glitazars is underway, data determining their safety for clinical use are awaited. In this perspective, it would be interesting to conduct *post hoc* analysis on the PROactive study patients receiving fibrates (8.6% = 207 patients).

SPPARMs

To circumvent the adverse effects of TZDs, PPARγ activators are being designed that do not show the negative effect of oedema formation caused by existing TZDs. Selective PPARγ modulators (SPPARMs) are a class of compounds under development that are intended to possess the positive effects of TZDs, such as insulin sensitisation and reduction of inflammation, but without oedema formation and body weight gain [78, 79]. Recently, the angiotensin receptor-1 blocker telmisartan was identified to be a SPPARM, activating PPARγ, and improving insulin resistance without inducing weight gain in diet-induced obese mice [80]. In a clinical study, telmisartan decreased the triglyceride level as well as total- and LDL-cholesterol levels, and increased HDL-cholesterol as compared to placebo and eprosartan-treated patients [81]. Interestingly, no changes were observed with respect to fasting plasma glucose and insulin and glycosylated HbA1c, which may call into debate the activation of PPARγ by telmisartan in humans. Other SPPARMs are under development, such as RWJ-348260 [82], nTZDpa [83], GW1929 [84], GW0072 [85], LG100641 [86], L-796,449 [87], PA-082 [88], although no data in humans are available for these compounds.

The effects induced by SPPARMs are thought to be the result of differential recruitment of transcriptional co-activators such as peroxisome proliferator activated receptor γ coactivator-1 α (PGC-1α) [89] and steroid receptor coactivator-1 (SRC-1) and corepressors like nuclear receptor corepressor (NCoR) [86] as compared to full agonists.

SUMMARY

Activators of PPARγ and PPARα have been shown in clinical trails not only to improve plasma lipids and insulin sensitivity but also reduce CVD. This chapter attempts to provide an overview of the current status and future developments in the pharmacology of these receptors. However, other detailed aspects of PPARγ and PPARα are beyond the scope of this chapter. Apart from the PPARα and γ isoforms, PPARβ/δ is also increasingly being recognised as a promising target in obesity and diabetes therapy (GW501516, Phase II, GlaxoSmithKline). The combined efforts of basic and clinical scientists in drug discovery processes should yield potential therapeutic agents acting through PPARγ and PPARα for the treatment of patients with obesity, diabetes and additional cardiovascular disease.

ACKNOWLEDGMENTS

This work was supported in part by the Region Nord-Pas de Calais/FEDER, the Fondation Coeur et Arteres and the European Vascular Genomics Network.

REFERENCES

1. Issemann I, Green S. Activation of a member of the steroid hormone receptor superfamily by peroxisome proliferators. *Nature* 1990; 347:645–650.
2. Staels B, Fruchart JC. Therapeutic roles of peroxisome proliferator-activated receptor agonists. *Diabetes* 2005; 54:2460–2470.
3. Mangelsdorf DJ, Thummel C, Beato M *et al.* The nuclear receptor superfamily: the second decade. *Cell* 1995; 83:835–839.
4. Mukherjee R, Jow L, Noonan D *et al.* Human and rat peroxisome proliferator activated receptors (PPARs) demonstrate similar tissue distribution but different responsiveness to PPAR activators. *J Steroid Biochem Mol Biol* 1994; 51:157–166.
5. Auboeuf D, Rieusset J, Fajas L *et al.* Tissue distribution and quantification of the expression of mRNAs of peroxisome proliferator-activated receptors and liver X receptor-alpha in humans: no alteration in adipose tissue of obese and NIDDM patients. *Diabetes* 1997; 46:1319–1327.
6. Escher P, Braissant O, Basu-Modak S *et al.* Rat PPARs: quantitative analysis in adult rat tissues and regulation in fasting and refeeding. *Endocrinology* 2001; 142:4195–4202.
7. Zhang Z, Burch PE, Cooney AJ *et al.* Genomic analysis of the nuclear receptor family: new insights into structure, regulation, and evolution from the rat genome. *Genome Res* 2004; 14:580–590.
8. Krey G, Braissant O, L'Horset F *et al.* Fatty acids, eicosanoids, and hypolipidemic agents identified as ligands of peroxisome proliferator-activated receptors by coactivator-dependent receptor ligand assay. *Mol Endocrinol* 1997; 11:779–791.
9. Kliewer SA, Sundseth SS, Jones SA *et al.* Fatty acids and eicosanoids regulate gene expression through direct interactions with peroxisome proliferator-activated receptors alpha and gamma. *Proc Natl Acad Sci USA* 1997; 94:4318–4323.
10. Forman BM, Chen J, Evans RM. Hypolipidemic drugs, polyunsaturated fatty acids, and eicosanoids are ligands for peroxisome proliferator-activated receptors alpha and delta. *Proc Natl Acad Sci USA* 1997; 94:4312–4317.
11. Gearing KL, Gottlicher M, Teboul M *et al.* Interaction of the peroxisome-proliferator-activated receptor and retinoid X receptor. *Proc Natl Acad Sci USA* 1993; 90:1440–1444.
12. Staels B, Koenig W, Habib A *et al.* Activation of human aortic smooth-muscle cells is inhibited by PPARalpha but not by PPARgamma activators. *Nature* 1998; 393:790–793.
13. Ricote M, Li AC, Willson TM *et al.* The peroxisome proliferator-activated receptor-gamma is a negative regulator of macrophage activation. *Nature* 1998; 391:79–82.
14. Elbrecht A, Chen Y, Cullinan CA *et al.* Molecular cloning, expression and characterization of human peroxisome proliferator activated receptors gamma 1 and gamma 2. *Biochem Biophys Res Commun* 1996; 224:431–437.
15. Vidal-Puig AJ, Considine RV, Jimenez-Linan M *et al.* Peroxisome proliferator-activated receptor gene expression in human tissues. Effects of obesity, weight loss, and regulation by insulin and glucocorticoids. *J Clin Invest* 1997; 99:2416–2422.
16. Tontonoz P, Hu E, Spiegelman BM. Stimulation of adipogenesis in fibroblasts by PPAR gamma 2, a lipid-activated transcription factor. *Cell* 1994; 79:1147–1156.
17. Semple RK, Chatterjee VK, O'Rahilly S. PPAR gamma and human metabolic disease. *J Clin Invest* 2006; 116:581–589.
18. Barroso I, Gurnell M, Crowley VE *et al.* Dominant negative mutations in human PPARgamma associated with severe insulin resistance, diabetes mellitus and hypertension. *Nature* 1999; 402:880–883.
19. Savage DB, Tan GD, Acerini CL *et al.* Human metabolic syndrome resulting from dominant-negative mutations in the nuclear receptor peroxisome proliferator-activated receptor-gamma. *Diabetes* 2003; 52:910–917.
20. Barak Y, Nelson MC, Ong ES *et al.* PPAR gamma is required for placental, cardiac, and adipose tissue development. *Mol Cell* 1999; 4:585–595.
21. Jones JR, Barrick C, Kim KA *et al.* Deletion of PPARgamma in adipose tissues of mice protects against high fat diet-induced obesity and insulin resistance. *Proc Natl Acad Sci USA* 2005; 102:6207–6212.
22. He W, Barak Y, Hevener A *et al.* Adipose-specific peroxisome proliferator-activated receptor gamma knockout causes insulin resistance in fat and liver but not in muscle. *Proc Natl Acad Sci USA* 2003; 100:15712–15717.
23. Zhang J, Fu M, Cui T *et al.* Selective disruption of PPARgamma2 impairs the developement of adipose tissue and insulin sensitivity. *Proc Natl Acad Sci USA* 2004; 101:10703–10708.

24. Koutnikova H, Cock TA, Watanabe M *et al.* Compensation by the muscle limits the metabolic consequences of lipodystrophy in PPAR gamma hypomorphic mice. *Proc Natl Acad Sci USA* 2003; 100:14457–14462.

25. Hevener AL, He W, Barak Y *et al.* Muscle-specific PPAR gamma deletion causes insulin resistance. *Nat Med* 2003; 9:1491–1497.

26. Norris AW, Chen L, Fisher SJ *et al.* Muscle-specific PPARgamma-deficient mice develop increased adiposity and insulin resistance but respond to thiazolidinediones. *J Clin Invest* 2003; 112:608–618.

27. Fujita T, Sugiyama Y, Taketomi S *et al.* Reduction of insulin resistance in obese and/or diabetic animals by 5-[4-(1-methylcyclohexylmethoxy)benzyl]-thiazolidine-2,4-dione (ADD-3878, U-63,287, ciglitazone), a new antidiabetic agent. *Diabetes* 1983; 32:804–810.

28. Chang AY, Wyse BM, Gilchrist BJ *et al.* Ciglitazone, a new hypoglycemic agent. I. Studies in ob/ob and db/db mice, diabetic Chinese hamsters, and normal and streptozotocin-diabetic rats. *Diabetes* 1983; 32:830–838.

29. Yki-Jarvinen H. Thiazolidinediones. *N Engl J Med* 2004; 351:1106–1118.

30. Tamori Y, Masugi J, Nishino N *et al.* Role of peroxisome proliferator-activated receptor-gamma in maintenance of the characteristics of mature 3T3-L1 adipocytes. *Diabetes* 2002; 51:2045–2055.

31. Coort SL, Coumans WA, Bonen A *et al.* Divergent effects of rosiglitazone on protein-mediated fatty acid uptake in adipose and in muscle tissues of Zucker rats. *J Lipid Res* 2005; 46:1295–1302.

32. Roden M. Muscle triglycerides and mitochondrial function: possible mechanisms for the development of type 2 diabetes. *Int J Obes (Lond)* 2005; 29(suppl 2):S111–S115.

33. Yang WS, Jeng CY, Wu TJ *et al.* Synthetic peroxisome proliferator-activated receptor-gamma agonist, rosiglitazone, increases plasma levels of adiponectin in type 2 diabetic patients. *Diabetes Care* 2002; 25:376–380.

34. Vionnet N, Hani El H, Dupont S *et al.* Genomewide search for type 2 diabetes-susceptibility genes in French whites: evidence for a novel susceptibility locus for early-onset diabetes on chromosome 3q27-qter and independent replication of a type 2-diabetes locus on chromosome 1q21-q24. *Am J Hum Genet* 2000; 67:1470–1480.

35. Tiikkainen M, Hakkinen AM, Korsheninnikova E *et al.* Effects of rosiglitazone and metformin on liver fat content, hepatic insulin resistance, insulin clearance, and gene expression in adipose tissue in patients with type 2 diabetes. *Diabetes* 2004; 53:2169–2176.

36. Yamauchi T, Kamon J, Minokoshi Y *et al.* Adiponectin stimulates glucose utilization and fatty-acid oxidation by activating AMP-activated protein kinase. *Nat Med* 2002; 8:1288–1295.

37. Suganami T, Nishida J, Ogawa Y. A paracrine loop between adipocytes and macrophages aggravates inflammatory changes: role of free fatty acids and tumor necrosis factor alpha. *Arterioscler Thromb Vasc Biol* 2005; 25:2062–2068.

38. Constant VA, Gagnon A, Landry A *et al.* Macrophage-conditioned medium inhibits the differentiation of 3T3-L1 and human abdominal preadipocytes. *Diabetologia* 2006; 49:1402–1411.

39. Permana PA, Menge C, Reaven PD. Macrophage-secreted factors induce adipocyte inflammation and insulin resistance. *Biochem Biophys Res Commun* 2006; 341:507–514.

40. Di Gregorio GB, Yao-Borengasser A, Rasouli N *et al.* Expression of CD68 and macrophage chemoattractant protein-1 genes in human adipose and muscle tissues: association with cytokine expression, insulin resistance, and reduction by pioglitazone. *Diabetes* 2005; 54:2305–2313.

41. Staels B, Dallongeville J, Auwerx J *et al.* Mechanism of action of fibrates on lipid and lipoprotein metabolism. *Circulation* 1998; 98:2088–2093.

42. Staels B. PPARgamma and atherosclerosis. *Curr Med Res Opin* 2005; 21(suppl 1):S13–S20.

43. Marx N, Froehlich J, Siam L *et al.* Antidiabetic PPAR gamma-activator rosiglitazone reduces MMP-9 serum levels in type 2 diabetic patients with coronary artery disease. *Arterioscler Thromb Vasc Biol* 2003; 23:283–288.

44. Marx N, Imhof A, Froehlich J *et al.* Effect of rosiglitazone treatment on soluble CD40L in patients with type 2 diabetes and coronary artery disease. *Circulation* 2003; 107:1954–1957.

45. Pfutzner A, Marx N, Lubben G *et al.* Improvement of cardiovascular risk markers by pioglitazone is independent from glycemic control: results from the pioneer study. *J Am Coll Cardiol* 2005; 45:1925–1931.

46. Sidhu JS, Cowan D, Kaski JC. The effects of rosiglitazone, a peroxisome proliferator-activated receptor-gamma agonist, on markers of endothelial cell activation, C-reactive protein, and fibrinogen levels in non-diabetic coronary artery disease patients. *J Am Coll Cardiol* 2003; 42:1757–1763.

47. Martens FM, Visseren FL, de Koning EJ *et al.* Short-term pioglitazone treatment improves vascular function irrespective of metabolic changes in patients with type 2 diabetes. *J Cardiovasc Pharmacol* 2005; 46:773–778.
48. Dormandy JA, Charbonnel B, Eckland DJ *et al.* Secondary prevention of macrovascular events in patients with type 2 diabetes in the PROactive Study (PROspective pioglitAzone Clinical Trial In macroVascular Events): a randomised controlled trial. *Lancet* 2005; 366:1279–1289.
49. Robinson JG, Smith B, Maheshwari N *et al.* Pleiotropic effects of statins: benefit beyond cholesterol reduction? A meta-regression analysis. *J Am Coll Cardiol* 2005; 46:1855–1862.
50. Al-Mallah MH, Tleyjeh IM, Abdel-Latif AA *et al.* Angiotensin-converting enzyme inhibitors in coronary artery disease and preserved left ventricular systolic function: a systematic review and meta-analysis of randomized controlled trials. *J Am Coll Cardiol* 2006; 47:1576–1583.
51. Zhang H, Zhang A, Kohan DE *et al.* Collecting duct-specific deletion of peroxisome proliferator-activated receptor gamma blocks thiazolidinedione-induced fluid retention. *Proc Natl Acad Sci USA* 2005; 102:9406–9411.
52. Staels B. Fluid retention mediated by renal PPARgamma. *Cell Metab* 2005; 2:77–78.
53. Marceille JR, Goins JA, Soni R *et al.* Chronic heart failure-related interventions after starting rosiglitazone in patients receiving insulin. *Pharmacotherapy* 2004; 24:1317–1322.
54. Scheen AJ. Combined thiazolidinedione-insulin therapy: should we be concerned about safety? *Drug Saf* 2004; 27:841–856.
55. Rosenstock J, Goldstein BJ, Vinik AI *et al.* Effect of early addition of rosiglitazone to sulphonylurea therapy in older type 2 diabetes patients (>60 years): the Rosiglitazone Early vs. SULphonylurea Titration (RESULT) study. *Diabetes Obes Metab* 2006; 8:49–57.
56. Lefebvre P, Chinetti G, Fruchart JC *et al.* Sorting out the roles of PPAR alpha in energy metabolism and vascular homeostasis. *J Clin Invest* 2006; 116:571–580.
57. Verges B. Role for fibrate therapy in diabetes: evidence before FIELD. *Curr Opin Lipidol* 2005; 16:648–651.
58. Keech A, Simes RJ, Barter P *et al.* Effects of long-term fenofibrate therapy on cardiovascular events in 9795 people with type 2 diabetes mellitus (the FIELD study): randomised controlled trial. *Lancet* 2005; 366:1849–1861.
59. Lalloyer F, Vandewalle B, Percevault F *et al.* Peroxisome proliferator-activated receptor {alpha} improves pancreatic adaptation to insulin resistance in obese mice and reduces lipotoxicity in human islets. *Diabetes* 2006; 55:1605–1613.
60. Gilde AJ, van der Lee KA, Willemsen PH *et al.* Peroxisome proliferator-activated receptor (PPAR) alpha and PPARbeta/delta, but not PPARgamma, modulate the expression of genes involved in cardiac lipid metabolism. *Circ Res* 2003; 92:518–524.
61. Carmona MC, Louche K, Nibbelink M *et al.* Fenofibrate prevents rosiglitazone-induced body weight gain in ob/ob mice. *Int J Obes (Lond)* 2005; 29:864–871.
62. Wagner JA, Larson PJ, Weiss S *et al.* Individual and combined effects of peroxisome proliferator-activated receptor and {gamma} agonists, fenofibrate and rosiglitazone, on biomarkers of lipid and glucose metabolism in healthy nondiabetic volunteers. *J Clin Pharmacol* 2005; 45:504–513.
63. Buse JB, Rubin CJ, Frederich R *et al.* Muraglitazar, a dual (alpha/gamma) PPAR activator: a randomized, double-blind, placebo-controlled, 24-week monotherapy trial in adult patients with type 2 diabetes. *Clin Ther* 2005; 27:1181–1195.
64. Saad MF, Greco S, Osei K *et al.* Ragaglitazar improves glycemic control and lipid profile in type 2 diabetic subjects: a 12-week, double-blind, placebo-controlled dose-ranging study with an open pioglitazone arm. *Diabetes Care* 2004; 27:1324–1329.
65. Nissen SE, Wolski K, Topol EJ. Effect of muraglitazar on death and major adverse cardiovascular events in patients with type 2 diabetes mellitus. *JAMA* 2005; 294:2581–2586.
66. Wierzbicki AS. Lipid-altering agents: the future. *Int J Clin Pract* 2004; 58:1063–1072.
67. Secondary prevention by raising HDL cholesterol and reducing triglycerides in patients with coronary artery disease: the Bezafibrate Infarction Prevention (BIP) study. *Circulation* 2000; 102:21–27.
68. Elkeles RS, Diamond JR, Poulter C *et al.* Cardiovascular outcomes in type 2 diabetes. A double-blind placebo-controlled study of bezafibrate: the St. Mary's, Ealing, Northwick Park Diabetes Cardiovascular Disease Prevention (SENDCAP) Study. *Diabetes Care* 1998; 21:641–648.
69. Goldberg RB, Kendall DM, Deeg MA *et al.* A comparison of lipid and glycemic effects of pioglitazone and rosiglitazone in patients with type 2 diabetes and dyslipidemia. *Diabetes Care* 2005; 28:1547–1554.

70. Fagerberg B, Edwards S, Halmos T *et al.* Tesaglitazar, a novel dual peroxisome proliferator-activated receptor alpha/gamma agonist, dose-dependently improves the metabolic abnormalities associated with insulin resistance in a non-diabetic population. *Diabetologia* 2005; 48:1716–1725.

71. Decochez K, Rippley RK, Miller JL *et al.* A dual PPAR alpha/gamma agonist increases adiponectin and improves plasma lipid profiles in healthy subjects. *Drugs R D* 2006; 7:99–110.

72. Devasthale PV, Chen S, Jeon Y *et al.* Design and synthesis of N-[(4-methoxyphenoxy) carbonyl]-N-[[4-[2-(5- methyl-2-phenyl-4-oxazolyl)ethoxy]phenyl]methyl]glycine [Muraglitazar/BMS-298585], a novel peroxisome proliferator-activated receptor alpha/gamma dual agonist with efficacious glucose and lipid-lowering activities. *J Med Chem* 2005; 48:2248–2250.

73. Oleksiewicz MB, Thorup I, Nielsen HS *et al.* Generalized cellular hypertrophy is induced by a dual-acting PPAR agonist in rat urinary bladder urothelium *in vivo. Toxicol Pathol* 2005; 33:552–560.

74. Egerod FL, Nielsen HS, Iversen L *et al.* Biomarkers for early effects of carcinogenic dual-acting PPAR agonists in rat urinary bladder urothelium *in vivo. Biomarkers* 2005; 10:295–309.

75. Sakamoto J, Kimura H, Moriyama S *et al.* A novel oxyiminoalkanoic acid derivative, TAK-559, activates human peroxisome proliferator-activated receptor subtypes. *Eur J Pharmacol* 2004; 495:17–26.

76. Willson TM, Brown PJ, Sternbach DD *et al.* The PPARs: from orphan receptors to drug discovery. *J Med Chem* 2000; 43:527–550.

77. Doebber TW, Kelly LJ, Zhou G *et al.* MK-0767, a novel dual PPARalpha/gamma agonist, displays robust antihyperglycemic and hypolipidemic activities. *Biochem Biophys Res Commun* 2004; 318:323–328.

78. Rangwala SM, Lazar MA. The dawn of the SPPARMs? *Sci STKE* 2002; 2002:PE9.

79. Berger JP, Akiyama TE, Meinke PT. PPARs: therapeutic targets for metabolic disease. *Trends Pharmacol Sci* 2005; 26:244–251.

80. Schupp M, Clemenz M, Gineste R *et al.* Molecular characterization of new selective peroxisome proliferator-activated receptor {gamma} modulators with angiotensin receptor blocking activity. *Diabetes* 2005; 54:3442–3452.

81. Derosa G, Ragonesi PD, Mugellini A *et al.* Effects of telmisartan compared with eprosartan on blood pressure control, glucose metabolism and lipid profile in hypertensive, type 2 diabetic patients: a randomized, double-blind, placebo-controlled 12-month study. *Hypertens Res* 2004; 27:457–464.

82. Chen X, Osborne MC, Rybczynski PJ *et al.* Pharmacological profile of a novel, non-TZD PPARgamma agonist. *Diabetes Obes Metab* 2005; 7:536–546.

83. Berger JP, Petro AE, Macnaul KL *et al.* Distinct properties and advantages of a novel peroxisome proliferator-activated protein [gamma] selective modulator. *Mol Endocrinol* 2003; 17:662–676.

84. Brown KK, Henke BR, Blanchard SG *et al.* A novel N-aryl tyrosine activator of peroxisome proliferator-activated receptor-gamma reverses the diabetic phenotype of the Zucker diabetic fatty rat. *Diabetes* 1999; 48:1415–1424.

85. Oberfield JL, Collins JL, Holmes CP *et al.* A peroxisome proliferator-activated receptor gamma ligand inhibits adipocyte differentiation. *Proc Natl Acad Sci USA* 1999; 96:6102–6106.

86. Mukherjee R, Hoener PA, Jow L *et al.* A selective peroxisome proliferator-activated receptor-gamma (PPARgamma) modulator blocks adipocyte differentiation but stimulates glucose uptake in 3T3-L1 adipocytes. *Mol Endocrinol* 2000; 14:1425–1433.

87. Pereira MP, Hurtado O, Cardenas A *et al.* The nonthiazolidinedione PPARgamma agonist L-796,449 is neuroprotective in experimental stroke. *J Neuropathol Exp Neurol* 2005; 64:797–805.

88. Burgermeister E, Schnoebelen A, Flament A *et al.* A novel partial agonist of peroxisome proliferator-activated receptor-gamma (PPAR{gamma}) recruits PPAR{gamma}-coactivator-1 alpha (PGC1{alpha}), prevents triglyceride accumulation and potentiates insulin signaling *in vitro. Mol Endocrinol* 2006; 20:809–830.

89. Burgermeister E, Schnoebelen A, Flament A *et al.* A novel partial agonist of peroxisome proliferator-activated receptor-gamma (PPARgamma) recruits PPARgamma-coactivator-1alpha, prevents triglyceride accumulation, and potentiates insulin signaling *in vitro. Mol Endocrinol* 2006; 20:809–830.

6

Incretin hormones and diabetes mellitus

T. Vilsbøll, F. K. Knop, C. F. Deacon, J. J. Holst

INTRODUCTION

Type 2 diabetes mellitus is characterised by insulin resistance, impaired glucose-induced insulin secretion and inappropriately elevated glucagon concentrations, which eventually result in hyperglycaemia [1, 2]. Thus, type 2 diabetes represents a complex disease, and the current treatment modalities for type 2 diabetes (metformin, thiazolidinedione [TZD] insulin sensitisers, sulphonylureas) are often unsatisfactory in getting patients to reach their glycaemic goals. Furthermore, as the glycaemic targets recommended by international guidelines are lowered, many patients are failing to achieve adequate glycaemic control, even when multidrug approaches are used, necessitating the eventual use of insulin therapy to control hyperglycaemia (i.e. 50% of patients with type 2 diabetes reach a haemoglobin A1c [HbA1c] level <7 %). Efficacy of available therapies, even when used appropriately, diminishes as the disease progresses because of a steady, relentless decline in pancreatic β-cell function. Additionally, current treatments are often limited by inconvenient dosing regimens, safety and tolerability issues, the latter including hypoglycaemia, body weight gain, oedema and gastrointestinal intolerance. Therefore, new medical therapies that offer improved efficacy and/or durability, better convenience and an improved safety and tolerability profile are absolutely imperative, and these should target not only glycaemic control, but also the prevention of the disease, its progression and its associated complications.

Recently, improved understanding of the role of the incretin hormones in the pathophysiology of type 2 diabetes has led to the development of a new approach for the treatment of the disease [3]. This treatment is based upon the effects of the incretin hormone glucagon-like peptide-1 (GLP-1) and glucose-dependent insulinotropic polypeptide (GIP). These are gastrointestinal peptides, released to the bloodstream from endocrine mucosal cells following food ingestion. Both hormones strongly enhance meal-induced insulin secretion. In addition, GLP-1 has a spectrum of other effects thought to be desirable in an antidiabetic agent, including trophic effects on the β-cell, inhibition of glucagon secretion and suppression of appetite and food intake. The native incretin peptides cannot easily be used thera-

Tina Vilsbøll, MD, DMSc, Physician, Diabetes Research Division, Department of Internal Medicine, Gentofte Hospital, University of Copenhagen, Copenhagen, Denmark.

Filip K. Knop, MD, PhD, Physician and Clinical Researcher, Diabetes Research Division, Department of Internal Medicine, Gentofte Hospital, University of Copenhagen, Copenhagen, Denmark.

Carolyn F. Deacon, PhD, DMSc, Senior Lecturer, Department of Biomedical Sciences, The Panum Institute, University of Copenhagen, Copenhagen, Denmark.

Jens Juul Holst, MD, DMSc, Professor, Department of Biomedical Sciences, The Panum Institute, University of Copenhagen, Copenhagen, Denmark.

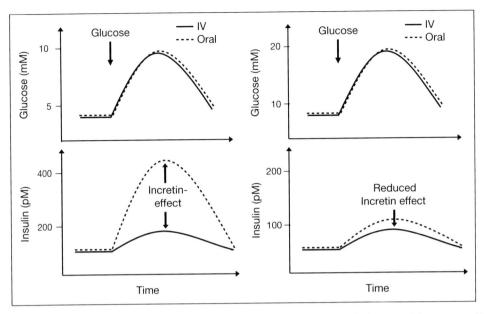

Figure 6.1 Upper panel: Glucose concentrations following administration of oral glucose and intravenous (IV) isoglycaemic glucose infusion, respectively, in healthy subjects (left) and patients with type 2 diabetes (right). Lower panel: The corresponding insulin responses in a healthy subject and patients with type 2 diabetes, respectively, showing the reduced incretin effect in patients with type 2 diabetes.

peutically because they are rapidly degraded *in vivo* by the enzyme dipeptidyl peptidase-4 (DPP-4), resulting in the loss of their insulinotropic activity [4].

INCRETIN HORMONES AND GLUCOSE REGULATION IN HEALTHY SUBJECTS

THE INCRETIN EFFECT

The incretin effect refers to the phenomenon that oral ingestion of glucose elicits a significantly higher insulin response than intravenous glucose infusions resulting in similar glycaemic excursions. The scientific history of the incretin effect extends back more than 100 years, but the scientific interest surrounding it has intensified considerably in recent years [5, 6]. In 1906, extracts of mucosa from porcine small intestine were used as a treatment for diabetes mellitus, hoping that '*the pancreas secretion might be stimulated by the substance of the nature of a hormone yielded by the duodenal mucosa membrane*' [7], but it was not until 1964 that it was demonstrated that orally administered glucose evokes a greater insulin response than intravenously administered glucose, and it was hypothesised that gut-derived factors could have potentiating effects on insulin secretion after oral ingestion of glucose [8]. Later, the incretin effect was confirmed by scientists who administered oral glucose and, on a separate day, copied the blood glucose excursion using an isoglycaemic intravenous glucose infusion in patients with diabetes mellitus and in healthy control subjects [9] (Figure 6.1). In healthy subjects, the incretin effect accounts for ~70% of the total amount of insulin released in response to an oral 75 g glucose load and can be entirely explained by the release of GLP-1 and GIP [10]. Although GLP-1 is more potent than GIP in this respect, GIP circulates in higher concentrations, with the net effect

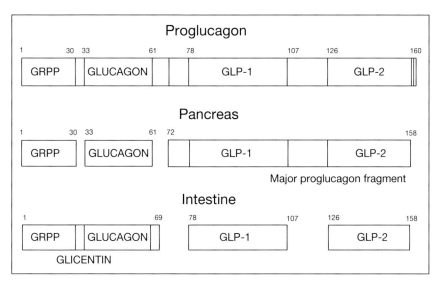

Figure 6.2 Proglucagon processing in human pancreatic alpha-cells and in mucosal endocrine L-cells in the small intestine.
GLP = glucagon-like peptide; GRPP = glicentin-related pancreatic peptide.

that both hormones contribute almost equally to the incretin effect in healthy subjects [11].

THE INCRETIN HORMONES

In 1970, gastric inhibitory polypeptide, secreted from small intestinal endocrine K-cells in response to ingestion of nutrients, was discovered and the 42-amino acid polypeptide was eventually shown to be insulinotropic at elevated glucose concentrations – a true incretin hormone – and renamed glucose-dependent insulinotropic polypeptide (GIP) [12, 13]. Later, experimental and clinical studies suggested that the gut produces more than a single insulinotropic hormone. In 1983, the gene encoding the human pancreatic hormone glucagon was cloned and the structure of its precursor, proglucagon was, surprisingly, shown to include the sequence of two glucagon-like peptides in addition to glucagon itself [14]. As expected, the gene was found to be expressed in both pancreatic α-cells and mucosal endocrine L-cells in the small intestine [15]. The primary transcripts and translation products of the gene in the two types of cells are identical, but the post-translational processing was shown to differ in the two tissues. In the pancreas, proglucagon is cleaved by prohormone convertase 2 (PC2) to glucagon, glicentin-related pancreatic peptide (GRPP) and a major proglucagon fragment (Figure 6.2). Apart from glucagon, these fragments seem to be biologically inactive. In contrast, in the intestinal L-cells, proglucagon is processed by prohormone convertase 1 (PC1) to GLP-1, glucagon-like peptide-2 (GLP-2) and glicentin. The 30-amino acid peptide, GLP-1, was found to be secreted in response to ingestion of nutrients and to be strongly insulinotropic – a true incretin hormone – and GLP-2, also secreted in response to ingestion of nutrients, turned out to be a key regulator of small intestinal growth [16].

Many hormones have been suspected to contribute to the incretin effect but, today, the evidence suggests that the incretin effect is mainly conveyed by the two incretin hormones, GIP and GLP-1.

SECRETION AND DEGRADATION OF THE INCRETIN HORMONES

In the fasting state, the plasma concentrations of the incretin hormones are very low, although they are not immeasurable, and it has been demonstrated that they can be further reduced with somatostatin in humans, suggesting that there is a certain basal rate of secretion [17]. Both incretin hormones are secreted rapidly (within 10–20 minutes) in response to ingestion of nutrients, with lipids and simple carbohydrates being potent stimulators of secretion [5]. Peak concentrations of GIP and GLP-1 are reached as soon as 15–30 and 30–45 minutes, respectively, after ingestion of glucose, for example. The rapid secretion following ingestion of nutrients – long before the bulk of substrates ingested have reached at least the distal parts of the small intestine – has led to the notion of vagus-mediated stimulation of secretion. As mentioned, GLP-1 is secreted from the L-cells, which are most numerous in the distal part of the small intestine, whereas GIP is released from the K-cells, situated primarily in the duodenum and proximal jejunum. Recent observations, however, indicate that GIP and GLP-1 are co-localised in a subset of endocrine cells throughout the gastrointestinal tract. This finding may explain the fast secretory responses following ingestion of nutrients, but other mechanisms – paracrine interaction between the two incretin hormones as indicated by data in dogs, and intrinsic neuroendocrine mechanisms, for instance – may be involved [18]. However, the bulk of evidence suggests that it is the contact between luminal subtrates and the 'open-type' endocrine cells of the intestinal mucosa that represents the predominant mechanism for release.

After secretion of GIP and GLP-1, both hormones are degraded by the enzyme dipeptidyl peptidase-4 (DPP-4) [19]. This enzyme, in addition to its localisation at sites such as the intestinal and renal brush border membranes, is also found on capillary surfaces and in a soluble form in plasma. It cleaves off the two N-terminal amino acids of its substrates, and for the incretin hormones, this abolishes their insulinotropic activity [19]. While GLP-1 is rapidly degraded in the circulation, resulting in a clearance that exceeds cardiac output and an apparent half-life of 1–1.5 minutes [20], GIP is degraded more slowly, with a half-life for the intact hormone of 7 minutes [21]. The truncated metabolites are eliminated more slowly through the kidneys, with half-lives of 4–5 and 17 minutes, respectively [20, 21].

ACTIONS OF GLP-1 AND GIP

Effects on insulin and glucagon secretion

The insulinotropic activities of GLP-1 and GIP are strictly glucose-dependent, meaning that the insulinotropic effect is apparent at elevated blood glucose concentrations and declines as normoglycaemia is approached. It is often claimed that both hormones require elevated plasma glucose concentrations to stimulate insulin secretion – for GIP, glucose levels may be as high as 8 mmol/l. The insulinotropic potential of GLP-1 and GIP was, therefore, reinvestigated in recent human experiments involving clamping of plasma glucose at fasting and postprandial levels and exact copying of the meal-induced concentrations of both GLP-1 and GIP by intravenous infusions [11]. The results showed that both hormones are active with respect to enhancing insulin secretion from the beginning of a meal (even at fasting glucose levels), and that they contribute almost equally, with the effect of GLP-1 predominating at higher glucose levels [11]. The effects of the two hormones with respect to insulin secretion have been shown to be additive in humans [22].

It should be noted that only GLP-1, but not GIP, caused inhibition of glucagon secretion from the α-cells exceeding that elicited by glucose clamping. The combined effects on insulin and glucagon secretion have been demonstrated to significantly decrease hepatic glucose production. The mechanism of GLP-1 induced inhibition of glucagon secretion is not completely elucidated. Notably, the glucagonostatic effect of GLP-1 is also glucose-dependent, in the sense that elevated GLP-1 concentrations have been demonstrated not to impair the glucagon counter-regulatory response to hypoglycaemia. The glucose-dependency of the effects on both insulin and glucagon secretion is important because it implies that treatment with GLP-1 will not lead to an increased risk of hypoglycaemia.

In agreement with their documented effects, studies in genetically modified mice with deletions of the incretin hormone receptors have demonstrated that both GIP and GLP-1 are essential for a normal glucose tolerance. Furthermore, the effect of deletion of one receptor was 'additive' to the effect of deleting the other [23, 24]. Thus, there is little doubt that the incretin effect plays an important role in postprandial insulin secretion and therefore in glucose tolerance in both humans and animals.

The incretin receptors and the effects of the incretin hormones on the beta cells

The antihyperglycaemic activity of GLP-1 is exerted via its interaction with a specific membrane-located receptor belonging to the type 2 G protein-coupled receptor superfamily, which also includes receptors for glucagon, GIP, pituitary adenylate cyclase-activating polypeptide, secretin and vasoactive intestinal peptide, and which is expressed in the pancreatic β-cell as well as in extrapancreatic sites [25]. Receptor activation leads to increases in intracellular cAMP with subsequent activation of protein kinase A, culminating in a series of events that alter ion channel activity and intracellular calcium handling and result in the stimulation of exocytosis of insulin-containing granules. Importantly, this cascade is glucose-dependent; i.e. a certain amount of glucose is a prerequisite for incretin hormone enhancement of insulin secretion [25]. Moreover, it appears that GLP-1 receptor signalling is necessary to facilitate β-cell responses to glucose itself, i.e. GLP-1 may act as a glucose sensitiser and impart glucose competence to the β-cell. In addition, GLP-1 upregulates the genes for the cellular machinery involved in insulin secretion, such as the glucokinase and GLUT2 genes [26]. The GIP receptor (GIPR) is also expressed in both pancreatic and extrapancreatic sites. In general, GIPR signalling leads to increases in cAMP and intracellular calcium concentrations, which in the β-cell culminates in insulin secretion [25].

In animal and *in vitro* studies, GLP-1 enhances β-cell proliferation and differentiation and inhibits apoptosis, leading to expansion of β-cell mass, which is of clinical interest since, under normal circumstances, an adequate number of β-cells is maintained in a balance between apoptosis and proliferation [27]. These observations raise the possibility that GLP-1 could be useful as a therapeutic agent in conditions with increased β-cell apoptosis, which would include type 1 diabetes mellitus as well type 2 diabetes [28]. Thus, treatment of mice with the GLP-1 agonist, exendin-4, reduced β-cell apoptosis induced by streptozotocin (while GLP-1 receptor knockout mice were abnormally susceptible to streptozotocin induced β-cell apoptosis) [29]. In spite of the fact that it has not yet been technically possible to demonstrate these trophic actions of GLP-1 in humans, the possibility arises that GLP-1 may be able to halt the deterioration in β-cell mass or even to give rise to new β-cells in patients with an insufficient number of functioning cells.

As mentioned with respect to GIP, the insulinotropic effect of the peptide when infused to result in physiological elevations of the plasma concentration in healthy subjects is comparable to that of GLP-1, but GIP has little effect on glucagon release, appears to have no physiological effect on the gastrointestinal tract, appetite or food intake, but may play a role in lipid metabolism.

Effects of GLP-1 on the gastrointestinal tract, appetite and body weight

Further important effects of GLP-1 include inhibition of gastrointestinal secretion and motility. GLP-1 has been shown to inhibit meal-induced acid secretion, as well as gastric emptying and pancreatic secretion [30]. The effect on pancreatic exocrine secretion was first suspected to be secondary to the inhibition of gastric emptying, but in subsequent studies, GLP-1 was demonstrated to also inhibit pancreatic secretion in response to intraduodenal stimulation [31]. The inhibitory effect of GLP-1 on acid secretion could be elicited by physiological elevations of the GLP-1 concentrations in plasma, and was, remarkably, additive to the inhibitory effects of peptide YY (PYY), which is released from the L-cell in parallel with GLP-1 [32]; these two peptides are the likely mediators of the 'ileal brake effect', i.e. the endocrine inhibition of upper gastrointestinal motility elicited by the presence of unabsorbed nutrients in the ileum [33–35]. In recent studies, Schirra and colleagues [36] were able to demonstrate the importance of endogenous GLP-1 for the regulation of antroduodenal motility (and pancreatic endocrine secretion) by administration of the GLP-1 receptor antagonist exendin-9-39. The physiological relevance of the 'ileal brake effect' of GLP-1 in humans thus seems established.

GLP-1 receptors are expressed in many regions of the brain involved in the regulation of food intake [37] and early studies with GLP-1 indicated an effect on appetite and food intake [38, 39]. Subsequently, more detailed studies in rodents confirmed these effects after intracerebroventricular administration of low doses of the peptide [40, 41]. However, most of the cerebral receptors are likely to be targets for GLP-1 produced by certain neurons in the brainstem, projecting to the hypothalamus and other regions of the brain.

Together, these effects of GLP-1 result in a curtailing of postprandial glucose excursions, promotion of satiety, and in humans, the GLP-1 satiating effects may, in the longer term, lead to significant weight loss.

Other effects of GLP-1

GLP-1 receptors are also found in the heart and a physiological role for these was recently shown in mice lacking the GLP-1 receptor. The animals exhibited impaired left ventricular contractility and diastolic functions, as well as impaired responses to exogenous epinephrine [42]. Recent studies indicate that GLP-1 protects the ischaemic and reperfused myocardium in rats (independent of effects on insulin and/or glucose) [43]. Additionally, left ventricular function improved following GLP-1 infusions in patients with chronic heart failure and in patients with acute myocardial infarction after successful reperfusion [44, 45]. In the basal state, GLP-1 may inhibit contractility, but after cardiac injury, it has consistently been shown to increase myocardial performance both in experimental animals and in patients [44, 46]. As GLP-1 also enhances insulin secretion, the improvement in myocardial performance may be mediated *via* both direct and indirect effects. In addition, GLP-1 has been found to reduce the postprandial rise in triglycerides and lower the concentration of free fatty acids in healthy subjects [47], and improve endothelial dysfunction in patients with type 2 diabetes and coronary heart disease [48]. These effects of GLP-1 are encouraging, since improved glycaemic control is often associated with an increase in body weight and thereby increased risk of cardiovascular (CV) morbidity, which is currently the major cause of mortality in patients with type 2 diabetes.

Finally, GLP-1 may also possess neurotropic effects. Thus, intracerebroventricular GLP-1 administration was associated with improved learning and memory in rats and also displayed neuroprotective effects [49, 50]. GLP-1 has also been proposed as a new therapeutic agent for neurodegenerative diseases including Alzheimer's disease [51].

INCRETIN PATHOPHYSIOLOGY IN TYPE 2 DIABETES MELLITUS

In 1986, it was shown that the incretin effect is severely impaired in patients with type 2 diabetes (estimated to be only 30% as compared to 70% in healthy subjects, corresponding to an amplification of insulin secretion in these patients by about 50% compared to 300% in healthy subjects) [52], and it is now well established that this undoubtedly contributes to the inappropriate insulin secretion that characterises the disease (Figure 6.1). The reduced incretin effect in type 2 diabetes is characterised by:

1. Impaired postprandial secretion of GLP-1 (whereas secretion of GIP is normal or only slightly impaired) [53].
2. Impaired β-cell sensitivity to GLP-1, although its efficacy is at least partially preserved [54].
3. A near-abolition of the effect of GIP on second-phase insulin secretion particularly [55].

Thus, defects in the secretion and actions of the incretin hormones are responsible for the reduced incretin effect and hence the inadequate insulin secretion seen in patients with type 2 diabetes [5]. From dose–response studies, it appears that the *potency* of GLP-1 with respect to enhancing glucose induced insulin secretion is greatly reduced in patients compared to healthy controls [54], whereas the loss of the GIP effects was independent of dose. The molecular mechanisms underlying these pathophysiological traits are currently unknown. The question arises as to whether these defects are primary or secondary in relation to diabetes, but the evidence to date suggests that the abnormalities are secondary to the development of diabetes and/or insulin resistance [5, 6]. Thus, the secretion of both GIP and GLP-1 is normal in glucose tolerant first-degree relatives of individuals with type 2 diabetes. On the other hand, the insulinotropic effects of GIP were found to be impaired in 50% of healthy first-degree relatives of patients with type 2 diabetes, suggesting that defective GIP action may have a genetic component [56]. However, another study examining patients with diabetes of different aetiologies (patients with diabetes mellitus secondary to chronic pancreatitis, lean patients with type 2 diabetes [body mass index (BMI) <25 kg/m^2], patients with latent autoimmune diabetes in adults [LADA], patients with mutations in the *HNF-1α* gene [maturity-onset diabetes of the young, MODY3], and patients with newly diagnosed type 1 diabetes) from those of the classic obese patient with type 2 diabetes demonstrated that all groups displayed the same absent late-phase insulin response to GIP. This suggests that the GIP defect is a consequence of the diabetic state *per se*, rather than being genetically predetermined [57]. Subsequent reinterpretation of the study in first-degree relatives concluded that the GIP defect in the relatives is likely to be indicative of general impairments of β-cell function that are not specific to GIP [56].

It is believed that several of the many actions of GLP-1 are involved in its antidiabetic effects [58]. One important mechanism is of course the restoration of the β-cell responsiveness to glucose itself, which is reduced in patients with type 2 diabetes, but can be normalised by pharmacological infusions of GLP-1. Generally, peripheral insulin levels do not increase during chronic GLP-1 treatment, but are maintained in spite of the concomitant reductions of plasma glucose by up to 5–6 mmol/l [39]. Upon intravenous infusion of GLP-1 to fasting patients with type 2 diabetes, insulin secretion first rises, but then, as plasma glucose concentrations are lowered, decreases again to baseline levels [59]. The reduced sensitivity to GLP-1 in type 2 diabetes may arise as a consequence of the deranged diabetic metabolism, possibly the elevated blood glucose levels, because correction of the hyperglycaemia helps improve β-cell responsiveness to GLP-1 [60].

IMPORTANCE OF GLUCAGON IN THE PATHOPHYSIOLOGY OF DIABETES

As noted, only GLP-1, but not GIP, causes inhibition of glucagon secretion from the α-cells exceeding that elicited by glucose clamping. Thereby, the glucagon-induced hepatic glucose production significantly decreases. The mechanism of GLP-1 induced inhibition of glucagon secretion is not completely elucidated. Notably, the glucagonostatic effect (and the insulinotropic properties) of GLP-1 also is glucose-dependent, meaning that elevated GLP-1 concentrations are unlikely to impair the glucagon counter-regulatory response to hypoglycaemia.

Recent studies have shown that patients with type 2 diabetes respond to oral glucose ingestion with initial hypersecretion of glucagon followed by a delayed glucagon suppression whereas their glucagon secretion during isoglycaemic intravenous glucose infusion is, surprisingly, suppressed in a perfectly normal way [61, 62]. Due to the incretin effect, even in type 2 diabetes insulin is secreted more rapidly and in larger amounts during oral glucose as compared to isoglycaemic intravenous glucose infusion. Thus, differences in plasma glucose (isoglycaemia) or plasma insulin concentrations seem not to explain this newly described phenomenon. The paradoxical glucagon response to oral glucose (and meals) in type 2 diabetes can be speculated to originate from luminal stimulation of endocrine cells in the mucosa of the small intestine. In other words, the incretin hormones (or other intestinal-released hormones, e.g. GLP-2) [63] may be responsible for the characteristic postprandial hyperglucagonaemia in type 2 diabetes by exhibiting a changed functional pattern on pancreatic α-cells (reduced glucagonostatic effect of GLP-1 and/or enhanced glucagonotropic effect of GIP) – in parallel with their inappropriate functionality on pancreatic β-cells in type 2 diabetes (see above).

INCRETIN HORMONE-BASED THERAPY FOR THE TREATMENT OF TYPE 2 DIABETES

The fact that GLP-1 concentrations are reduced in patients with type 2 diabetes raises the possibility that the impaired incretin effect in type 2 diabetes may be partly due to a greater degradation of GLP-1 (and possibly GIP) in these patients. However, elimination of intact (biologically active) GLP-1 and GIP does not differ between healthy subjects and patients with type 2 diabetes. The extreme degradation of GLP-1 in particular renders the native form unsuitable as a therapeutic agent for the treatment of type 2 diabetes [64, 65]. It could be hypothesised, therefore, that inhibition of the degradation of the incretin hormones might significantly impact incretin hormone action by elevating levels of the endogenous biologically active peptides to the range shown to be therapeutically useful [66].

Two approaches have been attempted to accomplished this:

1. Inhibition of DPP-4 using low molecular weight inhibitors, the so-called incretin enhancers, to elevate levels of the endogenously released active forms of both incretin hormones.
2. Development of long-acting stable analogues of GLP-1, the so-called incretin mimetics [4].

Both approaches take advantage of the actions of GLP-1, and because both α- and β-cell dysfunction is targeted, not only is insulin secretion enhanced, but the disrupted insulin–glucagon ratio is also improved. Since type 2 diabetes is characterised by progressive structural and functional β-cell deterioration this, together with the possible β-cell protective and trophic effects, may lead to improvements in long-term pancreatic islet health.

DPP-4 INHIBITORS FOR THE TREATMENT OF TYPE 2 DIABETES

The enzyme DPP-4 and its inhibition

DPP-4, also known as the T-cell antigen CD26, is a serine peptidase found in numerous sites including the kidney, intestinal brush-border membranes, hepatocytes and vascular endothelium, as well as in a soluble form in plasma [67]. It cleaves an N-terminal dipeptide from susceptible peptides and *in vitro* kinetic studies revealed that both GLP-1 and GIP are substrates [68]. A physiological role for DPP-4 in incretin hormone metabolism was demonstrated when DPP-4 inhibition was shown to prevent the N-terminal degradation of GLP-1 and GIP that normally occurs *in vivo* [66]. Cleavage of GLP-1 in particular is very rapid, resulting in an apparent plasma half-life of only 1–1.5 minutes [20]. DPP-4 is thought to contribute to T-cell activation and proliferation via interactions with other membrane-expressed antigens such as CD45, but its presence may not be essential for normal immune function, with the evidence to date indicating that DPP-4's role in the immune system is independent of its enzymatic action and that its absence can be compensated for. However, non-selective inhibitors and inhibitors selective for the closely related enzymes DPP-8 and DPP-9 do have an adverse impact, suggesting that the catalytic activity of these other enzymes may have a role in the immune system [69]. Long-term studies with the DPP-4 inhibitors in clinical development have, to date, proved these to be safe and well tolerated and not to be associated with adverse immune effects.

DPP4 inhibition and treatment of type 2 diabetes

Initial studies showed that DPP-4 inhibition enhances levels of endogenously released GLP-1 and GIP, and this inhibition has subsequently been demonstrated to be associated with improved glucose tolerance in animal models of insulin resistance, impaired glucose tolerance (IGT) and type 2 diabetes, respectively [70].

Sitagliptin [71] (Januvia®, Merck & Co., Inc.) was recently approved as the first DPP-4 inhibitor for treatment of type 2 diabetes in the USA (2006) and Europe (2007), and vildagliptin [72] (Galvus®, Novartis AG) reached the market in Europe in 2008. Many others are in late-stage clinical development. Most are competitive reversible inhibitors of DPP-4, with good oral bioavailability and a relatively long duration of action, such that once-daily dosing gives 70–90% inhibition of plasma DPP-4 activity over a 24-hour period [70]. Most data are available for sitagliptin and vildagliptin. Sitagliptin, which is longer acting than vildagliptin, is rapidly absorbed; steady-state plasma concentrations are attained within 2 days after once-daily dosing. Sitagliptin is not appreciably metabolised *in vivo* and ~90% of the dose is excreted renally, unchanged as the parent drug. Vildagliptin is rapidly absorbed and is suitable for both once- and twice-daily dosing. It has low protein binding; the predominant route of metabolism is hydrolysis to produce a pharmacologically inactive metabolite, with 85% of the dose being excreted as this metabolite in the urine. More than ten additional DPP-4 inhibitors are in different stages of development and several are expected to reach the market in the years to come.

Efficacy as monotherapy

When given as monotherapy over 12 weeks, sitagliptin (5–50 mg bd) dose-dependently reduced fasting plasma glucose (FPG) by up to 1.0 mmol/l and HbA1c levels by up to 0.8% with the highest dose, compared with placebo, from a baseline of 7.9 %. In another 12-week study, sitagliptin (100 mg qd) reduced HbA1c levels by 0.6% relative to placebo (baseline, 7.8%). The efficacy of sitagliptin as monotherapy has also been demonstrated in longer duration studies, giving reductions in HbA1c of 0.6% (baseline, 8.1%) and 0.8% (baseline, 8%) after 18 and 24 weeks respectively, together with improvements in markers of β-cell function. Similar results were obtained with vildagliptin both with respect to fasting glucose and HbA1c [73]. The reductions in HbA1c concentrations are sustainable for at least 24 and 52 weeks with sitagliptin and vildagliptin respectively [73, 74]. Of note is the finding that, with both sitagliptin and vildagliptin, patients with higher baseline HbA1c levels (8–9.5%), reflecting poorer metabolic control and seemed to show the greatest improvements, with reductions averaging 1.2–1.5%, suggesting that the benefits of DPP-4 inhibition may not be restricted to those patients with mild diabetes [74, 75].

Efficacy as combination therapy

DPP-4 inhibitors have been investigated for their utility in combination therapy. The first of these studies examined vildagliptin (50 mg qd) as add-on therapy in patients with type 2 diabetes treated with metformin (≥1500 mg/day) in a double-blinded, placebo-controlled trial. HbA1c levels in subjects receiving placebo (i.e. metformin alone) began to deteriorate by week 12, reaching 8.3% at week 52 (baseline, 7.9%). In contrast, addition of vildagliptin to ongoing metformin treatment reduced FPG and postprandial glucose concentrations, leading to a reduction by 0.7% in HbA1c at week 12, which was maintained until the end of the study, giving a between-group difference of -1.1%. After 52 weeks, ~ 40% of patients receiving vildagliptin and metformin achieved HbA1c levels of <7% compared to only 10% of patients on metformin alone [76]. Similar efficacy and sustained effect was seen with sitagliptin (100 mg qd) when combined with metformin [77]. Initial combination therapy with sitagliptin and metformin in drug-naïve patients was demonstrated to give greater improvements in glycaemic control than either sitagliptin or metformin monotherapy, even with an open-label cohort (baseline HbA1c, 11.2%) achieving reductions of 2.9% after 24 weeks of combination therapy [78].

The efficacy of DPP-4 inhibitors has also been examined when used in combination with TZDs with similar improvements in glycaemic control as seen when added on to metformin treatment [79]. The combination was generally well tolerated, although there was a modestly higher incidence of gastrointestinal adverse effects compared with placebo. Addition of the DPP-4 inhibitor had no additional effect on body weight relative to TZDs alone, which caused a weight gain of ~1.5 kg [79].

A single study has looked at the combination of DPP-4 inhibitors with insulin treatment (>30 U/day). Vildagliptin (50 mg bd) added to insulin treatment (~ 80 U/day), reduced HbA1c levels by 0.5% (baseline, 8.5%) versus a reduction of 0.2% with placebo. Interestingly, despite the improvements in glycaemic control, there were significantly fewer hypoglycaemic events in the patients receiving the combination therapy [80].

INCRETIN MIMETICS FOR THE TREATMENT OF TYPE 2 DIABETES

The clinical results with GLP-1 receptor activators, now often designated *incretin mimetics*, are promising and suggest that one can expect lasting improvement of glycaemic control as evidenced by improved levels of HbA1c [81]. Synthetic exendin-4 (exenatide) was approved for diabetes treatment in 2005 and is commercially available under the trade name Byetta®. Exendin-4 was isolated from the venom of the lizard, *Heloderma suspectum*, in a systematic search for biologically active peptides [82] and is a full agonist of the GLP-1 receptor with the same affinity as native GLP-1 [83]. Unlike GLP-1, it is not degraded by DPP-4 and is cleared primarily in the kidneys by glomerular filtration [84], resulting in a plasma half-life for the peptide of approximately 30 minutes after intravenous administration [85]. After subcutaneous injection of the maximally tolerated dose, a significant elevation of its plasma concentration may be observed for 5–6 h [86]. Another incretin mimetic under clinical development is liraglutide, which is based on the structure of native human GLP-1, but modified to include an amino acid substitution and an attachment of a C16 acyl chain [87], enabling the molecule to bind to albumin, thereby preventing renal elimination. Liraglutide is slowly absorbed and has a half-life of approximately 11–13 h after subcutaneous administration [88] making it suitable for once-daily injection. Clinically, the molecule has similar actions as continuously infused GLP-1 [89], and appears to have a similar clinical potential as exendin-4 [90]. Liraglutide will be available in the EU in 2009 under the trade name Victoza®.

Efficacy of incretin mimetics in the treatment of type 2 diabetes

Clinical studies using GLP-1 analogues have demonstrated sustained effects on HbA1c, body weight and β-cell function in patients with type 2 diabetes mellitus.

Combining data from studies comparing exenatide as add-on therapy to currently available antidiabetic treatment with placebo injection showed a statistically significant difference in HbA1c decline of approximately 1% from baseline in favour of exenatide (baseline HbA1c, 8.2%) [91]. In the same trials, a significant weight loss was observed during treatment with exenatide. The weight loss was progressive, dose-dependent, and without apparent plateau by week 30 (mean difference of 2.3 kg, randomised trials), although a plateau appeared to be reached in completers at years 2–3.5. By 3.5 years, the body weight decrease from baseline averaged 5.3 kg in the open-label trial [92]. Side-effects were primarily dose-dependent nausea and vomiting occurring in as many as 57 and 17% of cases respectively, although nausea was generally mild to moderate and declined with time.

Data demonstrated that liraglutide as monotherapy is capable of decreasing fasting plasma glucose levels up to 3.4 mmol/l (1.90 mg dose) on average when compared to placebo [93]. Interestingly, in the same study, a decrease in HbA1c of up to 1.7% (baseline HbA1c, 8.0%) was seen and almost 50% of the patients with type 2 diabetes managed to reached the goal level of <7% HbA1c. In the highest liraglutide dose group (1.9 mg), the change from baseline in body weight was -2.99 kg (-1.21 kg compared with placebo) [93]. As for exenatide, gastrointestinal side-effects were reported when using liraglutide. Thus transient and mild nausea was reported in the liraglutide treated subjects (liraglutide, 10%; placebo, 3%) [93]. Recently the Liraglutide Effect and Action in Diabetes (LEAD) programme evaluated the safety and efficacy of liraglutide and demonstrated an improved level of glycemic control relative to currently used oral antidiabetics [94, 95]. The data suggest that, at doses of 1.2 mg or 1.8 mg, the drug offers glycemic control superior to that of glimepiride, while preliminary findings from the LEAD studies confirm its suitability for combination therapy with traditional oral antidiabetics. CV risk factors commonly associated with type 2 diabetes include obesity and high systolic blood pressure, and early evidence suggests that GLP-1 based therapy may cause clinical relevant reductions in both.

The most exciting aspect of the incretin-based therapies (both incretin mimetics and DPP-4 inhibitors) is the possibility that they – perhaps especially because of their trophic effects on the pancreatic β-cells – may halt the progression of disease that inevitably seems to accompany conventional treatment. So far, this has not been established in any clinical trials but animal studies with GLP-1 analogues and DPP-4 inhibitors show that β-cell proliferation and cytoprotection is seen, and the recent results of *in vivo* studies using liraglutide, evaluating human β-cell function upon chronic administration, are promising [58]. Whether the improvement of *in vivo* β-cell function during treatment with incretin-based therapy will persist remains unclear, but the available data could indicate the GLP-1 based therapy should be started as early in the clinical course as possible, before β-cell function has deteriorated to perhaps incurable levels.

SUMMARY

Oral glucose elicits a much greater insulin response than when glucose is administered intravenously (the incretin effect). This is caused by the incretin hormones GLP-1 and GIP augmenting the glucose-induced insulin secretion. In patients with type 2 diabetes, this effect is severely impaired, such that the (already impaired) action of glucose alone accounts for almost all of the insulin response to an oral glucose challenge, and it is probable that this incretin defect contributes to the deficient insulin secretion that characterises type 2 diabetes. The deficient incretin effect in type 2 diabetes is characterised by impaired postprandial secretion of GLP-1, impaired β-cell sensitivity to GLP-1 and an almost abolished effect of GIP [6].

DPP-4 inhibitors are a new class of oral antidiabetic agents with an exciting potential for the treatment of type 2 diabetes. They seem likely to be as efficacious as currently available oral antidiabetic agents, although further trials powered for efficacy will help determine their likely clinical success. By enhancing incretin hormone action, DPP-4 inhibitors help restore the natural physiology of glucose homeostasis, improving the impaired insulin and inappropriate glucagon secretion to correct the imbalance in the insulin–glucagon ratio, thereby improving glucose uptake and reducing hepatic glucose output. They target fasting and postprandial glucose concentrations, which are both believed to contribute to the development of many diabetic complications. As a class, the DPP-4 inhibitors appear to have a good safety profile, with little or no risk for hypogly-caemia, no weight gain, and the potential benefit of addressing the islet dysfunction that characterises type 2 diabetes.

The clinical results with GLP-1 receptor activators, designated as *incretin mimetics*, are very promising and appear to result in lasting improvement of glycaemic control as evidenced by much improved levels of HbA1c. The use of GLP-1 analogues in the treatment of type 2 diabetes is a new and interesting approach that targets not only relative insulin deficiency and the glucagon hypersecretion, but also the overeating and obesity that represents a major problem in up to 90% of patients with type 2 diabetes. Incretin mimetics have so far been demonstrated to be safe, with mild to moderate and transient nausea being the most prominent side-effects.

If the β-cell preserving potential of the incretin-based therapies can also be sufficiently demonstrated in humans, the DPP-4 inhibitors and GLP-1 analogues may be able to address one of the underlying causes of progression of type 2 diabetes; the gradual loss of β-cell mass and function. Taking all these factors into consideration, incretin-based therapy may offer the unique possibility of being used not only to treat the symptoms of type 2 diabetes, but also as disease-modifying drugs. Furthermore, in the future, if the long-term safety of the new treatment modalities is confirmed, there is the real possibility that these drugs will not be confined to treating only patients with established diabetes but DPP-4 inhibitors may even be used to prevent the development or progression of type 2 diabetes in people with IGT or at high risk of developing the disease. The injectable incretin mimetics are probably more likely to be used after the diagnosis of type 2 diabetes is established, unless their β-cell protective potential eventually turns out to exceed that of other therapeutic approaches.

REFERENCES

1. Defronzo RA. Lilly lecture 1987. The triumvirate: beta-cell, muscle, liver. A collusion responsible for NIDDM. *Diabetes* 1988; 37:667–687.
2. Kahn SE, Halban PA. Release of incompletely processed proinsulin is the cause of the disproportionate proinsulinemia of NIDDM. *Diabetes* 1997; 46:1725–1732.
3. Drucker DJ, Nauck MA. The incretin system: glucagon-like peptide-1 receptor agonists and dipeptidyl peptidase-4 inhibitors in type 2 diabetes. *Lancet* 2006; 368:1696–1705.
4. Deacon CF. Therapeutic strategies based on glucagon-like peptide 1. *Diabetes* 2004; 53:2181–2189.
5. Vilsbøll T. On the role of the incretin hormones GIP and GLP-1 in the pathogenesis of type 2 diabetes mellitus. *Dan Med Bull* 2004; 51:364–370.
6. Vilsbøll T, Holst JJ. Incretins, insulin secretion and type 2 diabetes mellitus. *Diabetologia* 2004; 47:357–366.
7. Moore B: On the treatment of diabetus mellitus by acid extract of duodenal mucous membrane. *Biochem J* 1906; 1:28–38.
8. Mclintyre N, Holdsworth C, Turner DS. New interpretation of oral glucose tolerance. *Lancet* 1964; 2:20–21.
9. Perley MJ, Kipnis DM. Plasma insulin responses to oral and intravenous glucose: studies in normal and diabetic sujbects. *J Clin Invest* 1967; 46:1954–1962.
10. Nauck MA, Homberger E, Siegel EG *et al*. Incretin effects of increasing glucose loads in man calculated from venous insulin and C-peptide responses. *J Clin Endocrinol Metab* 1986; 63:492–498.
11. Vilsbøll T, Krarup T, Madsbad S, Holst JJ. Both GLP-1 and GIP are insulinotropic at basal and postprandial glucose levels and contribute nearly equally to the incretin effect of a meal in healthy subjects. *Regul Pept* 2003; 114:115–121.
12. Brown JC, Mutt V, Pederson RA. Further purification of a polypeptide demonstrating enterogastrone activity. *J Physiol* 1970; 209:57–64.
13. Elahi D, Andersen DK, Brown JC *et al*. Pancreatic alpha- and beta-cell responses to GIP infusion in normal man. *Am J Physiol* 1979; 237:E185–E191.

14. Bell G, Sanchez P, Laybourn P, Najarian R. Exon duplication and divergence in the human preproglucagon gene. *Nature* 1983; 304:368–371.
15. Orskov C, Holst JJ, Poulsen SS, Kirkegaard P. Pancreatic and intestinal processing of proglucagon in man. *Diabetologia* 1987; 30:874–881.
16. Drucker DJ. Biologic actions and therapeutic potential of the proglucagon-derived peptides. *Nat Clin Pract Endocrinol Metab* 2005; 1:22–31.
17. Toft-Nielsen M, Madsbad S, Holst JJ. The effect of glucagon-like peptide I (GLP-I) on glucose elimination in healthy subjects depends on the pancreatic glucoregulatory hormones. *Diabetes* 1996; 552–556.
18. Dube PE, Brubaker PL. Nutrient, neural and endocrine control of glucagon-like peptide secretion. *Horm Metab Res* 2004; 36:755–760.
19. Deacon CF, Nauck MA, Toft-Nielsen M, Pridal L, Willms B, Holst JJ. Both subcutaneously and intravenously administered glucagon-like peptide I are rapidly degraded from the NH2-terminus in type II diabetic patients and in healthy subjects. *Diabetes* 1995; 44:1126–1131.
20. Vilsbøll T, Agerso H, Krarup T, Holst JJ. Similar elimination rates of glucagon-like peptide-1 in obese type 2 diabetic patients and healthy subjects. *J Clin Endocrinol Metab* 2003; 88:220–224.
21. Vilsbøll T, Agerso H, Lauritsen T *et al.* The elimination rates of intact GIP as well as its primary metabolite, GIP 3–42, are similar in type 2 diabetic patients and healthy subjects. *Regul Pept* 2007; 137:168–172.
22. Nauck MA, Bartels E, Orskov C, Ebert R, Creutzfeldt W. Additive insulinotropic effects of exogenous synthetic human gastric inhibitory polypeptide and glucagon-like peptide-1-(7-36) amide infused at near-physiological insulinotropic hormone and glucose concentrations. *J Clin Endocrinol Metab* 1993; 76:912–917.
23. Flock G, Baggio LL, Longuet C, Drucker DJ. Incretin receptors for glucagon-like peptide 1 and glucose-dependent insulinotropic polypeptide are essential for the sustained metabolic actions of vildagliptin in mice. *Diabetes* 2007; 56:3006–3013.
24. Hansotia T, Maida A, Flock G *et al.* Extrapancreatic incretin receptors modulate glucose homeostasis, body weight, and energy expenditure. *J Clin Invest* 2007; 117:143–152.
25. Drucker DJ. The biology of incretin hormones. *Cell Metab* 2006; 3:153–165.
26. Buteau J, Roduit R, Susini S, Prentki M. Glucagon-like peptide-1 promotes DNA synthesis, activates phosphatidylinositol 3-kinase and increases transcription factor pancreatic and duodenal homeobox gene 1 (PDX-1) DNA binding activity in beta (INS-1)-cells. *Diabetologia* 1999; 42:856–864.
27. Bonner-Weir S. Beta-cell turnover: its assessment and implications. *Diabetes* 2001; 50(suppl 1):S20–S24.
28. Butler AE, Janson J, Bonner-Weir S, Ritzel R, Rizza RA, Butler PC. Beta-cell deficit and increased beta-cell apoptosis in humans with type 2 diabetes. *Diabetes* 2003; 52:102–110.
29. Li Y, Hansotia T, Yusta B, Ris F, Halban PA, Drucker DJ. Glucagon-like peptide-1 receptor signaling modulates beta cell apoptosis. *J Biol Chem* 2003; 278:471–478.
30. Wettergren A, Schjoldager B, Mortensen PE, Myhre J, Christiansen J, Holst JJ. Truncated GLP-1 (proglucagon 78–107-amide) inhibits gastric and pancreatic functions in man. *Dig Dis Sci* 1993; 38:665–673.
31. Groger G, Unger A, Holst JJ, Goebell H, Layer P. Ileal carbohydrates inhibit cholinergically stimulated exocrine pancreatic secretion in humans. *Int J Pancreatol* 1997; 22:23–29.
32. Wettergren A, Maina P, Boesby S, Holst JJ. Glucagon-like peptide-1 7-36 amide and peptide YY have additive inhibitory effect on gastric acid secretion in man. *Scand J Gastroenterol* 1997; 32:552–555.
33. Read N, French S, Cunningham K. The Role of the gut in regulation food intake in man. *Nutrition Reviews* 1994; 52:1–10.
34. Holst JJ. Enteroglucagon. *Annu Rev Physiol* 1997; 59:257–71.
35. Layer P. [Intestinal regulation of pancreatic enzyme secretion: stimulatory and inhibitory mechanisms] Intestinale Regulation der Pankreasenzymsekretion: Stimulatorische und inhibitorische Mechanismen. *Z Gastroenterol* 1992; 30:495–497.
36. Schirra J, Nicolaus M, Roggel R *et al.* Endogenous glucagon-like peptide 1 controls endocrine pancreatic secretion and antro-pyloro-duodenal motility in humans. *Gut* 2006; 55:243–251.
37. Goke R, Larsen PJ, Mikkelsen JD, Sheikh SP. Distribution of GLP-1 binding sites in the rat brain: evidence that exendin-4 is a ligand of brain GLP-1 binding sites. *Eur J Neurosci* 1995; 7:2294–2300.
38. Flint A, Raben A, Ersboll AK, Holst JJ, Astrup A. The effect of physiological levels of glucagon-like peptide-1 on appetite, gastric emptying, energy and substrate metabolism in obesity. *Int J Obes Relat Metab Disord* 2001; 25:781–792.

39. Zander M, Madsbad S, Madsen JL, Holst JJ. Effect of 6-week course of glucagon-like peptide 1 on glycaemic control, insulin sensitivity, and beta-cell function in type 2 diabetes: a parallel-group study. Lancet 2002; 359:824–830.

40. Tang-Christensen M, Larsen PJ, Goke R et al. Central administration of GLP-1-(7-36) amide inhibits food and water intake in rats. Am J Physiol 1996; 271:R848–R856.

41. Turton MD, O'Shea D, Gunn I et al. A role for glucagon-like peptide-1 in the central regulation of feeding [see comments]. Nature 1996; 379:69–72.

42. Gros R, You X, Baggio LL et al. Cardiac function in mice lacking the glucagon-like peptide-1 receptor. Endocrinology 2003; 144:2242–2252.

43. Bose AK, Mocanu MM, Carr RD, Brand CL, Yellon DM. Glucagon-like peptide 1 can directly protect the heart against ischemia/reperfusion injury. Diabetes 2005; 54:146–151.

44. Nikolaidis LA, Mankad S, Sokos GG et al. Effects of glucagon-like peptide-1 in patients with acute myocardial infarction and left ventricular dysfunction after successful reperfusion. Circulation 2004; 109:962–965.

45. Sokos GG, Nikolaidis LA, Mankad S, Elahi D, Shannon RP. Glucagon-like peptide-1 infusion improves left ventricular ejection fraction and functional status in patients with chronic heart failure. J Card Fail 2006; 12:694–699.

46. Nikolaidis LA, Elahi D, Shen YT, Shannon RP. Active metabolite of GLP-1 mediates myocardial glucose uptake and improves left ventricular performance in conscious dogs with dilated cardiomyopathy. Am J Physiol Heart Circ Physiol 2005; 289:H2401–H2408.

47. Meier JJ, Gethmann A, Gotze O et al. Glucagon-like peptide 1 abolishes the postprandial rise in triglyceride concentrations and lowers levels of non-esterified fatty acids in humans. Diabetologia 2006; 49:452–458.

48. Nystrom T, Gutniak MK, Zhang Q et al. Effects of glucagon-like peptide-1 on endothelial function in type 2 diabetes patients with stable coronary artery disease. Am J Physiol Endocrinol Metab 2004; 287:E1209–E1215.

49. Perry T, Haughey NJ, Mattson MP, Egan JM, Greig NH. Protection and reversal of excitotoxic neuronal damage by glucagon-like peptide-1 and exendin-4. J Pharmacol Exp Ther 2002; 302:881–888.

50. During MJ, Cao L, Zuzga DS et al. Glucagon-like peptide-1 receptor is involved in learning and neuroprotection. Nat Med 2003; 9:1173–1179.

51. Perry TA, Greig NH. A new Alzheimer's disease interventive strategy: GLP-1. Curr Drug Targets 2001; 5:565–571.

52. Nauck M, Stockmann F, Ebert R, Creutzfeldt W. Reduced incretin effect in type 2 (non-insulin-dependent) diabetes. Diabetologia 1986; 29:46–52.

53. Vilsbøll T, Krarup T, Deacon CF, Madsbad S, Holst JJ. Reduced postprandial concentrations of intact biologically active glucagon-like peptide 1 in type 2 diabetic patients. Diabetes 2001; 50:609–613.

54. Kjems LL, Holst JJ, Volund A, Madsbad S. The influence of GLP-1 on glucose-stimulated insulin secretion: effects on beta-cell sensitivity in type 2 and nondiabetic subjects. Diabetes 2003; 52:380–386.

55. Vilsbøll T, Krarup T, Madsbad S, Holst JJ. Defective amplification of the late phase insulin response to glucose by GIP in obese Type II diabetic patients. Diabetologia 2002; 45:1111–1119.

56. Meier JJ, Hucking K, Holst JJ, Deacon CF, Schmiegel WH, Nauck MA. Reduced insulinotropic effect of gastric inhibitory polypeptide in first-degree relatives of patients with type 2 diabetes. Diabetes 2001; 50:2497–2504.

57. Vilsbøll T, Knop FK, Krarup T et al. The pathophysiology of diabetes involves a defective amplification of the late-phase insulin response to glucose by glucose-dependent insulinotropic polypeptide-regardless of etiology and phenotype. J Clin Endocrinol Metab 2003; 88:4897–4903.

58. Holst JJ. Glucagon-like peptide-1: from extract to agent. The Claude Bernard Lecture, 2005. Diabetologia 2006; 49:253–260.

59. Nauck MA, Kleine N, Orskov C, Holst JJ, Willms B, Creutzfeldt W. Normalization of fasting hyperglycaemia by exogenous glucagon-like peptide 1 (7-36 amide) in type 2 (non-insulin-dependent) diabetic patients. Diabetologia 1993; 36:741–744.

60. Højberg PV, Zander M, Vilsbøll T et al. Near normalisation of blood glucose improves the potentiating effect of GLP-1 on glucose-induced insulin secretion in patients with type 2 diabetes. Diabetologia 2008; 51:632–640.

61. Knop FK, Vilsbøll T, Madsbad S, Holst JJ, Krarup T. Inappropriate suppression of glucagon during OGTT but not during isoglycaemic i.v. glucose infusion contributes to the reduced incretin effect in type 2 diabetes mellitus. Diabetologia 2007; 50:797–805.

62. Knop FK, Vilsbøll T, Hojberg PV et al. Reduced incretin effect in type 2 diabetes – cause or consequence of the diabetic state? *Diabetes* 2007; 56:1951–1959.

63. de HJ, Pedersen J, Orskov C, Holst JJ. The alpha cell expresses glucagon-like peptide-2 receptors and glucagon-like peptide-2 stimulates glucagon secretion from the rat pancreas. *Diabetologia* 2007; 50:2135–2142.

64. Deacon CF, Johnsen AH, Holst JJ. Degradation of glucagon-like peptide-1 by human plasma *in vitro* yields an N-terminally truncated peptide that is a major endogenous metabolite *in vivo*. *J Clin Endocrinol Metab* 1995; 80:952–957.

65. Deacon CF, Danielsen P, Klarskov L, Olesen M, Holst JJ. Dipeptidyl peptidase IV inhibition reduces the degradation and clearance of GIP and potentiates its insulinotropic and antihyperglycemic effects in anesthetized pigs. *Diabetes* 2001; 50:1588–1597.

66. Holst JJ, Deacon CF. Inhibition of the activity of dipeptidyl-peptidase IV as a treatment for type 2 diabetes. *Diabetes* 1998; 47:1663–1670.

67. Lambeir AM, Durinx C, Scharpé S, De Meester I. Dipeptidyl-peptidase IV from bench to bedside: an update on structural properties, functions, and clinical aspects of the enzyme DPP IV. *Crit Rev Clin Lab Sci* 2003; 40:209–294.

68. Mentlein R, Gallwitz B, Schmidt WE. Dipeptidyl-peptidase IV hydrolyses gastric inhibitory polypeptide, glucagon-like peptide-1(7-36) amide, peptide histidine methionine and is responsible for their degradation in human serum. *Eur J Biochem* 1993; 214:829–835.

69. Lankas GR, Leiting B, Roy RS et al. Dipeptidyl peptidase IV inhibition for the treatment of type 2 diabetes: potential importance of selectivity over dipeptidyl peptidases 8 and 9. *Diabetes* 2005; 54:2988–2994.

70. Deacon CF, Holst JJ. Dipeptidyl peptidase IV inhibitors: a promising new therapeutic approach for the management of type 2 diabetes. *Int J Biochem Cell Biol* 2006; 38:831–844.

71. Kim D, Kowalchick JE, Edmondson SD et al. Triazolopiperazine-amides as dipeptidyl peptidase IV inhibitors: close analogs of JANUVIA trade mark (sitagliptin phosphate). *Bioorg Med Chem Lett* 2007; 17:3373–3377.

72. Villhauer EB, Brinkman JA, Naderi GB et al. 1-[[(3-hydroxy-1-adamantyl)amino]acetyl]-2-cyano-(S)-pyrrolidine: a potent, selective, and orally bioavailable dipeptidyl peptidase IV inhibitor with antihyperglycemic properties. *J Med Chem* 2003; 46:2774–2789.

73. Schweizer A, Couturier A, Foley JE, Dejager S. Comparison between vildagliptin and metformin to sustain reductions in HbA(1c) over 1 year in drug-naive patients with type 2 diabetes. *Diabet Med* 2007; 24:955–961.

74. Aschner P, Kipnes MS, Lunceford JK, Sanchez M, Mickel C, Williams-Herman DE. Effect of the dipeptidyl peptidase-4 inhibitor sitagliptin as monotherapy on glycemic control in patients with type 2 diabetes. *Diabetes Care* 2006; 29:2632–2637.

75. Pratley RE, Jauffret-Kamel S, Galbreath E, Holmes D. Twelve-week monotherapy with the DPP-4 inhibitor vildagliptin improves glycemic control in subjects with type 2 diabetes. *Horm Metab Res* 2006; 38:423–428.

76. Ahren B, Gomis R, Standl E, Mills D, Schweizer A. Twelve- and 52-week efficacy of the dipeptidyl peptidase IV inhibitor LAF237 in metformin-treated patients with type 2 diabetes. *Diabetes Care* 2004; 27:2874–2880.

77. Nauck MA, Meininger G, Sheng D, Terranella L, Stein PP. Efficacy and safety of the dipeptidyl peptidase-4 inhibitor, sitagliptin, compared with the sulfonylurea, glipizide, in patients with type 2 diabetes inadequately controlled on metformin alone: a randomized, double-blind, non-inferiority trial. *Diabetes Obes Metab* 2007; 9:194–205.

78. Goldstein B et al. Effect of initial combination therapy with sitagliptin, a dipeptidyl peptidase-4 inhibitor, and metformin on glycemic control in patients with type 2 diabetes. *Diabetes Care* 2007; 30:1979–1987.

79. Rosenstock J, Brazg R, Andryuk PJ, Lu K, Stein P. Efficacy and safety of the dipeptidyl peptidase-4 inhibitor sitagliptin added to ongoing pioglitazone therapy in patients with type 2 diabetes: a 24-week, multicenter, randomized, double-blind, placebo-controlled, parallel-group study. *Clin Ther* 2006; 28:1556–1568.

80. Fonseca V, Schweizer A, Albrecht D, Baron MA, Chang I, Dejager S. Addition of vildagliptin to insulin improves glycaemic control in type 2 diabetes. *Diabetologia* 2007; 50:1148–1155.

81. Blonde L, Klein EJ, Han J et al. Interim analysis of the effects of exenatide treatment on A1C, weight and cardiovascular risk factors over 82 weeks in 314 overweight patients with type 2 diabetes. *Diabetes Obes Metab* 2006; 8:436–447.

82. Eng J, Kleinman WA, Singh L, Singh G, Raufman JP. Isolation and characterization of exendin-4, an exendin-3 analogue, from *Heloderma suspectum* venom. Further evidence for an exendin receptor on dispersed acini from guinea pig pancreas. *J Biol Chem* 1992; 267:7402–7405.

83. Thorens B, Porret A, Buhler L, Deng SP, Morel P, Widmann C. Cloning and functional expression of the human islet GLP-1 receptor. Demonstration that exendin-4 is an agonist and exendin- (9-39) an antagonist of the receptor. *Diabetes* 1993; 42:1678–1682.

84. Simonsen L, Holst JJ, Deacon CF. Exendin-4, but not glucagon-like peptide-1, is cleared exclusively by glomerular filtration in anaesthetised pigs. *Diabetologia* 2006; 49:706–712.

85. Edwards CM, Stanley SA, Davis R et al. Exendin-4 reduces fasting and postprandial glucose and decreases energy intake in healthy volunteers. *Am J Physiol Endocrinol Metab* 2001; 281:E155–E161.

86. Kolterman OG, Kim DD, Shen L et al. Pharmacokinetics, pharmacodynamics, and safety of exenatide in patients with type 2 diabetes mellitus. *Am J Health Syst Pharm* 2005; 62:173–181.

87. Knudsen LB, Nielsen PF, Huusfeldt PO et al. Potent derivatives of glucagon-like peptide-1 with pharmacokinetic properties suitable for once daily administration. *J Med Chem* 2000; 43:1664–1669.

88. Agerso H, Jensen LB, Elbrond B, Rolan P, Zdravkovic M. The pharmacokinetics, pharmacodynamics, safety and tolerability of NN2211, a new long-acting GLP-1 derivative, in healthy men. *Diabetologia* 2002; 45:195–202.

89. Degn KB, Juhl CB, Sturis J et al. One week's treatment with the long-acting glucagon-like peptide 1 derivative liraglutide (NN2211) markedly improves 24-h glycemia and alpha- and beta-cell function and reduces endogenous glucose release in patients with type 2 diabetes. *Diabetes* 2004; 53:1187–1194.

90. Vilsbøll T, Zdravkovic M, Le-Thi T et al. Liraglutide significantly improves glycemic control, and lowers body weight without risk of either major or minor hypoglycemic episodes in subjects with type 2 diabetes (Abstract). *Diabetes* 2006; 55:A27–A28.

91. Amori RE, Lau J, Pittas AG. Efficacy and safety of incretin therapy in type 2 diabetes: systematic review and meta-analysis. *JAMA* 2007; 298:194–206.

92. Buse JB, MacConell L, Stonehouse A et al. Exenatide maintained glycemic control with associated weight reduction over three years in patients with type 2 diabetes (Abstract). *Diabetes* 2007.

93. Vilsbøll T, Zdravkovic M, Le-Thi T et al. Liraglutide, a long-acting human glucagon-like peptide-1 analog, given as monotherapy significantly improves glycemic control and lowers body weight without risk of hypoglycemia in patients with type 2 diabetes. *Diabetes Care* 2007; 30:1608–1610.

94. Nauck M, Frid A, Hermansen K et al.; LEAD-2 Study Group. Efficacy and safety comparison of liraglutide, glimepiride, and placebo, all in combination with metformin, in type 2 diabetes: the LEAD (liraglutide effect and action in diabetes)-2 study. *Diabetes Care* 2009; 32:84–90.

95. Garber A, Henry R, Ratner R et al.; LEAD-3 (Mono) Study Group. Liraglutide versus glimepiride monotherapy for type 2 diabetes (LEAD-3 Mono): a randomised, 52-week, phase III, double-blind, parallel-treatment trial. *Lancet* 2009; 373:473–481.

Part 2

Cardiovascular considerations

7

An overview of current lipid-lowering treatments

J. P. D. Reckless

INTRODUCTION

In the last decades in the Westernised world cardiovascular disease has become the major cause of adult premature morbidity and mortality. At the same time, recognition of the main risk factors predisposing to macrovascular disease, and increasing evidence of the benefits gained from their reduction have emerged. The role of lowering cholesterol and low-density lipoprotein-cholesterol (LDL-C), and correction of dyslipidaemia by diet, lifestyle change and pharmacotherapy has become increasingly clear. However, this should be as part of a global risk assessment including age, sex, tobacco use, blood pressure, lipids, diabetes and family history.

The epidemiological relationships between lipids (cholesterol, LDL-C, high-density lipoprotein-cholesterol [HDL-C], non-HDL-C and triglycerides) and cardiovascular risk in both sexes and across all ages have been well documented. The Prospective Studies Collaboration [1] has examined data in 900 000 individuals for LDL-C and 150 000 for HDL-C. Risk increases markedly with increasing age, but although the risk is much lower at younger age, the effect of increasing LDL-C has a very much steeper effect on risk. The ratio of cholesterol to HDL-C has the strongest relationship with risk, but non-HDL-C (while able to be measured in non-fasting samples as a measure of all the atherogenic apoprotein-B-containing lipoproteins) is around 40% less sensitive.

It has been the 3-hydroxy-3-methyl-glutaryl (HMG)-CoA reductase inhibitors, the statins, which have established themselves as highly effective, well tolerated, low adverse event profile treatments of LDL-C to reduce total cardiovascular disease (CVD) comprising coronary heart disease (CHD) and cerebrovascular disease. This has come from very extensive randomised controlled trials [2–4], in both males and females, with and without CVD, up to age 85 years, and in those with hypertension or diabetes. The statin Health Technology Assessment (HTA) by the National Institute for Health and Clinical Excellence (NICE) [5] has advised their use in individuals with CVD or at a CVD risk of ≥20% over 10 years, together with the NICE Guideline Development Group recommendations [6].

STRATEGIES FOR CVD PREVENTION

How should we decide who to treat, and how do we identify them? This should always be in the context of addressing all modifiable risk factors contributing to global risk. Prevention of CVD requires integration of management advice for all risk factors and categorisation of

John P. D. Reckless, DSc, MD, FRCP, Consultant Endocrinologist, Department of Endocrinology, Royal United Hospital, Bath; Honorary Reader in Medicine, School of Health, University of Bath, Bath, UK.

patients by absolute risk, and has come from various international sources [7–9]. Where risk is sufficiently high, patients should be counselled and treatments offered in relation to the individuals' general health, a potential life expectancy of 2–3 years being appropriate to initiate a statin.

The third report of the Adult Treatment Panel of the National Cholesterol Education Program (NCEP-ATP III) [7] has recommended different targets for LDL-C of 160 mg/dl (4.16 mmol/l), 130 mg/dl (3.38 mmol/l) and 100 mg/dl (2.60 mmol/l) depending on the individual's cardiovascular risk. Subsequently, a modification has been proposed to treat to a lower target of 70 mg/dl (1.82 mmol/l) in the highest risk individuals [8].

The InterHeart study [10] has suggested that up to 90% of risk can be accounted for by nine primary risk factors. However, even with effective prevention strategies there is still very considerable residual risk with 60–70% of disease persisting in the major risk factor intervention trials.

DIABETES AND CARDIOVASCULAR DISEASE

Diabetes has become a world epidemic, the prevalence in some areas being more than 20% [11]. By 2025 it is estimated that the number of individuals with diabetes worldwide will have doubled to 340 million [12]. In the USA, the Centers for Disease Control and Prevention (CDC) has shown that the prevalence of type 2 diabetes increased between 1963 and 1975 (from 1.36% to 2.58%) at 5.1% per year. Between then and 1990, prevalence changed little, but prevalence since (1990 to 2005) has increased markedly at 4.6% per year (from 2.64% to 5.45%) [13]. Part of this rise is related to the increasingly sedentary lifestyle of individuals and their increasing adiposity, the more rapid rise in prevalence of obesity having started around 1986. In England and Wales over 20% of the adult population are now obese (body mass index >30 kg/m^2) [14], which is likely in turn to disproportionately increase diabetes [15], increase vascular risk and decrease life expectancy in the obese. Along with the increase in diabetes there is an associated increase in impaired glucose handling, either as impaired fasting glycaemia (IFG) or impaired glucose tolerance (IGT). These individuals also have increased vascular risk, while about one in fifteen each year will progress to overt diabetes [16].

Unfortunately, the β-cell failure of type 2 diabetes continues to progress [17], and glycaemic control continues to deteriorate despite increasing medication [18].

Diabetes has clearly been shown to increase CVD risk over that expected from accompanying recognised risk factors [19]. The great majority of individuals with type 2 diabetes are at high or very high cardiovascular risk, a risk that is in part but not entirely related to their glycaemia, blood pressure and lipids (together with other factors such as smoking). The risk is such that diabetic patients without CVD approach (for their first event) the level of risk seen in non-diabetic individuals with CVD for a further event [20]. The classical dyslipidaemia of type 2 diabetes is a low HDL-C and moderately raised triglycerides [21]. In type 1 diabetes HDL-C levels tend to be high but, unusually, these levels do not protect against CVD risk. Reasons for this are unclear, but protection by HDL against CVD would require normal quality and normal functioning of HDL molecules that may not always relate to HDL-C concentrations. While there will be individuals with diabetes whose CVD risk is currently not very high, the great majority will be at significant risk and management advice should now proceed from an assumption that they will require intervention for all elevated modifiable CVD risk factors unless there are reasons not so to do.

In diabetes, the levels of LDL-C may not be very different to those in the general population, albeit giving significant risk and being higher than desirable. Nonetheless, initial treatment of the dyslipidaemia of diabetes is still to address the LDL-C by diet and lifestyle change and by pharmacology. This reflects the high levels of LDL in man compared with other animals, the near-obligatory nature of LDL in atherogenesis with thrombotic risk being low when LDL-C is very low. Within the levels of LDL-C, HDL-C (inverse) and triglycerides normally encountered there may be no entirely safe profile. Therefore, residual lipid disturbances may need addressing as secondary targets, while in some individuals, severe hypertriglyceridaemia will be a primary problem.

CVD prevention requires attention to *all* modifiable risk factors. Treatments in diabetes that improve outcomes include management of blood pressure and reducing glycaemic load, both for microvascular and macrovascular complications, but for the reduction of CHD and CVD, a reduction of LDL-C is essential. For the latter, the most successful measure with the largest evidence base is treatment with a statin. Since the publication of the first results from the landmark Scandinavian Simvastatin Survival Study (4S Study) in 1994 [2], statin therapy has become an integral part of the modern management of patients with diabetes. The diabetes data from 4S is described in Chapter 8, but it is worth remembering that the typical dyslipidaemia of diabetes and the metabolic syndrome is raised triglycerides and low HDL cholesterol [22]. Because of a 3 to 4-fold increased risk, individuals with diabetes are now considered to have a risk level approaching that of stable coronary disease patients and require risk factor modification.

WHO IS AT HIGH CARDIOVASCULAR RISK THROUGH LIPID ABNORMALITIES?

Various groups of individuals can be identified to be at high risk [5, 6, 9, 22]. Some individuals have severe genetic predispositions such as familial hypercholesterolaemia (FH), affecting about 0.2% of the population, where perhaps 50% of males will have had an event or died by age 50 years, with a similar risk in women about a decade or so older [23, 24]. A large fall in the standardised mortality ratio for FH patients has occurred since statins became available in the late 1980s [23]. Diet and smoking change in FH appears to have reduced malignancy risk [24], which is of relevance to other at-risk groups.

In the second Joint British Societies'Guidelines (JBS2) [9] three groups of sufficient risk to warrant treatment were proposed:

1. Individuals with established atherosclerosis.
2. Individuals with diabetes.
3. Asymptomatic individuals without established CVD who have risk factor combinations putting them at high global risk (estimated CVD risk ≥20%/10 years) of developing atherosclerotic CVD.

The largest group of people qualifying for statins are asymptomatic individuals whose global CVD risk is ≥20% per 10 years. The cholesterol–HDL-C ratio is used. Charts from the second JBS guidelines [9] allow calculation of an individual's approximate risk and adjustment for some additional factors (family history, ethnicity, other dyslipidaemias). Finding these individuals is a much greater challenge. Some subgroups, such as hypertensive individuals and those with diabetes, will be known from clinical registers or searching of drug prescription databases.

STATINS AND DIABETES

While other agents are available for managing dyslipidaemia in general and diabetic populations, statins have become the mainstay of management, primarily addressing LDL-C. A meta-analysis of 14 trials published in the previous decade considered data from 90 056 individuals of whom 50% were statin-treated [25]. A linear relationship was found between LDL-C and CVD risk without evidence of heterogeneity of response across subgroups (including diabetes) and in individuals with initially low levels of LDL-C <2.6 mmol/l. There was a 12% reduction in all-cause mortality per mmol/l of LDL-C reduction, a 23% reduction

(26% in diabetic subjects) in first coronary events, a 24% reduction in coronary revascularisation and a 17% reduction in stroke. Numbers needed to treat (NNT) were 34.5 (over 4.3 years) and 13.8 (4.9 years) for primary and secondary prevention respectively. Another meta-analysis considered 14 studies of 17 749 individuals with type 2 diabetes using statins and fibrates, and gave similar results [26]. NICE published a Technology Appraisal (TA 94) for statins [27]. For details on the individual statin trials, the reader is referred to Chapter 8.

With the increased CVD risk for individuals with diabetes, and these results, statin therapy has been recommended routinely in individuals with diabetes and elevated lipid levels. The continuous epidemiological relationship between LDL-C and CVD risk does not appear to have an apparent lower LDL-C for risk. Trials in high-risk individuals with acute coronary syndrome have shown benefit when LDL-C is lowered further in the general population and in the diabetes subpopulations [28]. Target LDL-C levels have been recommended therefore between 1.8–2.0 mmol/l (70–77 mg/dl) [6, 8, 9].

OTHER DIABETES TREATMENTS AND CVD RISK

DIET AND LIFESTYLE

Dietary advice is essential for individuals with diabetes, influencing glucose, blood pressure and lipids. While following the principles of limiting excess simple sugars, reducing total fat (and especially saturated fat), increasing fibre and reducing salt, advice also needs to recognise an individual's needs and choices, their cultural and ethnic background and their readiness to change. Moderate amounts of physical exercise, weight loss and pharmacotherapy have all been shown to reduce progression of impaired glucose handling (IFG, IGT) to diabetes [29–31]. After the diagnosis of type 2 diabetes, dietary effort and moderate weight loss improve hyperglycaemia [32]. Loss of 5–10% of body weight can have major metabolic benefit. While the number of subjects was relatively low, multiple lifestyle approaches to CVD have been shown to be beneficial [33].

METFORMIN AND SULPHONYLUREAS

Improvement of glycaemic control and weight loss (which tends to be facilitated by metformin) will tend to improve accompanying hypertriglyceridaemia, but major changes in the lipid profile are not apparent. Partly as a result of the weight loss, metformin remains the initial treatment of choice for glycaemic control in type 2 diabetes. The evidence for CVD reduction is limited, since the number of patients on metformin alone in the United Kingdom Prospective Diabetes Study (UKPDS) was too small for the apparent reduction in CVD risk to be reliable, while the patients treated with metformin and a sulphonylurea had excess vascular disease. Elsewhere, sulphonylurea treatment was associated with better CVD outcomes than with metformin [34].

GLITAZONES

The glitazones, rosiglitazone and pioglitazone, are modulators of the peroxisome prolifera-tor-activated receptor (PPAR)-γ nuclear receptor family and improve glycaemia by improving insulin sensitivity. Can they also influence atherosclerotic risk? The PROactive (PROspective pioglitAzone Clinical Trial In macroVascular Events) study was designed to answer this question, comparing pioglitazone or placebo added to usual diabetes therapy [35]. Over 3 years in 5238 type 2 diabetic patients there was a non-significant 10% reduction ($P = 0.095$) in the primary endpoint, although a chance early excess of lower limb revascularisation in the pioglitazone group may have influenced the result. The secondary endpoint of all-cause mortality, non-fatal myocardial infarct and stroke was significantly reduced by piolitazone by 16% ($P = 0.027$). Progression to permanent insulin use was markedly reduced (odds ratio 0.47 [0.39, 0.56]; P <0.001). Contributions to the CVD benefits may have been from an associated HbA1c fall of 0.5%, a fall in systolic blood pressure of 3 mmHg, a reduction in triglycerides of 13% and a rise in HDL-C of 9%.

No large formal CVD outcome study has been completed for rosiglitazone, but a meta-analysis by Nissen and colleagues has suggested that, in contrast to pioglitazone, there was a borderline significant 43% *increase* in myocardial infarction (P = 0.03) and a non-significant 64% increase in cardiovascular death (P = 0.06) [36]. In the ADOPT (A Diabetes Outcome Progression Trial) study [34], rosiglitazone had longer glycaemic control than metformin or the sulphonylurea glyburide, but with more weight gain and oedema. There were more cardiovascular events with rosiglitazone than glyburide. These data were considered in detail by the US Food and Drug Administration (FDA) without change to the licence, but there may be moves to require harder outcomes than glycaemia to allow new diabetes drugs to be licensed [37]. The rosiglitazone outcome study, RECORD, suggested non-inferiority for coronary events, but with a low event rate was underpowered, and as expected it did show an increase in cardiac failure and in limb fractures [38]. Reasons for differences between the two glitazones are unclear but may be related to better effects of pioglitazone on the lipid profile.

WEIGHT REGULATION

Weight loss is an important objective in improving glycaemia in diabetic patients. Orlistat partly inhibits digestion and absorption of residual dietary fat and over 4 years reduced by 39% the progression from IGT to diabetes [36]. Orlistat also improves glycaemia, lipid profile and blood pressure in type 2 diabetes patients [39]. The centrally acting appetite suppressant, sibutramine, also reduces glycaemia and improves the lipid profile, but may increase blood pressure significantly in some patients [40]. Similarly, rimonabant, a CB_1 receptor antagonist working centrally and in peripheral tissues, led to weight reduction and improved metabolic control, but was withdrawn because of increased depression [41]. Major weight reduction with bariatric surgery (gastric banding or bypass procedures) can lead to regression of type 2 diabetes in 40% of individuals.

FIBRATES, DIABETES AND CARDIOVASCULAR RISK

Fibric acid derivatives have been available for more than 30 years, and while clofibrate has been withdrawn, bezafibrate, ciprofibrate, fenofibrate and gemfibrozil remain in the market. While gemfibrozil has been used in major outcome studies [42–44], side-effects are probably greater than for the other agents and there are significant interactions with statins making concurrent use of gemfibrozil and a statin contraindicated.

The fibrates have only moderate effects in lowering LDL-C as the main target of lipid treatment for CVD prevention. They do have significant greater effects on triglyceride lowering while increasing HDL-C. Because of these latter effects, there are also significant changes in the quality of LDL and HDL molecules [45]. With elevated triglyceride-rich lipoproteins, clearance of these particles (chylomicrons and very low density lipoproteins) takes longer and may be impaired where lipoprotein lipase (LPL) activity in peripheral tissues is decreased (as in type 2 diabetes). As a result, there is increased interchange between the lipoproteins of cholesterol ester and triglyceride. As a result, LDL and HDL become relatively triglyceride-enriched as part of a continuing, gradual process. At the same time as LPL may be low, the activity of hepatic lipase tends to be increased and LDL- and HDL-triglycerides are therefore removed. This leads to small dense LDL, which is poorly recognised by the LDL receptor and more avidly taken up by the scavenger receptor, for example in the arterial wall macrophage. Similarly, small dense HDLs are formed that may be functionally impaired. One of the major effects of a fibrate is to partly correct these abnormalities and they are, therefore, theoretically able to reduce CVD risk. This leads to the question as to whether a fibrate should be added to other LDL-C lowering therapy in type 2 diabetes, or in some circumstances be used as a first-line therapy or monotherapy.

Various studies have examined statin and fibrate combinations and some studies have examined CVD outcomes: for details the reader is referred to Chapter 8. Overall, fibrates do show evidence for CVD protection in type 2 diabetes, although the evidence is less firm than for statins. Fenofibrate tolerability and adverse event profile are good even when given with a statin. There may be risks of pancreatitis at high triglyceride levels, although individuals with such levels may still need fibrate treatment. At triglyceride levels ≥ 1.5 mmol/l, the quality of LDL moves towards small dense LDL, and the threshold to consider intervention in the USA has been set at 1.7 mmol/l (150 mg/dl). For the majority of individuals with type 2 diabetes, after primary statin treatment to a target LDL-C, consideration should be given to the addition of a fibrate where residual triglyceride levels are above 1.7 mmol/l and particularly when in the 2.3–4.5 mmol/l range. Fenofibrate is likely to be the agent of first choice. While gemfibrozil has outcome data, it has higher adverse event and drug interaction rates, while fenofibrate has more outcome evidence and is well tolerated. Bezafibrate has lesser lipid modifying effect, although it is cheaper than fenofibrate, while ciprofibrate has limited data.

OTHER LIPID MODULATORS, CARDIOVASCULAR RISK AND DIABETES

EZETIMIBE

Ezetimibe is a specific inhibitor of cholesterol absorption across the gut enterocyte and its main action is to reduce LDL-C return to the liver. As a result, there is increased LDL-C uptake from plasma by the liver through upregulation of hepatic LDL-receptors. At a dose of 10 mg, this will lead to a reduction in plasma LDL-C of around 18–25%. Ezetimibe is well tolerated, with limited adverse events reported and it is as effective in individuals with diabetes as in those without. It provides additional LDL-C lowering when added to statin therapy and will therefore allow more patients to reach particular LDL-C targets [46]. Ezetimibe has become quite widely used as an addition to statin therapy or as therapy in individuals intolerant of statins, although long-term safety and CVD outcome studies are not yet available.

ANION-EXCHANGE RESINS

Cholestyramine and colestipol have been available for more than 30 years and remove biliary and dietary cholesterol. They are non-absorbed. As a result of reduced cholesterol absorption, hepatic LDL-receptor uptake of plasma LDL-C is upregulated. Arterial atheroma regression studies have demonstrated less progression and some regression compared to placebo. These agents are not easy to take, as powders need to be suspended in water, and are associated with significant local gastrointestinal side-effects, so that few individuals are able to take substantial doses longer term. They will have additional LDL-C lowering effect added to statin therapy.

NICOTINIC ACID DERIVATIVES

Nicotinic acid in pharmacological doses has potent lipid modifying effect, reducing triglycerides and LDL-C and raising HDL-C. However, flushing is a major side-effect only slightly reduced by careful initiation and titration and by prior aspirin administration, although laropiprant, a specific prostaglandin inhibitor to minimise this flushing, is in development. Nicotinic acid would be a desirable agent to correct the mixed dyslipidaemia of type 2 diabetes, but there may be some deterioration in glycaemia to offset this, and pruritis, gastrointestinal side-effects and liver function abnormality may also occur.

Various relatively small placebo-controlled studies of nicotinic acid in immediate or delayed release formulations have been undertaken [47–50], showing improvements in the dyslipidaemic profile at doses of ≥1500 mg/day, but with modest increases in g;ycosylated haemoglobin (HbA1c), fasting glucose and uric acid. For example, HbA1c rose by 8% ($P = 0.03$) and fasting plasma glucose by 26% ($P = 0.02$), while in the non-diabetic populations there were no changes in plasma glucose, but a 4% rise in HbA1c ($P = 0.02$) [50]. With these mixed clinical and biochemical effects, nicotinic acid is not an indicated treatment in most individuals with type 2 diabetes, but may be indicated by specialists in a small number of individuals with severe dyslipidaemia. With a specific inhibitor of nicotinic acid flushing, addition of nicotinic acid to statin therapy may have a role and a major CVD outcome study has been initiated.

OMEGA-3 FISH OILS

It has been well established that saturated fatty acids increase LDL-C levels. In contrast, omega-3 fatty acids can improve dyslipidaemic profiles (at eicosapentaenoic acid (EPA) amounts of 2–4 g/day), separate to the potential antithrombotic effects of somewhat lower doses (<2 g/day of EPA) [51–53], some studies being in type 2 diabetes and some showing mixed results [53]. Omega-3 oils can be taken as pharmacological supplements or as increased oily fish intake. Triglyceride reductions are greater in markedly hypertriglyceridaemic subjects than in those with normal levels, although LDL-C concentrations may then rise somewhat. Fish oil supplements at high concentrations are relatively expensive. Widespread intake of high-dose pharmacological supplements of fish oils (EPA and docosahexaenoic acid [DHA]) in type 2 diabetes patients is therefore not recommended, but oily fish intake as part of a normal diet should be considered. After acute coronary syndrome a role of moderate (1 g/day) omega-3 oils may be considered.

HOW LOW SHOULD WE LOWER LDL-CHOLESTEROL?

How low should LDL-C be taken? The NICE type 2 diabetes guideline [54] has recommended intensified treatment where individuals are at a particular risk with existing CVD, with target organ damage (such as microalbuminuria) or where risk of a first CVD event prior to statin therapy is >20% over the next ten years. In these individuals, therapy should be increased if LDL-C is >2.0 mmol/l or the cholesterol is >4.0 mmol/l (as long as the HDL-C is not high). Where the diabetic subject's risk is 'high but not very high', intensification of treatment should be considered if LDL-C or cholesterol are >3.0 or 5.0 mmol/l respectively.

Several comparative studies of statins have indicated, after an initial LDL-C reduction with the entry dose of a statin, that doubling of any statin dose leads to a further reduction of approximately 5–6% in LDL-C [55, 56]. In efficacy terms, on a milligram-per-milligram basis, LDL-C lowering efficacies are approximately: fluvastatin/pravastatin < (5–6%) simvastatin < (5–6%) atorvastatin < (8–9%) rosuvastatin.

Some statins have come off patent (pravastatin, simvastatin) and others will follow. Use of generic statins will provide major improvements in cost-effectiveness and allow access for wider populations, although maximum LDL-cholesterol lowering would require transfer to non-generic statins and/or adding the cholesterol absorption inhibitor ezetimibe. The incremental cost-effectiveness of such changes in therapy will depend on the strategy, the incremental efficacy and the absolute risk and benefit of the individual patient. In its calculations of cost-effectiveness, the NICE statin technology appraisal [6] considered the use of a 'basket' of statins.

WHEN TO TREAT

In managing primary and secondary CVD prevention in diabetes all modifiable risk factors should be addressed. Dietary and lifestyle changes should be recommended and stressed in all individuals. Smoking cessation must have a high priority. Hypertension and hypergly-caemia require control.

For lipid management, all individuals with diabetes should be considered to need treat-ment, including pharmacological treatment, unless there is clear evidence that they are at particularly low risk with lipid levels close to target. In some individuals, particularly those below age 40 years with shorter duration of diabetes and limited other risk factors, absolute CVD risk in the next ten years may be <20%, but these individuals should be reassessed annually as their life-long risk is very high.

From the very strong evidence base, the prime treatment is to normalise LDL-C and a statin is first choice therapy. From a health economic viewpoint this should be with a generic statin at a dose shown to have outcome benefits in large randomised, controlled trials (usu-ally with simvastatin 40 mg or pravastatin 40 mg daily). Where statins are advised to women of childbearing potential, they must be advised to stop their statin from conception planning to the end of breast-feeding. Relatively few women with type 2 diabetes are likely to become pregnant as nearly all will be >40 years of age, but as type 2 diabetes becomes increasingly common at a younger age, associated with increasing obesity and inactivity, this precaution will become more relevant. Abnormal liver transaminases are not a contraindication to sta-tin therapy once primary causes of liver disease have been excluded, as non-alcoholic fatty liver disease is common in type 2 diabetes.

While there is no observed lower level of LDL-C at which CVD risk stabilises, it is of pragmatic and practical value to have a lipid target that allows, for population groups, a criterion against which an audit standard can be set. As the main atherogenic particle, LDL is the most appropriate target although, in the future, specific apoprotein components of lipoproteins (such as apoprotein B or apoprotein-B–apoprotein-A ratio) may come to the fore. An LDL-C of <2.0 mmol/l (or total cholesterol <4.0 mmol/l) is appropriate.

WHAT SHOULD BE THE PRIMARY TARGETS AND TREATMENTS?

The primary target for the management of dyslipidaemia in diabetes should be the concen-tration of LDL-C. The ideal target is to achieve an LDL-C <2.0 mmol/l (cholesterol <4.0 mmol/l).

WHAT SHOULD BE SECONDARY TARGETS AND TREATMENTS?

Where individuals on a generic statin have an LDL-C remaining above 2.0 mmol/l (choles-terol >4.0 mmol/l) then titration of statin, change of statin, and/or addition of ezetimibe should be considered in those with existing CVD, with diabetes end-organ damage, or with very high CVD risk (>30–40%/10 years).

In other type 2 diabetic individuals, at high rather than very high risk, such treatment escalation would be advised if LDL-C remains >3.0 mmol/l (total cholesterol >5.0 mmol/l).

To assess efficiency of treatment provision for populations, percentage standards should be set for the number of patients expected to reach these LDL-C levels of <2.0 or <3.0 mmol/l.

In individuals with type 2 diabetes that have significant residual mixed dyslipidaemia (elevated triglycerides and low HDL-C) and have high or very high CVD risk, a fibrate should be considered in addition to a statin. Prior to addition of fibrate therapy to a statin, other secondary causes should be addressed. Prime among these will be glycaemic control and obesity will be a major exacerbator. Hypothyroidism and alcohol excess should be excluded. The addition of fibrate therapy should be considered where triglycerides are 2.3–4.5 mmol/l and HDL-C is low. Some individuals who have severe hypertriglyceridaemia but in whom total cholesterol is not greatly elevated may warrant fibrate treatment *before* statin treatment.

Ezetimibe does have limited data of tolerability with fibrates, and triple therapy of statin, ezetimibe and fenofibrate is used in specialist lipid services. Ezetimibe is subject to a Technology Appraisal by the National Institute for Health and Clinical Excellence [46].

TYPE 1 DIABETES

The evidence base for lipid management in type 1 diabetes is much more limited than for type 2 diabetes. While some patients with type 1 diabetes have been included in major randomised trials of statins, their numbers are very small. An exception is in the Heart Protection Study where over 700 individuals had type 1 diabetes. While this number is too small for independent subgroup analysis, there was no evidence of heterogeneity of response to statin therapy in the reduction of CVD risk. Patients with type 1 diabetes are at very high CVD risk. Their life expectancy is reduced by around 30% at any age of onset of diabetes. Individuals with onset of type 1 diabetes in childhood are likely to have up to a 50% risk of death or a CVD event by the age of 50 years, especially if microvascular complications have ensued. As chronic kidney disease has been better managed and as renal support for end stage renal disease has become universal, the risk of CVD becomes accelerated.

Patients with type 1 diabetes should have their CVD risk factors assessed and treated. While many individuals with type 1 diabetes have high levels of HDL-C, the HDL-C level does not, unfortunately, appear to protect against CVD risk. For many such patients, their risk may be better expressed by using an HDL-C value nearer 1.0 mmol/l. From the age of around 25 years it would be expected that elevated lipid levels would be treated with a statin as for type 2 diabetes. In individuals younger than 25 years, but with a duration of diabetes >10 years or with microalbuminuria, lipid management should again be instigated.

SUMMARY

The risk of a first cardiovascular event in diabetic patients is 2–4-fold greater than in a non-diabetic population, and thus approaches the CVD risk of non-diabetic individuals with existing CVD. As such, lipid management is essential in the diabetic population, and nearly all individuals aged over 40 years will require pharmacotherapy for lipids. A substantial number of type 2 diabetic patients under the age of 40 years will also have sufficient risk to warrant treatment, as will adult patients with type 1 diabetes. The primary target for treatment is the LDL-cholesterol level and the primary therapy is a statin. Cost-effectiveness makes a generic statin the initial treatment. Some individuals will need augmented therapy addressed towards further LDL-C lowering and/or the residual classical dyslipidaemia of diabetes, hypertriglyceridaemia and low HDL-C.

REFERENCES

1. Prospective Studies Collaboration. Blood cholesterol and vascular mortality by age, sex and blood pressure: meta-analysis of individual data from 61 prosepctive studies with 55,000 vascular deaths. *Lancet*; 2007; 370:1829–1839.
2. Scandinavian Simvastatin Survival Study Group. Randomised trial of cholesterol lowering in 4444 patients with coronary heart disease, the Scandinavian Survival Study. *Lancet* 1994; 344:1383–1389.
3. Heart Protection Study Collaborative Group. MRC/BHF heart protection study of cholesterol lowering with simvastatin in 20,536 high-risk individuals: a randomised, placebo-controlled trial. *Lancet* 2002; 360:7–22.
4. Cholesterol Treatment Trialists' Collaboration. Efficacy and safety of cholesterol-lowering treatment: prospective meta-analysis of data from 90,056 participants in 14 randomised trials of statins. *Lancet* 2005; 366:1267–1278.

5. National Institute for Health and Clinical Excellence. Statins for the prevention of cardiovascular events (TA94). National Institute for Health and Clinical Excellence, 2006 (*www.nice.org.uk*).

6. National Institute for Health and Clinical Excellence. Cardiovascular risk assessment and the modification of blood lipids for the primary and secondary prevention of cardiovascular disease (CG67). National Institute for Health and Clinical Excellence, 2008 (*www.nice.org.uk*).

7. National Cholesterol Education Program Adult Treatment Panel. Executive summary of the third report of the National Cholesterol Education Program (NCEP) Expert Panel on detection, evaluation, and treatment of high blood cholesterol in adults (Adult Treatment Panel III). *J Amer Med Assoc* 2001; 285:2486–2497.

8. Grundy SM, Cleeman JI, Merz CNB *et al*. Implications of recent trials for the National Cholesterol Education Program Adult Treatment Panel III guidelines. *Circulation* 2004; 110:227–239.

9. Joint British Societies. Joint British Societies' second guidelines for the prevention of cardiovascular disease. *Heart* 2005; 91(Supp V):1–52.

10. Yusuf S, Hawken S, Ounpuu S *et al*; INTERHEART Study Investigators. Effect of potentially modifiable risk factors associated with myocardial infarction in 52 countries (the INTERHEART study): case-control study. *Lancet* 2004; 364:937–952.

11. World Health Organization. Preventing chronic disease: a vital investment. 2005 (*www.who.int*).

12. International Diabetes Federation. World Atlas of Diabetes 2003 (*www.idf.org*).

13. Geiss LA, Chief of Diabetes Surveillance for CDC's Diabetes Program in the Division of Diabetes Translation. Data from an analysis of 1963–2005 data from the National Health Interview Study, presented at the 67th ADA, Chicago, 22–24 Jun 07 (reported in DOC (diabetes, obesity, CVD) News (*www.diabetes.org/docnews* August 2007).

14. Department of Health. Health Survey for England. 2002 (*www.dh.gov.uk*).

15. Hu FB, Manson JE, Stampfer MJ *et al*. Diet, lifestyle, and the risk of type 2 diabetes mellitus in women. *N Engl J Med* 2001; 345:790–797.

16. Haffner SM, Stern MP, Hazuda HP, Mitchell BD, Patterson JK. Cardiovascular risk factors in confirmed pre-diabetic individuals. Does the clock for coronary heart disease start ticking before the onset of clinical diabetes? *JAMA* 1990; 263:2893–2898.

17. Matthews DR, Cull CA, Stratton IM, Holman RR, Turner RC. UKPDS 26: Sulphonylurea failure in non-insulin-dependent diabetic patients over six years. UK Prospective Diabetes Study (UKPDS) Group. *Diabet Med* 1998; 15:297–303.

18. Matthews DR, Cull CA, Stratton IM, Holman RR, Turner RC, for the UK Prospective Diabetes Study (UKPDS) Group. UKPDS 26: Sulphonylurea failure in non-insulin-dependent diabetic patients over six years. *Diabet Med* 1998; 15:297–303.

19. Fox CS, Coady S, Sorlie PD *et al*. Trends in cardiovascular complications of diabetes. *JAMA* 2004; 292:2495–2499.

20. Haffner SM, Lehto S, Ronnemaa T *et al*. Mortality from coronary heart disease in subjects with type 2 diabetes and in nondiabetic subjects with and without prior myocardial infarction. *N Engl J Med* 1998; 339:229–234

21. Tuomilehto J, Rastenyte D. Epidemiology of macrovascular disease and hypertension in diabetes mellitus. International textbook of diabetes mellitus, 2nd edition. John Wiley 1997: 1559–1583.

22. Adiels M, Olofsson SO, Taskinen MR, Borén J. Diabetic dyslipidaemia. *Curr Opin Lipidol* 2006; 17:238–246.

23. Simon Broome Steering Committee on behalf of the Simon Broome Register Group. Mortality in treated heterozygous familial hypercholesterolaemia: implications for clinical management. *Atherosclerosis* 1999; 142:105–112.

24. Neil HAW, Hawkins MM, Durrington PN, Betteridge DJ, Capps NE, Humphries SE, for the Simon Broome Familial Hyperlipidaemia Register Group and Scientific Steering Committee. Non-coronary heart disease mortality and risk of fatal cancer in patients with treated heterozygous familial hypercholesterolaemia: a prospective registry study. *Atherosclerosis* 2005; 179:293–297.

25. Baigent C, Keech A, Kearney PM *et al*. Efficacy and safety of cholesterol-lowering treatment: prospective meta-analysis of data from 90,056 participants in 14 randomised trials of statins. *Lancet* 2005; 366:1267–1278.

26. Vijan S, Hayward RA. Pharmacologic lipid-lowering therapy in type 2 diabetes mellitus: background paper for the American College of Physicians. *Annals Intern Med* 2004; 140:650–658.

27. Statins for the prevention of cardiovascular events in patients at increased risk of developing cardiovascular disease or those with established cardiovascular disease. TA94, January 2006 (*www.nice.org.uk*).
28. Shepherd J, Barter P, Carmena R *et al*. Effect of lowering LDL-cholesterol substantially below recommended levels in patients with coronary heart disease and diabetes: the treating to new targets (TNT) study. *Diabetes Care* 2006; 29:1220–1226.
29. Diabetes Prevention Program Research Group. Reduction in the Incidence of Type 2 Diabetes with Lifestyle Intervention or Metformin. *N Engl J Med* 2002; 346:393–403.
30. Tuomilehto J, Lindstrom J, Eriksson JG *et al*. Prevention of type 2 diabetes mellitus by changes in lifestyle among subjects with impaired glucose tolerance. *N Engl J Med* 2001; 344:1343-1350.
31. Torgerson JS, Hauptman J, Boldrin MN, Sjöström L. XENical in the prevention of diabetes in obese subjects (XENDOS) study: a randomized study of orlistat as an adjunct to lifestyle changes for the prevention of type 2 diabetes in obese patients. *Diabetes Care* 2004; 27:155–161 (erratum in: *Diabetes Care* 2004; 27:856).
32. United Kingdom Prospective Diabetes Study Group. UKPDS7: Response of fasting plasma glucose to diet therapy in newly presenting type 2 diabetic patients. *Metabolism* 1990; 39:905–912.
33. Gaede P, Vedel P, Larsen N *et al*. Multifactorial intervention and cardiovascular disease in patients with type 2 diabetes. *N Engl J Med* 2003; 348:383–393.
34. Kahn SE, Haffner SM, Resse R *et al*. Glycaemic durability of rosiglitazone, metformin and glyburide therapy. *N Engl J Med* 2006; 355:2427–2443.
35. Dormandy JA, Charbonnel B, Eckland DJ *et al*. Secondary prevention of macrovascular events in patients with type 2 diabetes in the PROactive study (PROspective pioglitAzone Clinical Trial In macrovascular Events): a randomised controlled trial. *Lancet* 2005; 366:1279–1289.
36. Nissen SE and Wolski K. Effect of rosigltazone on the risk of myocardial infarction and death from cardiovascular causes. *N Engl J Med* 2007; 356:2457–2471.
37. Rosen CJ. The rosiglitazone story – lessons from an FDA advisory committee meeting. *N Engl J Med* 2007; 357:844–846.
38. Home PD, Pocock SJ, Beck-Nielsen H *et al*., for the RECORD Study Team. Rosiglitazone evaluated for cardiovascular outcomes in oral agent combination therapy for type 2 diabetes (RECORD): a multicentre, randomised, open-label trial. *Lancet* 2009; 373:2125–2135.
39. Miles JM, Leiter L, Hollander P *et al*. Effect of orlistat in overweight and obese patients with type 2 diabetes treated with metformin. *Diabetes Care* 2002; 25:1123–1128.
40. Vetter R, Serra R, Fabris R, Pagano C, Federspil G. Effect of sibutramine on weight management and metabolic control in type 2 diabetes: a meta-analysis of clinical studies. *Diabetes Care* 2005; 28: 942–949.
41. Sheen AJ, Finer N, Hollander P, Jensen MD, Van Gall LF. Efficacy and tolerability of rimonabant in overweight or obese patients with type 2 diabetes: a randomised controlled study. *Lancet* 2006; 368:1660–1672.
42. Rubins HB, Robins SJ, Collins D *et al*. Gemfibrozil for the secondary prevention of coronary heart disease in men with low levels of high-density lipoprotein cholesterol. Veterans Affairs High-Density Lipoprotein Cholesterol Intervention Trial Study Group. *N Engl J Med* 1999; 341:410–418.
43. Rubins HB, Robins SJ, Collins D *et al*. Diabetes, plasma insulin, and cardiovascular disease: subgroup analysis from the Department of Veterans Affairs high-density lipoprotein intervention trial (VA-HIT). *Arch Intern Med* 2002; 162:2597–2604.
44. Frick MH, Elo O, Haapa K *et al*. Helsinki Heart Study: primary prevention trial with gemfibrozil in middle-aged men with dyslipidaemia. Safety of treatment, changes in risk factors, and incidence of coronary heart disease. *N Engl J Med* 1987; 317:1237–1245.
45. Austin MA, Edwards KL. Small, dense low-density lipoproteins, the insulin resistance syndrome and non-insulin-dependent diabetes. *Curr Opin Lipidol* 1996; 7:167–171.
46. Identification and management of familial hypercholesterolaemia, Clinical Guideline CG71; August 2008 (*www.nice.org.uk*).
47. Elam MB, Hunninghake DB, Davis KB *et al*. Effect of niacin on lipid and lipoprotein levels and glycaemic control in patients with diabetes and peripheral arterial disease: the ADMIT study: a randomised trial. Arterial Disease Multiple Intervention Trial. *JAMA* 2000; 284:1263–1270.
48. Grundy SM, Vega GL, McGovern ME *et al*. Efficacy, safety, and tolerability of once-daily niacin for the treatment of dyslipidaemia associated with type 2 diabetes: results of the assessment of diabetes control and evaluation of the efficacy of niaspan trial. *Arch Intern Med* 2002; 162:1568–1576.

49. Garg A, Grundy SM. Nicotinic acid as therapy for dyslipidaemia in non-insulin-dependent diabetes mellitus. *JAMA* 1990; 264:723–726.
50. Tsalamandris C, Panagiotopoulos S, Sinha A *et al.* Complementary effects of pravastatin and nicotinic acid in the treatment of combined hyperlipidaemia in diabetic and non-diabetic patients. *J Cardiovasc Risk* 1994; 1:231–239.
51. Farmer A, Montori V, Dinneen S *et al.* Fish oil in people with type 2 diabetes mellitus. Cochrane Database of Systematic Reviews 2001; CD003205.
52. Hartweg J, Farmer AJ, Holman RR *et al.* Meta-analysis of the effects of n-3 polyunsaturated fatty acids on haematological and thrombogenic factors in type 2 diabetes. *Diabetologia* 2007; 50:250–258.
53. Hooper L, Thompson RL, Harrison RA *et al.* Risks and benefits of omega 3 fats for mortality, cardiovascular disease, and cancer: systematic review. *Br Med J* 2006; 332:752–760.
54. Type 2 diabetes: the management of type 2 diabetes (update), Clinical Guideline CG66. May 2008 (*www.nice.org.uk*).
55. Miller M, Dobs A, Yuan Z *et al.* Effectiveness of simvastatin therapy in raising HDL-C in patients with type 2 diabetes and low HDL-C. *Curr Med Res Opin* 2004; 20:1087–1094.
56. Berne C, Siewert-Delle A. Comparison of rosuvastatin and atorvastatin for lipid lowering in patients with type 2 diabetes mellitus: results from the URANUS study. *Cardiovasc Diabetol* 2007; 4:7.

8

Statins and fibrates in the treatment of diabetic dyslipidaemia

G. E. Marshall, M. Fisher, F. L. J. Visseren

INTRODUCTION

It has been established beyond any doubt that cardiovascular risk is increased in people with diabetes. There are now multiple measures that have been proven to reduce cardiovascular risk in a person with diabetes, including aggressive management of glycaemia and hypertension. The most successful measure, with the largest evidence base, is treatment with a statin. Since the publication of the first results from the landmark Scandinavian Simvastatin Survival Study (4S Study) in 1994 [1], statin therapy has become an integral part of the modern management of patients with diabetes. The diabetes data from 4S is described in detail below, but it is worth remembering that the typical dyslipidaemia of diabetes and the metabolic syndrome is raised triglycerides and low HDL-cholesterol (HDL-C) [2]. The entry criteria for 4S included serum triglycerides ≤2.5 mmol/l [1] and as a consequence, only around 5% of the study participants had diabetes. There were no results for diabetic subjects in the principal publication and it was 3 years later that data were first published from a *post hoc* analysis of diabetic patients [3].

Recent reviews of statin therapy in diabetes have tended to divide the evidence base into primary and secondary prevention studies, depending on the presence or absence of known vascular disease [4–7]. This is known to be an oversimplification, as many diabetic patients have cardiovascular disease that is clinically silent until it presents with a major, catastrophic vascular event. The most important factor is that vascular risk is increased in diabetes. In this chapter we have adopted a different approach, and examine the evidence for the benefits of statins firstly for the older statin preparations, and then for the newer, more potent preparations. We present evidence on further benefit from more aggressive cholesterol lowering with larger doses of the more potent statins and how much this evidence has been incorporated into recent diabetes guidelines on cardiovascular risk reduction in the diabetic patient.

Gillian E. Marshall, MBChB, MRCP, PhD, Specialist Registrar in Cardiology, Department of Cardiology, Glasgow Royal Infirmary, Glasgow, UK.

Miles Fisher, MD, FRCP, MBChB, Consultant Physician, Diabetes Clinic, Glasgow Royal Infirmary, Glasgow, UK.

Frank L. J. Visseren, MD, PhD, Professor in Vascular Medicine, Epidemiologist, Department of Vascular Medicine, University Medical Center Utrecht, The Netherlands.

OLDER STATINS

STUDIES WITH PRAVASTATIN (TABLE 8.1)

The Cholesterol and Recurrent Events (CARE) trial examined the effects of 40 mg pravastatin or placebo in 4159 patients with previous myocardial infarction and average cholesterol levels [8]. The primary endpoint of 'major coronary events' (fatal coronary event or a non-fatal myocardial infarction) was significantly reduced by 24% with pravastatin therapy [8]. There were 586 patients with diabetes (14% of the study population). Although they had similar LDL-cholesterol (LDL-C) levels at baseline, they were older, more obese and had more hypertension than non-diabetic subjects [9]. Treatment with pravastatin led to an insignificant 13% reduction in the primary endpoint, but a significant 25% reduction was observed in an extended endpoint that included revascularisations, with a larger absolute risk reduction of coronary events in the diabetic subgroup than in the study population as a whole (8.1% vs. 5.2%), reflecting the higher event rate in the diabetic group.

The Long-Term Intervention with Pravastatin in Ischaemic Disease (LIPID) trial examined the effects of 40 mg pravastatin or placebo in 9014 patients with previous myocardial infarction or hospitalisation for unstable angina [10]. The primary study outcome was mortality from coronary heart disease, which was reduced by 24% in the main study (relative risk [RR] 0.76, $P <0.001$). In the main publication there was a 19% reduction in the 782 patients with diabetes and there was no evidence of significant heterogeneity for the subgroup [10], but the reduction did not reach statistical significance because of the small numbers.

Information from detailed diabetic subgroup analysis was published 5 years later, when the diagnostic criteria for diabetes had changed, and thus included 1077 subjects with type 2 diabetes [11]. A 19% reduction in major coronary events (coronary heart disease [CHD] death or non-fatal myocardial infarction [MI]) was demonstrated in the diabetic subgroup and again this was not quite statistically significant when compared to placebo. An expanded endpoint of any cardiovascular event (CHD death or non-fatal MI, coronary artery bypass graft [CABG] or percutanerous transluminal coronary angioplasty [PTCA], or stroke) was significantly reduced (RR 0.79, $P <0.008$). The absolute risk of a first CHD event was higher in the diabetes placebo group (23.4% vs. 14.5%), and the estimated number needed to treat (NNT) with pravastatin therapy for 6 years to prevent one CHD-related event was 18 in the diabetes subgroup compared to 26 in the total study population.

The West of Scotland Coronary Prevention Study (WOSCOPS) included 6595 subjects and was the first study to demonstrate that statins reduced cardiovascular events in subjects without myocardial infarction [12]. Although it is often considered a primary prevention study, around one in six of the subjects had prior vascular disease but not infarction. A significant reduction was observed in major coronary events (non-fatal myocardial infarction or CHD death), but WOSCOPS contained only 76 known diabetic patients (1%) and subgroup analysis of diabetic patients was not possible. Some further interesting data about diabetes emerged from follow-up of the WOSCOPS cohort; non-diabetic subjects who received pravastatin had a 30% reduction in the chance of developing new onset diabetes [13] and baseline predictors of the development of new onset diabetes included body mass index (BMI), fasting triglyceride, fasting glucose and C-reactive protein concentrations [14].

The Prospective Study of Pravastatin in the Elderly at Risk (PROSPER) study examined the effects of pravastatin 40 mg or placebo in 5804 elderly patients aged 70–82 years with, or at high risk of developing, cardiovascular disease and stroke [15]. Nearly half of all subjects had a history of vascular disease. The primary endpoint, 'major cardiovascular events', a composite of coronary death, non-fatal MI, and fatal or non-fatal stroke, was reduced by 15% (RR 0.85; $P = 0.014$). There were only 320 diabetic patients in the active treatment group and 303 participants in the placebo group, and the primary endpoint was insignificantly increased in the treatment group (70 events; 23.1%) compared to the placebo group (59

Table 8.1 Diabetes results from studies with pravastatin. 'Major coronary events' is a composite of death from coronary heart disease, or non-fatal myocardial infarction.
'Major cardiovascular events' is a composite of death from coronary heart disease, non-fatal myocardial infarction, or non-fatal stroke

Study	Dose	Total subjects	Diabetic subjects (%)	Diabetes results
CARE	40 mg	4159	586 (14%)	Insignificant reduction in major coronary events, significant reduction in expanded endpoint (CHD death, MI, CABG, PCI)
LIPID	40 mg	9014	1077 (12%)	Insignificant reduction in major coronary events, significant reduction in any cardiovascular event (CHD death, MI, CABG, PCI, stroke)
PROSPER	40 mg	5804	623 (11%)	Insignificant increase in major cardiovascular events
ALLHAT-LLT	40 mg	10 355	3638 (35%)	Insignificant reduction in all-cause mortality, insignificant reduction in major coronary events

CABG = coronary artery bypass graft; CHD = coronary heart disease; MI = myocardial infarction; PCI = percutaneous coronary intervention.

events; 18.4%). As the authors indicated: *'the number of individuals with diabetes was too small to permit accurate interpretation of the treatment effect'*.

Although the Antihypertensive and Lipid-Lowering Treatment to Prevent Heart Attack Trial (ALLHAT-LLT) contained a large number of diabetic patients (3638; 35%), the use of pravastatin 40 mg compared with 'usual care' did not show any significant reduction in either the primary endpoint of all-cause mortality, or the secondary endpoint of CHD events (non-fatal MI or fatal CHD) [16]. This trial is difficult to interpret, as it was not a double-blind trial: around one-quarter of the pravastatin group stopped receiving the study drug, and around one-quarter of the usual care group received open-label statins, so that there was only a very modest reduction in cholesterol in the treatment group compared to the usual care group.

STUDIES WITH SIMVASTATIN (TABLE 8.2)

In the landmark 4S study the effects of simvastatin were examined in 4444 patients with angina or previous myocardial infarction and raised total cholesterol [1]. Most patients received 20 mg of simvastatin, but around one-third had the dose increased to 40 mg when the serum cholesterol was above the target range of 3.0–5.2 mmol/l. Treatment with simvastatin was associated with a significant reduction in the primary endpoint of total mortality, and a significant reduction in major coronary events (coronary heart disease related death and non-fatal MI).

Table 8.2 Diabetes results from studies with simvastatin

Study	Dose	Total subjects	Diabetic subjects (%)	Diabetes results
4S	20–40 mg	4444	202 (5%)	Insignificant reduction in total mortality, significant reduction in major coronary events
4S second diabetes analysis	20–40 mg	4444	483 (11%)	Insignificant reduction in total mortality, significant reduction in major coronary events
HPS	40 mg	20 536	5963 (29%)	Significant reduction in major coronary events, significant reduction in major cardiovascular events
HPS diabetes, primary	40 mg	5963	2912 (49%)	Significant reduction in major coronary events, significant reduction in major cardiovascular events

There were two *post hoc* subgroup analyses of the endpoint data from diabetic patients. The first examined patients with known diabetes at the start of the study, and revealed significant reductions in major coronary events [3]. Although there was a larger reduction in all-cause mortality in this group when compared to the whole trial population, this did not reach statistical significance as a result of the small size of the subgroup. The second *post hoc* analysis added people diagnosed using the new World Health Organization (WHO) criteria (i.e. fasting glucose ≥ 7.0 mmol/l), as well as known diabetic patients ($n = 483$; 11% of the total), and the reduction in major coronary events was similar [17]. Further diabetes publications from 4S showed that treatment with simvastatin reduced cardiovascular disease-related hospitalisations and total hospital days [18], and that estimates of cost per life-year gained were well within the range generally considered to be cost-effective [19].

The Heart Protection Study (HPS) was a large study designed to address the possible benefit of simvastatin 40 mg compared to placebo in 20 536 subjects who would not have been included in the early coronary studies [20]. Its aim was to study the effects of lipid lowering within subgroups for which there was limited existing evidence, including subjects with a cholesterol level below previously accepted thresholds for treatment, subjects with diabetes, females, the elderly and those with non-coronary occlusive arterial disease. HPS randomised patients with known CHD or risk factors such as peripheral vascular disease (PVD), stroke, diabetes and hypertension. It included patients who had random total cholesterol of >3.5 mmol/l, which was considerably lower than the levels previously used in the other major trials. The primary outcome for overall analysis was total mortality, and this was significantly reduced with simvastatin.

There were 5963 diabetic subjects (29% of the total) and most were classified as having type 2 diabetes [21]. Patients with diabetes and prior myocardial infarction or CHD had the highest event rate of any group in the study, with a first major vascular event rate (major coronary event, stroke or revascularisation) of 38% in 5 years in the placebo group that was reduced to 33% with simvastatin 40 mg, extending the results of the 4S, CARE and LIPID studies to diabetic patients with lower baseline cholesterol concentrations. This was also the first study to demonstrate a reduction in strokes with statins in addition to the reduction in coronary events in people with diabetes. 2912 diabetic patients (49% of diabetic subjects) had no prior occlusive vascular disease (primary prevention), and simvastatin significantly reduced the primary endpoint of first major cardiovascular event from 13.5% down to 9.3% in this group.

STUDIES WITH OTHER STATINS

The Air Force/Texas Coronary Atherosclerosis Prevention Study (AFCAPS/TexCAPS) was a primary prevention study in 6605 Texans [22]. Compared to placebo, lovastatin (20–40 mg) significantly reduced the primary endpoint of first major coronary events, defined as fatal or non-fatal myocardial infarction, unstable angina, or sudden cardiac death. The study included 155 people with known type 2 diabetes, and a further 84 subjects with a fasting glucose >7.0 mmol/l, totalling only 239 diabetic subjects (4%), so diabetic subgroup analysis was not possible.

The Post Coronary Artery Bypass Graft (Post-CABG) trial examined the effects of lovastatin in 1351 patients with previous coronary artery bypass grafts and at least one patent graft on angiography [23]. The intervention group received 20–40 mg lovastatin, and the control group 2.5 mg, which was essentially the same as a placebo. The primary outcome was progression of atherosclerosis on angiography, and was reduced with higher dose lovastatin. 'Clinical outcomes' were secondary endpoints, and were not significantly reduced. A *post hoc* analysis of 116 diabetic patients (9%) showed that the angiographic benefits were the same in diabetic and non-diabetic subjects [24]. As might be expected from other studies, the number of clinical events was higher in diabetic subjects compared to non-diabetic subjects and although there was a trend to reductions in clinical events with higher dose lovastatin therapy, there was no statistical power to perform this analysis.

The Lescol Intervention Prevention Study (LIPS) examined 1677 patients undergoing successful percutaneous coronary intervention (PCI) for stable or unstable angina or silent ischaemia [25]. Compared to placebo, fluvastatin 80 mg significantly reduced the survival time free of major adverse coronary events, which for this study was defined as cardiac death, non-fatal myocardial infarction, or a reintervention procedure. Subgroup analysis of 202 diabetic patients (12%) showed significant benefit [25].

Thus, of the older statins, there is a large evidence base for the use of simvastatin and pravastatin for both primary and secondary prevention in people with diabetes. Less evidence exists for lovastatin and fluvastatin. Together, these results suggest that with regard to efficacy, the benefits of statins are a probably a class effect.

NEWER STATINS

STUDIES WITH ATORVASTATIN (TABLE 8.3)

The Collaborative AtoRvastatin Diabetes Study (CARDS) was the first study to assess the benefits of cholesterol reduction solely in a cohort of subjects with diabetes and no previous cardiovascular disease, and randomised 2838 participants with type 2 diabetes to receive atorvastatin 10 mg or placebo [26]. All of the participants had a minimum of one other risk factor for cardiovascular disease. The median LDL-C level at entry was 3.1 mmol/l, which

Table 8.3 Diabetes results from studies with atorvastatin

Study	Dose	Total subjects	Diabetic subjects (%)	Diabetes results
CARDS	10 mg	2838	2838 (100 %)	Significant reduction in major cardiovascular events
ASCOT-LLA	10 mg	10 305	2532 (25%)	Significant reduction in major cardiovascular events
GREASE	10 mg uptitrated to 80 mg	1600	313 (20%)	Significant reduction in all cause and coronary mortality
ASPEN	10 mg	2410	2410 (100%)	Insignificant reduction in primary endpoint
German Diabetes and Dialysis Study	20 mg	1255	1255 (100%)	No effect on primary endpoint
SPARCL	80 mg	4731	794 (17%)	Diabetes results not reported

was not markedly elevated and was lower than the equivalent group in the Heart Protection Study [27].

CARDS was stopped early because of a significant reduction of 37% in the composite primary endpoint of major cardiovascular event (hazard ratio [HR] 0.63; confidence interval [CI] 0.48–0.83; $P = 0.001$), which equated to an absolute risk reduction of 3.2% [28]. This primary endpoint comprised all acute coronary heart disease events including resuscitated cardiac arrest, coronary revascularisation procedures and stroke. The largest benefit was seen in stroke prevention, with a 48% risk reduction. There was a non-significant 27% reduction in the secondary endpoint of all-cause mortality. These results were seen with initial LDL levels both above and below the median. *Post hoc* analysis of the data showed that atorvastatin significantly reduced major cardiovascular events as early as 18 months after initiation of treatment with a significant reduction in coronary heart disease events as early as 1 year [29].

Published shortly before CARDS, the Anglo-Scandinavian Cardiac Outcomes Trial Lipid Lowering Arm (ASCOT-LLA) was the lipid-lowering arm of a hypertension study [30]. This was another double-blind, placebo-controlled, primary prevention study in which participants were randomised to either atorvastatin 10 mg or placebo. All the subjects had uncontrolled hypertension with three or more prespecified cardiovascular risk factors including type 2 diabetes but no previous coronary heart disease. The average LDL concentration at entry was 3.4 mmol/l and random total cholesterol was 5.5 mmol/l.

ASCOT-LLA was stopped early after a mean follow up of 3.3 years (intended follow-up period was 5 years). Statin therapy lowered LDL-C to 2.3 mmol/l and total cholesterol to 4.2 mmol/l by the end of the study. The primary endpoint of non-fatal MI and fatal coronary heart disease occurred in 100 patients treated with atorvastatin compared to 154 patients on placebo, a 36% relative risk reduction with atorvastatin (HR 0.64; CI 0.5–0.83; $P = 0.0005$). There was also a significant reduction in the incidence of total coronary events, total cardiovascular events and procedures, and strokes. Surprisingly, the effects of lipid lowering in the

2532 subjects with type 2 diabetes did not show a benefit in the primary endpoint, with 38 events in the atorvastatin group compared to 46 events in the placebo group (HR 0.84; CI 0.55–1.29; $P = 0.4$). This may be explained by the fact the study was not powered to show a statistically different result with subgroup analysis and may also reflect the relatively high use of statins within the diabetic placebo group [31].

The GREek Atorvastatin Coronary heart disease Evaluation study (GREACE) was a randomised, open-label study of atorvastatin in patients with established coronary heart disease [32]. The aim of the study was to compare the use of atorvastatin, uptitrated to achieve LDL levels of <2.6 mmol/l, with usual care lipid therapy. In fact, the use of statins for secondary prevention was so poor this was effectively a placebo-controlled trial with only 12% of the usual care group receiving statins. Initial LDL and fasting total cholesterol levels were high in both groups at 6.6 and 4.6 mmol/l. By the end of the study, LDL was reduced to 2.5 mmol/l in the atorvastatin group and there were significant reductions in the primary endpoints, which included total mortality (43% reduction) and coronary mortality (47% reduction).

The GREASE study included 313 subjects with diabetes [33]. Initial lipid levels were even higher amongst this cohort, with LDL and total cholesterol levels of 4.9 and 7 mmol/l. There was a significant 52% reduction in all-cause mortality and 62% reduction in coronary mortality with atorvastatin, such huge reductions surely reflecting both the substantial reduction in LDL as well as the very high-risk nature of the population.

Published in 2006, but designed and recruited during the late 1990s, the Atorvastatin Study for Prevention of Coronary Heart Disease Endpoints in Non-Insulin-Dependent Diabetes Mellitus (ASPEN) was another randomised, placebo-controlled study of atorvastatin [34]. The study was originally designed as a secondary prevention study to look at lowering LDL levels below the guideline levels of that time. Due to changes in lipid treatment guidelines during the course of the study, recruitment was expanded to include patients without coronary disease and many patients had study medication discontinued and substituted for usual care. Initial mean LDL- and total-cholesterol levels were 3.0 and 5.0 mmol/l and treatment with 10 mg of atorvastatin lowered these to 2.1 and 4.1 mmol/l. There was no benefit seen with atorvastatin therapy in the composite primary endpoint of major cardiovascular events (HR 0.9; CI 0.73–1.12; $P = 0.3$) most likely reflecting the many changes made to the study protocol during the course of the trial, and the high use of open-label statins in the placebo group.

The German Diabetes and Dialysis Study examined atorvastatin 20 mg or placebo in 1255 subjects with type 2 diabetes on haemodialysis [35]. Many had a history of cardiovascular disease and intervention. There was no effect on major cardiovascular events, and the authors concluded that: 'the initiation of lipid-lowering therapy in patients with type 2 diabetes mellitus who already have end-stage renal disease may come too late to translate into consistent improvement of the cardiovascular outcome'.

Recently, the Stroke Prevention by Aggressive Reduction in Cholesterol Levels (SPARCL) study in 4731 patients with previous stroke or TIA has demonstrated that 80 mg of atorvastatin significantly reduced the primary endpoint of fatal or non-fatal stroke, and reduced the secondary outcome of major cardiovascular events (794 patients had diabetes, but subgroup analysis was not presented) [36].

STUDIES WITH ROSUVASTATIN

Rosuvastatin, one of the newest and most potent statins, does not yet have any positive endpoint trials to support its use in people with diabetes, although it does have some short-term comparative trials against other statins in people with diabetes, and an open label ultrasound study included some diabetic patients.

The cholesterol-lowering effects of rosuvastatin compared with atorvastatin in patients with type 2 diabetes (CORALL) study was a 24-week open-label, randomised study of 263 subjects with type 2 diabetes [37], comparing the ability of escalating doses of rosuvastatin and atorvastatin to lower the apoB–apoA1 ratio, a recognised predictor of myocardial infarction. Doses of 20 and 40 mg of rosuvastatin resulted in significant reductions in both the apoB–apoA1 ratio and LDL levels compared with 40 and 80 mg of atorvastatin. The Use of Rosuvastatin versus Atorvastatin in Type 2 Diabetes Mellitus (URANUS) study was a 16-week double-blind randomised study in 465 subjects with type 2 diabetes, comparing the ability of escalating doses of rosuvastatin and atorvastatin to reach European LDL-C targets (<3.0 mmol/l) [38]. Again, rosuvastatin was more effective than atorvastatin at reducing LDL-C and achieving European LDL-C goals. In some of the early registration studies with rosuvastatin a slight, temporary increase in tubular protein excretion was documented, and data from URANUS reassuringly demonstrated no change in urinary albumin excretion or glomerular filtration rate [39].

The open-label A Study To Evaluate the Effect of Rosuvastatin on Intravascular Ultrasound-Derived Coronary Atheroma Burden (ASTERIOD) trial was designed to determine whether aggressive lipid lowering with high dose rosuvastatin could regress coronary atherosclerosis as determined by intravascular ultrasound (IVUS) imaging [40]. Patients undergoing coronary angiography were treated with 40 mg of rosuvastatin for an average of 24 months and had IVUS measurements of coronary atheroma at the start and end of the treatment period. Sixty-nine percent (382 patients) completed the treatment phase and 349 had paired IVUS examinations and so completed the trail. Rosuvastatin resulted in a significant reduction in atheroma volume with an accompanying reduction in LDL-C from 3.4 to 1.5 mmol/l. Forty-six of the 349 patients completing the trial had diabetes, and similar reductions in atheroma volume were demonstrated in this subgroup.

STUDIES OF AGGRESSIVE CHOLESTEROL LOWERING

There is considerable evidence supporting the use of statins to lower cholesterol in patients with diabetes both in primary and secondary prevention. The question remains unclear as to what cholesterol targets we should be aiming for. This is a complex question as it inevitably has financial implications, and concerns have been raised as to as the safety of the more potent or high-dose statins required to achieve maximum reductions in cholesterol.

Several studies already discussed have shown a benefit of lowering LDL-C below previously accepted targets. The treatment groups in both CARDS and the diabetic subgroup of HPS achieved mean LDL levels of <2.6 mmol/l and the benefits of treatment were seen irrespective of initial LDL levels. More recent studies have compared different regimes and doses of statins in order to examine the possible benefits of even more intensive LDL lowering (Table 8.4).

The Pravastatin or Atorvastatin Evaluation and Infection Therapy – Thrombolysis in Myocardial Infarction 22 (PROVE-IT TIMI 22) trial [41] and phase Z of the Aggrastat to Zocor (A to Z) trial [42] were both designed to compare intensive versus more modest LDL lowering regimes in patients with recent acute coronary syndromes. PROVE-IT was a double-blind study and patients were randomised to either 40 mg of pravastatin or 80 mg of atorvastatin within 10 days of hospitalisation. At the start of the study they had modestly elevated total and LDL-C levels of 4.7 and 2.7 mmol/l respectively. After a mean follow-up period of 24 months the atorvastatin group achieved a 32% reduction in LDL-C (2.7 to 1.6 mmol/l) compared to minor reductions seen with pravastatin (2.7 to 2.4 mmol/l). There was a significant 16% relative risk reduction in the primary endpoint of time to first major cardiovascular event in the atorvastatin group (HR 0.84; CI 0.74–0.95; $P = 0.005$). This included death from any cause, MI, unstable angina, stroke and revascularisation procedures occurring more than 30 days after randomisation. This reduction in events with high-dose atorvastatin was evident as early as 30 days, reaching significance by 6 months. There were 978 subjects with diabetes in this study, representing 23% of the study group. The reduction in

Table 8.4 Diabetes results from studies comparing low-dose and high-dose statins

Study	Statins	Total subjects	Diabetic subjects (%)	Diabetes results
PROVE-IT	Atorvastatin 80 mg vs. pravastatin 40	4162	734 (18%)	Insignificant reduction in major cardiovascular events
A-Z	Simvastatin 40 mg then 80 mg vs. placebo then simvastatin 20 mg	4497	1059 (24%)	Insignificant reduction in primary endpoint
TNT	Atorvastatin 80 mg vs. atorvastatin 10 mg	10 001	1501 (15%)	Significant reduction in major cardiovascular events
IDEAL	Atorvastatin 80 mg vs. simvastatin 20–40 mg	8888	1069 (12%)	Diabetes results not reported

the primary endpoint was not statistically significant in the diabetes subgroup, presumably reflecting the relatively small number of patients with diabetes [43]. A significant reduction was observed in the triple endpoint of death, myocardial infarction and unstable angina requiring hospitalisation..

Phase Z of the A to Z trial randomised 4497 patients presenting with acute coronary syndromes to receive either an early intensive or a delayed less aggressive statin regime [42]. This consisted of 40 mg of simvastatin for 30 days followed by 80 mg of simvastatin thereafter or placebo for 4 months followed by 20 mg of simvastatin. Again, the lipid levels were not markedly elevated at the start of the study with mean total and LDL-C levels of 4.8 and 2.9 mmol/l in each group. A slightly higher proportion of patients with diabetes were included in this study, at 24% of the total population.

In comparison with PROVE-IT, treatment with the aggressive statin regimen in the A to Z trial did not result in a significant reduction in the primary endpoint, which, in this case, was a composite of cardiovascular death, non-fatal MI, readmission for ACS and stroke (HR 0.89; CI 0.76–1.04; $P = 0.14$). The reasons for the disparities between these two studies are not clear, although there are several possible explanations. The intensive treatment group in A to Z achieved similar reductions in LDL as the intensive group in PROVE-IT, with levels of 1.6 mmol/l after 8 months, but the LDL levels in the less aggressive treatment group were lower at 1.9 mmol/l despite 4 months of placebo. The A to Z trial had a high dropout rate and, despite recruiting the planned number of patients, had a lower-than-expected event rate. It is also possible that the higher reduction in C-reactive protein (CRP) levels seen with the aggressive treatment group in PROVE-IT reflected a different mechanism of action of the statin regime in that study beyond LDL lowering.

The Treatment to New Targets (TNT) study and the Incremental Decrease in End Points through Aggressive Lipid Lowering (IDEAL) trial were two other studies designed to look at the benefit of aggressive LDL lowering in a population with stable coronary heart disease. TNT compared low-dose (10 mg) against high-dose (80 mg) atorvastatin with the aim of studying the potential benefits of lowering LDL-C to below 2.6 mmol/l [44]. This was a large, open-label study that randomised 10 001 patients with coronary heart disease, 15 % of which had diabetes. The study design included a run-in period of 8 weeks in which all patients received 10 mg of atorvastatin. Following this, half of the patients then had their dose increased. By the end of the run-in period, the mean LDL in both patient groups was 2.6 mmol/l and this was reduced even further to a mean of 2.0 mmol/l in the 80 mg atorvastatin group by the end of the study (4.9-year follow-up). The high-dose statin regimen resulted in a significant 22% relative risk reduction in the primary endpoint of major cardiovascular events, which included death from coronary heart disease or stroke, non-fatal or procedural MI, resuscitated cardiac arrest or non-fatal stroke (HR 0.78; CI 0.69–0.89; P <0.001). There were also significant reductions in the secondary endpoints of any coronary event, any cardiovascular event, hospitalisation with a primary diagnosis of heart failure and stroke.

The diabetic population in the TNT study were slightly older, more overweight and had a higher prevalence of cardiovascular disease that the general study population [45]. They had similar lipid levels and achieved similar reductions in LDL compared to the study population as a whole. There was a 25% relative risk reduction in major cardiovascular events (HR 0.75; CI 0.58–0.97; P <0.026), which was seen for all quintiles of age, initial LDL or duration of diabetes and in patients with glycosylated haemoglobin (HbA1c) < or > 7%. There were too few subjects to see significant reductions in most of the secondary endpoints, although there was a significant reduction in the time to cerebrovascular event (HR 0.69; CI 0.48–0.98; P = 0.037) and time to cardiovascular event (HR 0.85; CI 0.73–1.0; P = 0.044) with high-dose atorvastatin.

The IDEAL trial was a large, open-label, blinded-endpoint trial [46]. In this study 8888 patients with a prior history of MI were randomised to either 20 mg of simvastatin or 80 mg of atorvastatin. Any patients on doses of statins equivalent to >20 mg of simvastatin prior to randomisation were excluded. The dose of simvastatin could be increased to 40 mg after 24 weeks if the total cholesterol was >5 mmol/l and the dose of atorvastatin could be reduced for adverse events. At baseline, the mean LDL and total cholesterols were 3.1 and 5.1 mmol/l and 12% of the patients in each group had diabetes. In comparison to TNT, the primary endpoint on this occasion was time to first major coronary event, including resuscitated cardiac arrest.

By the end of the follow-up period of 4.8 years, 23% of the simvastatin group were prescribed a dose of 40 mg and 13% of patients in the other group had their atorvastatin reduced to 40 mg. The intensive LDL lowering strategy with high-dose atorvastatin resulted in a mean LDL-C of 2.1 mmol/l by the end of the study, compared to 2.6 mmol/l in the usual care simvastatin group. These changes were associated with a borderline, non-significant, relative risk reduction of 11% in the primary endpoint with atorvastatin as compared to simvastatin (HR 0.89; CI 0.78–1.10; P = 0.07). There were significant reductions in the incidence of some of the prespecified secondary endpoints including reductions in cardiovascular and coronary heart disease events in the group taking atorvastatin. The effects of intensive LDL lowering in the diabetic subgroup were not reported.

SYSTEMATIC REVIEWS AND META-ANALYSES

The CARE, LIPID and WOSCOPS studies each compared pravastatin 40 mg with placebo, and the investigators initiated a pooling project shortly after the individual trails started and before the results of any of the trails were known [47]. The Prospective Pravastatin Pooling (PPP) Project included 19 768 patients, 102 559 person-years of follow-up, 2194 primary endpoints (coronary death or non-fatal myocardial infarction) and 3717 expanded endpoints (primary endpoint, CABG or PCI). Pravastatin significantly reduced relative risk in younger and older patients, men and women, smokers and non-smokers, and patients with or without diabetes or hypertension. In the diabetic subjects the 19% relative risk reduction in the primary endpoint was not statistically significant, but the 26% reduction in the expanded endpoint reached statistical significance. Results were similar when a pooled analysis was performed of CARE and LIPID without data from WOSCOPS [46].

The Evidence in Diabetes Enquiry Stem (EVIDENS) Research Group performed a systematic review of lipid lowering for primary prevention of coronary heart disease in diabetes, which mainly included data from WOSCOPS, AFCAPS/TexCAPS and HPS. In a brief publication they commented on the general lack of diabetes primary prevention data, but the review was performed before the results of the CARDS study were available [48].

The American College of Physicians performed a much larger meta-analysis of pharmacological lipid-lowering therapy in type 2 diabetes [49], and on the basis of this review recommended a clinical practice guideline [50]. They included data from AFCAPS/TexCAPS, ALLHAT-LLA, HPS (primary and secondary prevention), PROSPER, ASCOT-LLA, 4S, CARE, LIPID, LIPS, and Post-CABG. They found a similar relative risk reduction in diabetic subjects but more than twice the absolute risk reduction. They commented that most studies compared a lipid-lowering drug with placebo and did not evaluate the effect of reaching specific cholesterol levels, and that benefit appeared to be similar regardless of starting cholesterol concentrations [48]. More recently, a meta-analysis was performed by other authors of the same studies to specifically compare diabetic and non-diabetic subjects, and it was demonstrated that lipids were reduced to a similar degree in both groups, but that diabetic patients benefited more in both primary and secondary prevention because of the greater absolute risk reduction [51].

The Cholesterol Treatment Trialists' (CTT) Collaborators [52] performed a meta-analysis that included all of the statin studies that were in the American College of Physicians systematic review, with the addition of a few other studies, including WOSCOPS and CARDS. They included data for 90 056 participants, 8186 deaths and 14 348 major vascular events. Interestingly, the benefits were significant within the first year, but were greater in subsequent years. There were 18 686 diabetic subjects (21% of the total), with 776 major coronary events in the statin patients (8.3%) and 979 (10.5%) in the control groups, a relative risk reduction of 22%.

DIABETES GUIDELINES

The benefits of cholesterol lowering with statins are now well established for primary and secondary prevention of cardiovascular disease in diabetic patients with both elevated and relatively 'normal' serum cholesterol. This appears to hold true for a number of different statins suggesting that this is a class effect, and not simply dependent on the individual drugs used. However, evidence of efficacy is not the same as evidence of safety, and it should be remembered that cerivastatin was withdrawn because of unacceptable muscle side-effects when used widely in routine clinical practice. We suggest, therefore, that simvastatin, pravastatin or atorvastatin is prescribed for any diabetic patient with cardiovascular disease, regardless of baseline cholesterol concentration, as these drugs have both proven benefit and safety in large studies.

The role of statins in primary prevention of cerebrovascular disease in diabetic subjects has also been established in a number of studies, but this does not necessarily help decide which patients should be started on this therapy. Most risk estimation tables used for establishing cardiovascular risk and influencing both statin and antihypertensive treatments are based on Framingham data, which included few diabetic subjects, and so do not adequately represent the diabetic population [53]. This complicates the issue of which diabetic patients should be treated with statins in the primary prevention setting?

The high incidence of CHD within diabetic patients has led many to believe that diabetes should be considered as a CHD risk equivalent, and therefore all patients should receive a statin. Guidelines from the major international diabetes associations use this approach for patients over 40 years of age, with risk estimation for younger patients. The International Diabetes Federation (IDF) recommends the use of statins at standard dose in all diabetic patients aged ≥40 years, or all patients aged >20 years with microalbuminuria or assessed as being at particularly high risk. They suggest a target LDL-C <2.5 mmol/l [54]. This is similar to the older European guidelines produced by the Joint European Societies' Task

Force on Cardiovascular Disease Prevention in Clinical Practice, which included the European Association for the Study of Diabetes (EASD). They recommended statins for patients with type 2 diabetes and type 1 diabetes with microalbuminuria, with target total cholesterol <4.5 mmol/l and LDL-C <2.5 mmol/l [55]. The American Diabetes Association (ADA) recommends statin therapy for those aged >40 years with a goal of LDL-C <2.6 mmol/l and a 30–40% reduction, and similar for those aged <40 years but at increased risk due to other cardiovascular risk factors [56].

As described previously, there appears to be reasonable evidence to support the use of statins to aggressively lower LDL-C in patients with established vascular disease although there is less evidence within the diabetic population. These recent studies have, on the whole, provided further reassurance as to the safety of statins although notably in the A to Z trial there was a relatively high rate of myopathy associated with 80 mg of simvastatin, suggesting that this dose should only be used with caution. Given the results of these recent trials described above, the American Diabetes Association suggests that a lower LDL-C goal of <1.8 mmol/l using a high-dose statin may be an option for those with overt cardiovascular disease.

The American College of Physicians offer useful practical advice and suggest that for patients with type 2 diabetes who are taking statins, routine monitoring of liver function tests or muscle enzymes is not recommended except in specific circumstances (e.g. if the patient has symptoms or are taking other drugs that interact with statins to increase the risk for adverse events) [50] and we endorse that approach when using standard doses of statins. For patients on high-dose statins there is a much higher incidence of abnormalities, so routine testing of liver function tests and muscle enzymes is required.

FIBRATES IN THE TREATMENT OF DIABETIC DYSLIPIDAEMIA

The typical lipid disorder in patients with diabetes mellitus type 2 is characterised by low HDL-C and elevated triglyceride plasma concentrations, while, in general, LDL-C is not higher than in non-diabetic subjects. Given the fact that patients with type 2 diabetes are at elevated cardiovascular risk and that LDL-C is one of the most important modifiable risk factors, therapy influencing lipid metabolism is focused on lowering LDL-C. Therefore, treatment with statin as monotherapy or a combination therapy of statin with cholesterol absorption inhibition is the cornerstone of cardiovascular risk management in diabetic patients. It is now well established that lowering LDL-C with statins in patients with type 2 diabetes results in lower cardiovascular risk. Nevertheless, the residual cardiovascular risk in treated patients with type 2 diabetes remains high. The question remains whether raising HDL-C and/or lowering plasma triglycerides in patients with type 2 diabetes also lowers the cardiovascular risk. Studies are reviewed that investigate the effect of fibrates on cardiovascular risk in patients with diabetes mellitus type 2.

A low plasma concentration of HDL-C is an established independent risk factor for development of vascular diseases. Fibrates have peroxisome proliferator-activated receptor-α (PPAR-α) agonistic activity and increase HDL-C by 15–20%, lower plasma triglycerides by 20–30% and decrease LDL-C by 10–20%. Stimulation of the transcription factor PPAR-α increases lipoprotein lipase and apolipoprotein-CIII production, reduces very low-density lipoprotein (VLDL) production by the liver and stimulates apolipoprotein-AI and AII production. Fibrate therapy not only results in quantitative changes in plasma lipids but also in qualitative changes by reducing the plasma concentration of small dense LDL-C [57]. Small dense LDL-C is considered to be very atherogenic. In addition, fibrates may have anti-inflammatory properties, which may be relevant in preventing cardiovascular diseases [58].

The Helsinki Heart Study (HHS) was the first trial that investigated the effects of a fibrate, in this case gemfibrozil, on cardiovascular endpoints [59]. In that study, in 4081 participants without clinically manifest vascular diseases, only 135 had diabetes. The HHS reported a 10% increase in HDL-C and a 34% reduction in the combined endpoint of cardiovascular death and non-fatal MI compared to placebo during a mean follow up of 5 years. All-cause mortality was similar in patients treated with gemfibrozil or placebo. In the 135 patients with diabetes in HHS the event rate was 10.5% in placebo-treated patients and 3.4% in gemfibrozil-treated patients, resulting in a relative risk reduction of 68%.

In the Veterans Affairs High-Density Lipoprotein Cholesterol Intervention Trial (VA-HIT) 2531 men with coronary heart disease participated, of which 627 had diabetes [60, 61]. Participants were treated with gemfibrozil (1200 mg once daily) or placebo. After 5 years of follow–up, the HDL-C plasma concentration was 6% higher in the gemfibrozil-treated patients compared to placebo, plasma triglycerides were 33% lower and LDL-C was similar in the placebo group and in the gemfibrozil treated group. After 5 years the combined end-point of cardiovascular death, non-fatal MI or stroke was 23% lower in the gemfibrozil group compared to placebo. In patients with diabetes this was 22%.

The Bezafibrate Infarction Prevention (BIP) trial investigated the effect of bezafibrate (400 mg once daily) compared to placebo in 3090 patients with previous myocardial infarction or angina pectoris [62]. About 10% of the study population had diabetes but results for this group have not been published in detail. During a mean follow-up time of 6.2 years, sudden death and myocardial infarction were recorded. During the study the HDL-C concentration was 18% higher and triglycerides 21% lower in the bezafibrate group compared to placebo. In the bezafibrate group the endpoint was observed in 13.6% of the patients and in the placebo group this was 15.0%. Although there was a slightly lower event rate in the fibrate-treated patients, the conclusion of the BIP trial was that there was no significant reduction in vascular events in bezafibrate-treated patients compared to placebo.

The Diabetes Atherosclerosis Intervention Study (DAIS) trial only included patients with type 2 diabetes and compared treatment with micronized fenofibrate (200 mg once daily) to placebo on atherosclerosis progression on coronary angiography in 418 participants [63]. Patients had a good glycaemic control (HbA1c = 7.5%). Fenofibrate-treated patients had a smaller decrease in minimal lumen diameter than the placebo group. The study was not powered to investigate differences in the occurrence of clinical endpoints but during 3 years follow-up the incidence of clinical endpoints was also lower in the fenofibrate compared to placebo (38% vs. 50%).

The Fenofibrate Intervention and Event Lowering in Diabetes (FIELD) study is the largest lipid trial done exclusively in patients with diabetes mellitus thus far [64]. Fenofibrate was compared to placebo in 9795 participants with diabetes. The observed 5-year rates for the primary endpoint (coronary heart disease death or myocardial infarction) were 5.2% and 5.9% with fenofibrate and placebo, respectively ($P = 0.16$). The rate of total cerebrovascular disease events (composite of cardiovascular death, myocardial infarction, stroke, and coronary and carotid revascularisation) was lower in participants who received fenofibrate (12.5%) than in those who received placebo (13.9%) ($P = 0.035$). In the group of patients randomised to placebo a greater proportion started statin treatment during the study (17% vs. 8%), which may have masked a modest therapeutic effect of fenofibrate.

SUMMARY

The prescribing of statins to diabetic patients is a frequently used therapeutic strategy, and as was suggested by the CARDS investigators: 'the debate about whether all people with this disorder warrant statin treatment should now focus on whether any patients are at sufficiently low risk for this treatment to be withheld'. However, the age at which to begin statin therapy, and the optimum dosage and treatment targets for different groups of diabetic patients remain to be established.

Influencing diabetic dyslipidaemia, other than LDL-C lowering, remains controversial. In common with the statin trials, all fibrate cardiovascular endpoint studies were designed to evaluate the effect of monotherapy. The fibrate studies show little or no effect of fibrate treatment on the occurrence of cardiovascular events in patients with diabetes limiting the use of fibrates as cardioprotective agents. Fibrates may have a secondary role in reducing cardiovascular events in patients with diabetes in combination with statins. However, it remains to be determined whether the combination of a fibrate with a statin reduces the risk beyond that achieved with a statin alone. The lipid lowering arm of the Action to Control Cardiovascular Risk in Diabetes (ACCORD) trial, investigating the effect of fenofibrate and stringent blood pressure control in a 2 × 2 factorial design may give answers to remaining questions in managing dyslipidaemia in patients with diabetes mellitus [65]. This study will be undertaken in patients with diabetes already using statins. The combination of statin and fibrate has the potential for adverse effects, which has limited their use together in current clinical practice, but the results of the ACCORD trial may change this view. For now, the role for fibrate therapy is reserved as an adjunct to statin treatment for the prevention of pancreatitis in patients with very high plasma triglycerides at increased risk of developing pancreatitis and for preventing cardiovascular disease in patients with diabetes who are intolerant to statin treatment.

REFERENCES

1. Scandinavian Simvastatin Survival Study Group. Randomised trial of cholesterol lowering in 4444 patients with coronary heart disease: the Scandinavian Simvastatin Survival Study (4S). *Lancet* 1994; 344:1383–1389.
2. Colhoun HM, Betteridge JD. Treatment of lipd disorders in patients with diabetes. *Curr Treat Options Cardiovasc Med* 2006; 8:37–45.
3. Pyörälä K, Pedersen TR, Kjekshus J, Faergeman O, Olsson AG, Thorgeirsson G & the Scandinavian Simvastatin Survival Study (4S) Group. Cholesterol lowering with simvastatin improves prognosis of diabetic patients with coronary heart disease. A subgroup analysis of the Scandinavian Simvastatin Survival Study (4S). *Diabetes Care* 1997; 20: 614–620
4. Marshall G, McDougall C, Brady AJB, Fisher M. Should all diabetic patients receive a statin? Results from recent trials. *Br J Cardiol* 2004; 11: 455–460
5. Prisant LM. Clinical trials and lipid guidelines for type II diabetes. *J Clin Pharmacol* 2004; 44:423–430.
6. Plummer CJ. What's in the CARDS? *Diabet Med* 2006; 23:711–714.
7. Reckless JPD. Diabetes and lipid lowering: where are we? *Br Med J* 2006; 332:1103–1104.
8. Sacks FM, Pfeffer MA, Moye LA *et al*, for the Cholesterol and Recurrent Events Trial Investigators. The effect of pravastatin on coronary events after myocardial infarction in patients with average cholesterol levels. *N Engl J Med* 1996; 335:1001–1009.
9. Goldberg RB, Mellies MJ, Sacks FM *et al*, for the CARE Investigators. Cardiovascular events and their reduction with pravastatin in diabetic and glucose-intolerant myocardial infarction survivors with average cholesterol levels. Subgroup analyses in the Cholesterol And Recurrent Events (CARE) Trial. *Circulation* 1998; 98:2513–2519.
10. The Long-Term Intervention with Pravastatin in Ischaemic Disease (LIPID) Study Group. Prevention of cardiovascular events and death with pravastatin in patients with coronary heart disease and a broad range of initial cholesterol levels. *N Engl J Med* 1998; 339:1349–1357.
11. Keech A, Colquhoun D, Best J *et al*, for the LIPID Study Group. Secondary prevention of cardiovascular events with long-term pravastatin in patients with diabetes or impaired fasting glucose. Results from the LIPID trial. *Diabetes Care* 2003; 26:2713–2721.
12. Shepherd J, Cobbe SM, Ford I *et al*, for the West of Scotland Coronary Prevention Study Group. Prevention of coronary heart disease with pravastatin in men with hypercholesterolemia. *N Engl J Med* 1995; 333:1301–1307.
13. Freeman DJ, Norrie J, Sattar N *et al*. Pravastatin and the development of diabetes mellitus. Evidence for a protective effect in the West of Scotland Coronary Prevention Study. *Circulation* 2001; 103:357–362.

14. Freeman DJ, Norrie J, Caslake MJ et al, for the West of Scotland Coronary Prevention Study Group. C-reactive protein is an independent predictor of risk for the development of diabetes in the West of Scotland Coronary Prevention Study. *Diabetes* 2002; 51:1596–1600.

15. Shepherd J, Blaw GJ, Murphy MB et al, on behalf of the PROSPER study group. Pravastatin in elderly individuals at risk of vascular disease (PROSPER): a randomised controlled trial. *Lancet* 2002; 360:1623–1630.

16. The ALLHAT Officers and Coordinators for the ALLHAT Collaborative Research Group. Major outcomes in moderately hypercholesterolemic, hypertensive patients randomised to pravastatin vs usual care. The Antihypertensive and Lipid-Lowering Treatment to Prevent Heart Attack Trial (ALLHAT-LLT). *JAMA* 2002; 288:2998–3007.

17. Haffner SM, Alexander CM, Cook TJ et al, for the Scandinavian Simvastatin Survival Study Group. Reduced coronary events in simvastatin-treated patients with coronary heart disease and diabetes or impaired fasting glucose levels. Subgroup analyses in the Scandinavian Simvastatin Survival Study. *Arch Intern Med* 1999; 159:2661–2667.

18. Herman WH, Alexander CM, Cook JR et al, for Scandinavian Simvastatin Survival Study Group. Effect of simvastatin treatment on cardiovascular resource utilization in impaired fasting glucose and diabetes. Findings from the Scandinavian Simvastatin Survival Study. *Diabetes Care* 1999; 22:1771–1778.

19. Jonsson B, Cook JR, Pedersen TR. The cost-effectiveness of lipid lowering in patients with diabetes: results from the 4S trial. *Diabetologia* 1999; 42:1293–1301.

20. Heart Protection Study Collaborative Group. MRC / BHF Heart Protection Study of cholesterol lowering with simvastatin in 20 536 high-risk individuals: a randomised placebo-controlled trial. *Lancet* 2002; 360:7–22.

21. Heart Protection Study Collaborative Group. MRC / BHF Heart Protection Study of cholesterol-lowering with simvastatin in 5963 people with diabetes: a randomised placebo-controlled trial. *Lancet* 2003; 361:2005–2016.

22. Downs JR, Clearfield M, Weiss S et al, for the AFCAPS/TexCAPS Research Group. Primary prevention of acute coronary events with lovastatin in men and women with average cholesterol levels: results of AFCAPS/TexCAPS. *JAMA* 1998; 279:1615–1622.

23. The Post Coronary Artery Bypass Graft Trial Investigators. The effect of aggressive lowering of low-density lipoprotein cholesterol levels and low-dose anticoagulation on obstructive changes in saphenous-vein coronary-artery bypass grafts. *N Engl J Med* 1997; 336:153–162.

24. Hoogwerf BJ, Waness A, Cressman M et al, for the Post CABG Study Investigators. Effects of aggressive cholesterol lowering and low-dose anticoagulation on clinical and angiographic outcomes in patients with diabetes. The Post Coronary Artery Bypass Graft Trial. *Diabetes* 1999; 48:1289–1294.

25. Serruys PWJC, de Feyter P, Macaya C et al, for the Lescol Intervention Prevention Study (LIPS) Investigators. Fluvastatin for prevention of cardiac events following successful first percutaneous coronary intervention. A randomized controlled trial. *JAMA* 2002; 287:3215–3222.

26. Colhoun HM, Thomason MJ, Mackness MI et al and the CARDS Investigators. Design of the Collaborative AtoRvastatin Diabetes Study (CARDS) in patients with Type 2 diabetes *Diabet Med* 2002; 19:201–211.

27. Thomason MJ, Colhoun HM, Livingstone SJ et al and the CARDS Investigators. Baseline characteristics in the Collaborative AtoRvastatin Diabetes Study (CARDS) in patients with Type 2 diabetes *Diabet Med* 2004; 21:901–905.

28. Colhoun HM, Betteridge DJ, Durrington PN et al, on behalf of the CARDS investigators. Primary prevention of cardiovascular disease with atrovastatin in type 2 diabetes in the Collaborative AtoRvastatin Diabetes Study (CARDS): multicentre randomised placebo-controlled trial. *Lancet* 2004; 364:685–696.

29. Colhoun HM, Betteridge DJ, Durrington PN et al, on behalf of the CARDS Investigators. Rapid emergence of effect of atorvastatin on cardiovascular outcomes in the Collaborative AtoRvastatin Diabetes Study (CARDS). *Diabetologia* 2005; 48:2482–2485.

30. Sever PS, Dahlöf B, Poulter NR et al, for the ASCOT investigators. Prevention of coronary and stroke events with atorvastatin in hypertensive patients who have average or lower-than-average cholesterol concentrations, in the Anglo-Scandinavian Cardiac Outcomes Trial-Lipid Lowering Arm (ASCOT-LLA): a multicentre randomised controlled trial. *Lancet* 2003; 361:1149–1158.

31. Sever PS, Poulter NR, Dahlof B et al, for the ASCOT Investigators. Reduction in cardiovascular events with atorvastatin in 2,532 patients with type 2 diabetes: Anglo-Scandinavian Cardiac Outcomes Trial-lipid-lowering arm (ASCOT-LLA). *Diabetes Care.* 2005; 28:1151–1157.

32. Athyros VG, Papageorgiou AA, Mercouris BR et al. Treatment with atorvastatin to the National Cholesterol Educational Program goal versus 'usual' care in secondary coronary heart disease prevention. The GREek Atorvastatin and Coronary-heart-disease Evaluation (GREACE) study. Curr Med Res Opin 2002; 18:220–228.

33. Athyros VG, Papageorgiou AA, Symeonidis AN et al. Early benefit from structured care with atorvastatin in patients with coronary heart disease and diabetes mellitus. Angiology 2003; 54:679–690.

34. Knopp RH, d'Emden M, Smilde JG, Pocock SJ on behalf of the ASPEN Study Group. Efficacy and safety of atorvastatin in the prevention of cardiovascular end points in subjects with type 2 diabetes: the Atorvastatin Study for Prevention of Coronary Heart Disease Endpoints in Non-Insulin-Dependent Diabetes Mellitus (ASPEN). Diabetes Care 2006; 29:1478–1485.

35. Wanner C, Krane V, März W et al, for the German Diabetes and Dialysis Study Investigators. Atorvastatin in patients with type 2 diabetes mellitus undergoing hemodylasis. N Eng J Med 2005; 353:238–248 (erratum in: N Engl J Med 2005; 353:1640).

36. The Stroke Prevention by Aggressive Reduction in Cholesterol Levels (SPARCL) Investigators. High-dose atorvastatin after stroke or transient ischemic attack. N Engl J Med 2006; 355:549–559.

37. Wolffenbuttel BH, Franken AA, Vincent HH on behalf of the Dutch CORALL Study Group. Cholesterol-lowering effects of rosuvastatin compared with atorvastatin in patients with type 2 diabetes – CORALL study. J Intern Med 2005; 257:531–539.

38. Berne C, Siewert-Delle A, on behalf of the URANUS investigators. Comparison of rosuvastatin and atorvastatin for lipid lowering in patients with type 2 diabetes mellitus: results from the URANUS study. Cardiovasc Diabetol 2005; 4:7.

39. Sorof J, Berne C, Siewert-Delle, Jorgensen L, Sager P on behalf of the URANUS investigators. Effect of rosuvastatin or atorvastatin on urinary albumin excretion and renal function in type 2 diabetic patients. Diabetes Res Clin Pract 2006; 72:81–87.

40. Nissen SE, Nicholls SJ, Sipahi I et al, for the ASTERIOD Investigators. Effect of very high-intensity statin therapy on regression of coronary atherosclerosis: the ASTEROID trial. JAMA 2006; 295:1556–1565.

41. Cannon CP, Braunwald E, McCabe CH et al, for the Pravastatin or Atorvastatin Evaluation and Infection Therapy-Thrombolysis in Myocardial Infraction 22 Investigators. Intensive versus moderate lipid lowering with statins after acute coronary syndromes. N Engl J Med 2004; 350:1495–1504.

42. de Lemos JA, Blazing MA, Wiviott SD et al, for the A to Z investigators. Early intensive vs a delayed conservative simvastatin strategy in patients with acute coronary syndromes: phase Z of the A to Z trial. JAMA 2004; 292:1307–1316.

43. Ahmed S, Cannon CP, Murphy SA, Braunwald E. Acute coronary syndromes and diabetes: is intensive lipid lowering beneficial? Results of the PROVE IT-TIMI 22 trial. Eur Heart J 2006; 27:2323–2329.

44. LaRosa JC, Grundy SM, Waters DD et al, for the Treating to New Targets Investigators. Intensive lipid lowering with atorvastatin in patients with stable coronary disease. N Engl J Med 2005; 352:1425–1435.

45. Shepherd J, Barter P, Carmena R et al, for the Treating to New Targets Investigators. Effect of lowering LDL-C substantially below currently recommended levels in patients with coronary heart disease and diabetes: the Treating to New Targets (TNT) study. Diabetes Care 2006; 29:1220–1226.

46. Pedersen TR, Faergeman O, Kastelein JJ et al. For the Incremental Decrease in End Points through Aggressive Lipid Lowering (IDEAL) Study Group. High-dose atorvastatin vs usual-dose simvastatin for secondary prevention after myocardial infarction: the IDEAL study: a randomized controlled trial. JAMA 2005; 294:2437–2445.

47. Sacks FM, Tonkin AM, Shepherd J et al, for the Prospective Pravastatin Pooling Project Investigators Group. Effect of pravastatin on coronary disease events in subgroups defined by coronary risk factors. The Prospective Pravastatin Pooling Project. Circulation 2000; 102:1893–1900.

48. Game AS, Montori VM, Erwin PJ, Khan MA, Smith SA for the Evidence in Diabetes Enquiry System (EVIDENS) Research Group. Systematic review of lipid lowering for primary prevention of coronary heart disease in diabetes. Br Med J 2003; 326:528–529.

49. Vijan S, Hayward RA. Pharmacologic lipid-lowering therapy in type 2 diabetes mellitus: background paper for the American College of Physicians. Ann Intern Med 2004; 140:650–658.

50. Snow V, Aronson MD, Hornbake ER et al. Lipid control in the management of type 2 diabetes mellitus: a clinical practice guideline from the American College of Physicians. Ann Intern Med 2004; 140:644–649.

51. Costa J, Borges M, David C, Vaz Carneiro A. Efficacy of lipid lowering drug treatment for diabetic and non-diabetic patients: meta-analysis of randomised controlled trails. Br Med J 2006; 332:1115–1118.

52. The Cholesterol Treatment Trialists' (CTT) Collaborators. Efficacy of cholesterol-lowering therapy in 18686 people with diabetes in 14 randomised trials of statins; a meta-analysis. *Lancet* 2008; 371:117–125.

53. Winocour PH, Fisher M. Prediction of cardiovascular risk in people with diabetes. *Diabet Med* 2003: 20:515–527.

54. IDF Clinical Guidelines Task Force. Global Guideline for Type 2 Diabetes; recommendations for standard, comprehensive, and minimal care. *Diabet Med* 2006; 23:579–593.

55. De Backer G, Ambrosioni E, Borch-Johnsen *et al*. ESC European guidelines on cardiovascular disease prevention in clinical practice. Third Joint Task Force of European and Other Societies on Cardiovascular Disease Prevention in Clinical Practice. *Eur Heart J* 2003; 24:1601–1610.

56. American Diabetes Association. Standards of medical care in diabetes. *Diabetes Care* 2006; 29:S4–S42.

57. Tokuno A, Hirano T, Hayashi T *et al*. The effects of statin and fibrate on lowering small dense LDL-cholesterol in hyperlipidemic patients with type 2 diabetes. *J Atheroscler Thromb* 2007; 14:128–132.

58. Wu TJ, Ou HY, Chou CW, Hsiao SH, Lin CY, Kao PC. Decrease in inflammatory cardiovascular risk markers in hyperlipidemic diabetic patients treated with fenofibrate. *Ann Clin Lab Sci* 2007; 37:158–166.

59. Frick MH, Elo O, Haapa K *et al*. Helsinki Heart Study: primary-prevention trial with gemfibrozil in middleaged men with dyslipidemia. Safety of treatment, changes in risk factors, and incidence of coronary heart disease. *N Engl J Med* 1987; 317:1237–1245.

60. Rubins HB, Robins SJ, Collins D *et al*, for the Veterans Affairs High-Density Lipoprotein Cholesterol Intervention Trial Study Group. Gemfibrozil for the secondary prevention of coronary heart disease in men with low levels of high-density lipoprotein cholesterol. *N Engl J Med* 1999; 341:410–418.

61. Rubins HM, Davenport J, Babikian V *et al*. Reduction in stroke with gemfibrozil in men with coronary heart disease and low HDL cholesterol. The veteran affairs HDL intervention trial (VA-HIT). *Circulation* 2001; 103:2828–2833.

62. BIP Study Group. Secondary prevention by raising HDL cholesterol and reducing triglycerides in patients with coronary artery disease: the Bezafibrate Infarction Prevention (BIP) study. *Circulation* 2000; 102:21–27.

63. Diabetes Atherosclerosis Intervention Study Investigators. Effect of fenofibrate on progression of coronary-artery disease in type 2 diabetes: the Diabetes Atherosclerosis Intervention Study, a randomised study. *Lancet* 2001; 357:905–910.

64. Keech A, Simes RJ, Barter P *et al*, for the FIELD Study Investigators. Effects of long-term fenofibrate therapy on cardiovascular events in 9795 people with type 2 diabetes mellitus (the FIELD [Fenofibrate Intervention and Event Lowering in Diabetes] study): randomised controlled trial. *Lancet* 2005; 366:1849–1861.

65. ACCORD study group; Buse JB, Bigger JT, Byington RP *et al*. Action to Control Cardiovascular Risk in Diabetes (ACCORD) trial: design and methods. *Am J Cardiol* 2007; 99:21i-33i.

9

Managing blood pressure in diabetes

J. A. McKnight, P. L. Padfield, M. W. J. Strachan

INTRODUCTION

Diabetes is associated with widespread damage to the vascular system. Higher blood pressure is known to increase the risk of all vascular complications. This manifests clinically as increased macrovascular disease including ischaemic heart disease, cerebrovascular disease and peripheral vascular disease. Added to this is recognised microvascular damage including diabetic retinopathy, nephropathy and neuropathies. It has been estimated, for example, that there is a 15% reduction in the risk of cardiovascular (CV) disease death with each 10 mmHg reduction in systolic blood pressure [1]. The assessment and management of blood pressure is therefore recognised as important in diabetes care.

As the vascular risk associated with blood pressure is continuous, any cut-off target is, by its nature, arbitrary. It is therefore not surprising that guidelines [2] and position statements [3] differ slightly in the targets they set. The Scottish Intercollegiate Guidelines Network (SIGN) recommend a target of <140/80 mmHg and the American Diabetes Association (ADA) <130/80 mmHg. The Joint British Societies' guidelines (JBS 2) [4] suggest an audit standard of 140/80 mmHg in patient groups, such as those with diabetes, that are at higher vascular risk. The key message, however, is that those with diabetes benefit from having a lower blood pressure and, in addition, they may have added benefit from lower targets than that of the general population [5]. Targets may be useful as an overview of performance in populations, but assessment and treatment of the individual patient is influenced by many factors including age, overall risk, complications, side-effects and personal patient preferences.

CHOICE OF THERAPY

The drug or drugs chosen to lower blood pressure in any individual may be influenced by specific circumstances. It is reasonable otherwise to use combinations recommended in the JBS 2 guidelines (Figure 9.1) [6]. In younger (<55 years) patients with diabetes, high blood pressure and no other specific complications, angiotensin converting enzyme (ACE) inhibition or, if this is not tolerated, angiotensin II receptor blockers would be the drugs of choice. If blood

John A. McKnight, MB, BCh, BAO, MD, FRCP (Ed), Consultant Physician, Metabolic Unit, Western General Hospital; Honorary Reader, University of Edinburgh, Edinburgh, UK.

Paul L. Padfield, MB, BCh, FRCP (Edin), MBA, Professor of Hypertension, Consultant Physician, Metabolic Unit, Western General Hospital, Edinburgh, UK.

Mark W. J. Strachan, BSc(Hons), MBChB(Hons), MD, FRCP (Ed), Consultant Physician, Metabolic Unit, Western General Hospital; Honorary Senior Lecturer, University of Edinburgh, Edinburgh, UK.

pressure is not adequately controlled with this therapy, the addition of a thiazide or calcium channel blocker, or both would follow. Other factors that may influence therapeutic choice include the use of β-blockers in angina and α-blockers in benign prostatic hypertrophy. A clear message from many studies, however, is that more than one drug is required to adequately lower blood pressure.

In the remainder of this chapter we will consider some specific clinical situations that involve the assessment and treatment of blood pressure in a specialist diabetes unit.

Case Scenario 1

A 55-year-old female with type 2 diabetes of 5 years known duration is referred because her GP has recorded a blood pressure of 160/96 mmHg (average of three readings). The patient is asymptomatic, appears to manage her diabetes well (glycosylated haemoglobin [HbA1c] = 6.4%) and is taking only metformin 500 mg twice daily.

At her first visit to the diabetes centre, physical examination is unremarkable apart from a blood pressure of 162/102 mmHg. There is no microalbuminuria.

The doctor arranges for a 24-h ambulatory blood pressure recording to be performed. This is reported as showing an awake time average of 138/86 mmHg and a nighttime average of 132/80 mmHg.

THE CLINICAL DILEMMA – BLOOD PRESSURE MEASUREMENT

Higher blood pressure carries a greater risk of cardiovascular disease in the presence of diabetes and, although the evidence is mostly available for type 2 diabetes [1], the increased risks are also evident in type 1 [7]. One question that arises from the case above is: does this patient really have hypertension?

CLINIC BLOOD PRESSURE MEASUREMENT

Clinic measurement of blood pressure (BP) has changed little in 100 years and it is this methodology that has been used in trials that have demonstrated that lowering BP reduces cardiovascular events in patients with diabetes [8]. Blood pressure is extremely labile, however, such that, without any intervening changes in therapy, systolic BP can differ by as much as 30 mmHg over a 2-week period without a change in therapy [9]. Given this degree of inherent variability, it is axiomatic that decisions on blood pressure management should be made on the basis of multiple readings in any given patient. All guidelines stress this fact, but it remains unclear how rigid routine clinic practice is in this regard. It is probably unrealistic to expect that the inherent weaknesses of 'office' blood pressure measurements (patient–doctor interaction, terminal digit preference and other confounding factors) will change and thus there has been a tendency to move from conventional mercury manometry (accelerated by fears of mercury toxicity) to an increasing use of electronic devices, both within the surgery/clinic and in the patient's home environment.

'OUT-OF-OFFICE' BLOOD PRESSURE MEASUREMENT

There are numerous devices available now for the measurement of ambulatory or home BP (see *www.dableducational.com* or *www.bhsoc.org* for validated devices). The term 'ambulatory' is strictly a misnomer, as patients are advised to cease activity when warned (usually by a bleep) of impending cuff inflation. An ambulatory monitor is therefore a tool for obtaining multiple static readings. Self- or home-monitors offer less flexibility and cannot yet measure BP at night but are much cheaper to buy (Figure 9.2).

Ambulatory blood pressure (ABP) monitors are worn relatively unobtrusively and comfortably, usually for 24 hours (h), with blood pressure being recorded every 15–30 minutes during the day and usually every 30 minutes at night. This allows for the calculation of an

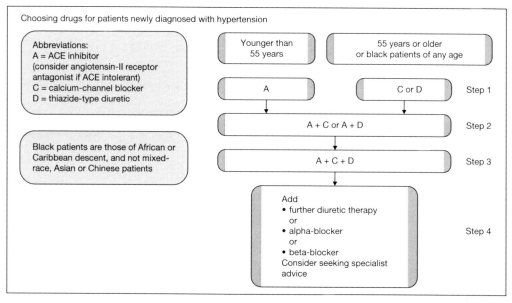

Choosing drugs for patients newly diagnosed with hypertension

Abbreviations:
A = ACE inhibitor
(consider angiotensin-II receptor antagonist if ACE intolerant)
C = calcium-channel blocker
D = thiazide-type diuretic

Black patients are those of African or Caribbean descent, and not mixed-race, Asian or Chinese patients

Younger than 55 years	55 years or older or black patients of any age	
A	C or D	Step 1
A + C or A + D		Step 2
A + C + D		Step 3

Add
• further diuretic therapy
or
• alpha-blocker
or
• beta-blocker
Consider seeking specialist advice — Step 4

Figure 9.1 Choosing a drug or drug combination to treat hypertension (with permission from [6]).

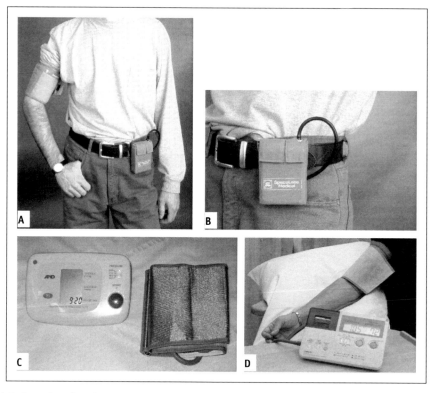

Figure 9.2 Examples of modern ambulatory and self-monitoring technology. **A, B.** Ambulatory monitor: **C.** Self-monitor that links directly to PC. **D.** Self-monitor with printer.

average 'awake time' and 'sleep time' BP. On average, an ambulatory awake time pressure is of the order of 7–10/5 mmHg lower than the clinic BP, but the variation is so great that for an individual patient this difference cannot be predicted.

In case scenario 1, this patient's clinic blood pressure is high by any standards but her ambulatory pressure is significantly lower. The difference between the clinic and the awake time average (24/16 mmHg for this patient) is often referred to as the 'white coat effect' [10]. The term 'white coat hypertension' is reserved for individuals whose clinic/office BP is abnormal (usually defined as ≥140/90 mmHg) but whose daytime ABP is <135/85 mmHg [11, 12]. Approximately 20% of patients with clinic hypertension are normotensive in their own environment [13] and can be described as having 'white coat hypertension'.

In this patient, it should also be noted that there is little difference between the awake- and sleep-time pressures (6/6 mmHg). In most individuals (whatever their level of BP) there is a significant fall of BP at night [13]. Patients in whom nocturnal BP does not fall by at least 10% of the daytime or awake values are usually described as 'non-dippers' [14]. Figure 9.3 shows examples of different ambulatory traces.

There are two polarised views regarding the use of 'out-of-office' BP measurements in clinical medicine. There is the purist's view that argues that, because most intervention trials have used 'clinic' measurements of BP as the guide to treatment, it is not possible to base a management decision on data obtained outside of a clinic setting. The contrary view holds that because both ABP and self blood pressure (SBP) monitoring provide a much better prediction (of future CV risk) than any clinic measurement [15], these 'out-of-office' readings should be considered when managing apparently hypertensive individuals. This observation assumes an even greater significance when one considers the group of individuals who have 'masked' or 'reverse white coat' hypertension [16]. This term describes individuals who have a normal BP in the clinic but who have a high ABP or SBP (Figure 9.3). In keeping with the general observation that it is the 'out-of-office' BP that best predicts risk, it may come as no surprise that such individuals are at greater risk than those with normal ABP/SBP [16]. Figure 9.4 gives a graphic description of the various combinations of ABP/SBP and clinic BP relationships. In summary, all aspects of ambulatory BP: awake, sleep and the dipping status have independent prognostic value that is greater than that obtained by clinic measurements [17, 18].

There is good evidence that the variability of blood pressure reduces dramatically when multiple measurements are averaged [9] and therein lies, perhaps, the major advantage of either ABP monitoring (ABPM) or SBP monitoring (SBPM). Electronic monitoring of blood pressure allows 'out-of-office' measurement on multiple occasions thus ensuring a robust average blood pressure.

While it is true that all published intervention trials have used clinic pressures as a marker of risk, the variability described above means that for individual patients it is difficult to establish a fixed baseline using clinic pressures. Indeed, there is good evidence that clinic measurements (even in the careful setting of a clinical trial) are fallible in the extreme [19].

Definitions of normality and abnormality for 'out-of-office' BP are as difficult as those for conventional blood pressure measurement, given that blood pressure is uniformly distributed throughout the population. Target pressures for intervention are therefore somewhat arbitrary but, given the increased cardiovascular risk in patients with diabetes, are set at lower levels than for management of the general population. Very few hypertension guidelines are explicit about ABP targets in any hypertensive groups, let alone those with diabetes, but the British Hypertension Society (BHS) in their 1999 guidelines [20] highlighted an 'optimal' target of <130/80 mmHg for daytime ABP in non-diabetic patients and <130/75 mmHg for those with diabetes (an audit standard of 140/85 mmHg and 140/80 mmHg respectively was also set).

Ambulatory blood pressure monitors remain expensive and it seems unlikely that their use will become widespread outside of secondary centres. An alternative way of recording blood

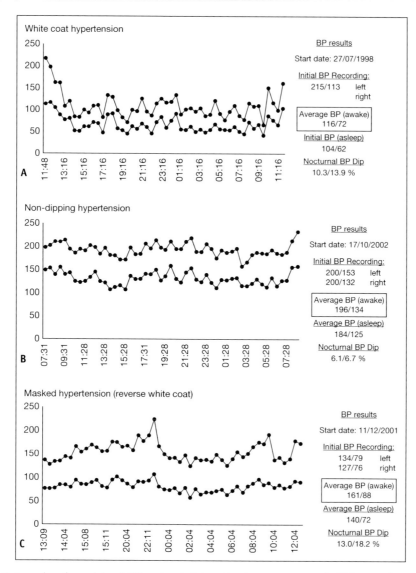

Figure 9.3 Examples of a variety of different ambulatory blood pressure traces. **A.** White coat hypertension; **B.** Non-dipping hypertension: **C.** Masked hypertension (reverse white coat).

pressure outside of the healthcare environment is to use one of the many electronic devices that are suitable for self-monitoring of blood pressure (*www.dableducational.com* or *www.bhsoc. org*). At the moment, these are not capable of measuring blood pressure during sleeping hours but are able to give an average blood pressure through multiple measurements during the waking period, which is broadly similar to that obtained with an ambulatory device. There are fewer data relating self-monitoring blood pressures to clinical outcome than there are for ambulatory pressures, but what information is available suggests that self-monitoring of blood pressure is a better predictor of outcome than clinic/office pressures [21].

Population studies would suggest that the upper limit of 'normal' for both the daytime average blood pressure and for self-monitored blood pressure is of the order of 135/85

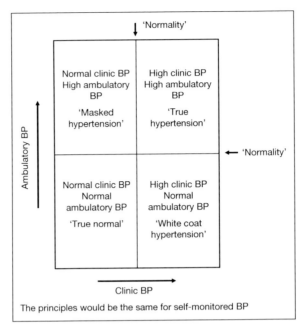

Figure 9.4 Schematic relationship between clinic and ambulatory BP. True hypertensives are at greatest risk of cardiovascular (CV) events; true normals at lowest risk. 'White coat hypertensives (WCH)' and masked hypertensives lie in between, with WCH having a risk close to true normals and masked hypertensives closer to true hypertensives.

mmHg, although this is often described as being (ideally) lower in patients with diabetes (130/80 mmHg). Given the high cardiovascular risk of patients with diabetes and the low level of blood pressure above which drug therapy is suggested, it is clear that most patients with type 2 diabetes will have a level of blood pressure that requires treatment. A recent study suggested that when careful measurement of a clinic BP is made, it is unusual for an ABP measurement to result in a different management decision [22].

In conclusion, the patient in case scenario 1 is hypertensive and warrants aggressive antihypertensive therapy. Future assessment would probably require the use of 'out-of-office' self-monitoring of BP in order to ensure adequate, but not excessive, control.

Case Scenario 2

A 32-year-old woman with a 16-year history of type 1 diabetes attends clinic for initial review. She has recently moved to the area, having been followed-up in another centre for many years. Her glycaemic control over the years has been relatively suboptimal with glycated haemoglobin (HbA1c) concentrations typically between 8–9% (non-diabetic range 5.0–6.5%). Six years ago she had pan-retinal photocoagulation for proliferative diabetic retinopathy and her eyes have been quiescent since then. Her only current medications are insulin lispro and glargine, which she administers in a basal bolus regimen. In the clinic, her blood pressure is 146/92 mmHg and this level is sustained over several repeated measurements. Estimated glomerular filtration rate (GFR) is >90 ml/min/1.73m². Dip-test urinalysis is normal, but the albumin–creatinine ratio is elevated at 21 mg/mmol (normal range 0–3.5 mg/mmol). Urine culture is negative and over the next three weeks she supplies two further urine samples that also demonstrate an elevated albumin–creatinine ratio. Her blood pressure remains elevated when rechecked by her general practitioner.

ANTIHYPERTENSIVE THERAPY IN DIABETIC KIDNEY DISEASE

Hypertension is more common in people with type 1 diabetes than in the general population and is strongly linked to the presence of diabetic kidney disease (DKD) [23]. There can be little doubt that the patient in case scenario 2 has DKD — she has persistent microalbuminuria (urine albumin excretion 30–300 mg/day) in the context of hypertension and proven microvascular disease (i.e. retinopathy). If left untreated, she is at substantial risk of progression to overt diabetic nephropathy (urinary albumin excretion >300mg/day) and is likely to develop end-stage chronic kidney disease [24]. Aside from the morbidity associated with renal replacement therapy, DKD is an independent risk factor for cardiovascular disease [25], although in this case the patient's 10-year cardiovascular risk remains modest because of her young age.

There are a plethora of data demonstrating the importance of blood pressure reduction in DKD, both in terms of reducing progression of the kidney disease and cardiovascular risk. The most studied classes of drugs in DKD are angiotensin-converting enzyme inhibitors (ACEI) and angiotensin II receptor antagonists (AIIRA). Indeed, in a recent Cochrane review, 50 studies (in a total of 13 215 individuals) examining one or other of these agents in patients with DKD were identified [26]. The ACEI studies included patients with either type 1 or type 2 diabetes, or both. However, with the exception of the rate of regression of microalbuminuria to normoalbuminuria, which was greater in people with type 2 diabetes, there was no evidence that the effects of ACEIs were influenced by the type of diabetes. Compared with placebo/no treatment, ACEIs reduced the risk of progression from micro- to macroalbuminuria by 55% (Figure 9.5) and increased by three-fold the chance of microalbuminuria regressing to normoalbuminuria. ACEIs also reduced the risk of progressing to end-stage kidney disease by 40%. Interestingly, ACEIs did not reduce overall mortality, but in a subgroup analysis, studies using ACEIs at the maximum tolerable dose compared to placebo were associated with a 22% reduction in mortality, while studies using ACEIs at half the maximum tolerable dose or less did not demonstrate a survival benefit. Studies involving AIIRAs have primarily been in people with type 2 diabetes and, in the main, they are equally effective, although no overall effect on mortality has been demonstrated.

Non-dihydropyridine calcium channel blockers also have an antiproteinuric effect in DKD and non-diabetic kidney disease [27] and so there is considerable debate as to whether the renoprotective actions of ACEIs and AIIRAs are a specific effect of blockade of the renin–angiotensin system, or whether they are simply a consequence of blood pressure reduction [23]. This is, in essence, a sterile argument though, because individuals with DKD invariably need multiple drugs to achieve the recommended blood pressure target of <130/80 mmHg [23]. Thus, the woman described in the case scenario above should be commenced on an ACEI as first-line therapy and the dose titrated to the maximum recommended (and tolerable) dose. If side-effects develop (e.g. cough), the ACEI should be substituted for an AIIRA. If blood pressure targets are not reached then additional agents should be added, along the lines recommended by the Joint British Societies' Guidelines [4].

ANTIHYPERTENSIVE THERAPY IN WOMEN OF REPRODUCTIVE AGE

There is, though, one crucial area that must additionally be considered in this case — the fact that she is a woman of reproductive age. It has been known for a considerable time that use of ACEIs in the second and third trimesters of pregnancy is associated with multiple abnormalities, including oligohydramnios, fetal renal failure and hypotension, and intra-uterine death [28]. However, recent data also suggest that ACEI use in the first trimester is associated with major congenital malformations of the cardiovascular and central nervous systems [29]. Thus, ACEIs should only be used in sexually active women of reproductive age if

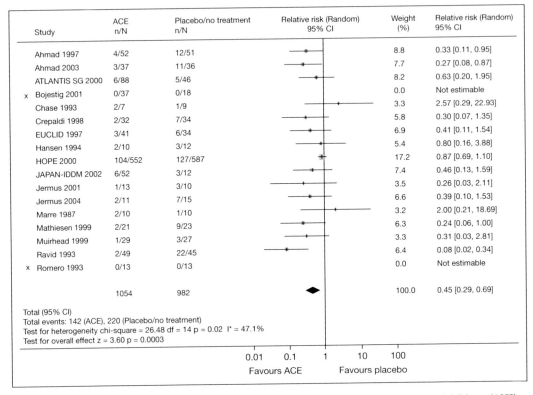

Study	ACE n/N	Placebo/no treatment n/N	Relative risk (Random) 95% CI	Weight (%)	Relative risk (Random) 95% CI
Ahmad 1997	4/52	12/51		8.8	0.33 [0.11, 0.95]
Ahmad 2003	3/37	11/36		7.7	0.27 [0.08, 0.87]
ATLANTIS SG 2000	6/88	5/46		8.2	0.63 [0.20, 1.95]
x Bojestig 2001	0/37	0/18		0.0	Not estimable
Chase 1993	2/7	1/9		3.3	2.57 [0.29, 22.93]
Crepaldi 1998	2/32	7/34		5.8	0.30 [0.07, 1.35]
EUCLID 1997	3/41	6/34		6.9	0.41 [0.11, 1.54]
Hansen 1994	2/10	3/12		5.4	0.80 [0.16, 3.88]
HOPE 2000	104/552	127/587		17.2	0.87 [0.69, 1.10]
JAPAN-IDDM 2002	6/52	3/12		7.4	0.46 [0.13, 1.59]
Jermus 2001	1/13	3/10		3.5	0.26 [0.03, 2.11]
Jermus 2004	2/11	7/15		6.6	0.39 [0.10, 1.53]
Marre 1987	2/10	1/10		3.2	2.00 [0.21, 18.69]
Mathiesen 1999	2/21	9/23		6.3	0.24 [0.06, 1.00]
Muirhead 1999	1/29	3/27		3.3	0.31 [0.03, 2.81]
Ravid 1993	2/49	22/45		6.4	0.08 [0.02, 0.34]
x Romero 1993	0/13	0/13		0.0	Not estimable
	1054	982		100.0	0.45 [0.29, 0.69]

Total (95% CI)
Total events: 142 (ACE), 220 (Placebo/no treatment)
Test for heterogeneity chi-square = 26.48 df = 14 p = 0.02 I² = 47.1%
Test for overall effect z = 3.60 p = 0.0003

0.01   0.1   1   10   100
Favours ACE   Favours placebo

Figure 9.5 Meta-analysis of studies comparing the effects of angiotensin converting enzyme inhibitors (ACEI) to placebo on the progression of micro- to macroalbuminuria in people with diabetes. CI = 95% confidence intervals. N = total number of individuals in treatment arm; n = number of individuals who progressed from micro- to macroalbuminuria. ACEI therapy was associated with a 55% reduction in the risk of progression (with permission from [26]).

adequate contraception is being utilised. AIIRAs should be regarded as posing the same risk to an unborn child as ACEIs [28].

If a woman is not using adequate contraception and/or fertility is required, the decision-making process is more difficult. Women with type 1 diabetes have a 4-fold increased risk of developing pre-eclampsia compared to the general population [30] and some studies have suggested that the risk may be even higher [31]. It is also well established that the risk of pre-eclampsia is higher in women with DKD compared to normoalbuminuric women with type 1 diabetes, and that the risk increases further with higher levels of proteinuria [32]. The evidence that determines the choice of antihypertensive agents to be used in pregnancy is, however, poor. β-blockers tend not to be used in pregnancy because of concerns that they might promote fetal intra-uterine growth retardation [28]. Diuretics are generally not favoured because of their potential to reduce intravascular volume, but in fact one review suggested a possible benefit in terms of reducing the development of pre-eclampsia [33]. Thus, the antihypertensive agents that tend to be used in pregnancy are methyldopa, calcium channel blockers (especially long-acting preparations of nifedipine), hydralazine and labetolol [23]. It is reasonable to use β-blockers, thiazide diuretics or calcium channel blockers for women who do not wish to conceive but are not using adequate contraception, as these are safe and could be reviewed if a pregnancy occurs.

Ideally, all pregnancies in women with diabetes should be planned and the pregnancy itself should be monitored closely in a joint clinic with an experienced obstetrician and diabetologist (Confidential Enquiry into Maternal and Child Health, CEMACH) [34]. Pre-pregnancy planning allows time for a full and frank discussion with the woman and her partner about the risks of pregnancy and, in the context of hypertension, allows appropriate alterations in antihypertensive therapy to be made prior to conception. In the case in question, if the woman is on an ACEI, this should be discontinued and replaced with methyl-dopa or nifedipine. A blood pressure target of <140/80 mmHg would be reasonable, as there are concerns that overly aggressive control of blood pressure can increase the risk of growth retardation of the foetus [35]. When pregnant, the woman and her baby will need to be monitored very closely, although there is limited evidence of the effectiveness of any one technique [2]. While meta-analysis of trials of antihypertensive therapy in pregnancy suggests that the risk of progression to severe hypertension is reduced, there are no significant data that antihypertensive therapy actually reduces the risk of pre-eclampsia [23]. The hope is, though, that antihypertensive therapy allows the pregnancy to progress further, so that if pre-term delivery is required, the baby has the best possible chance of survival.

Case Scenario 3

A 33-year-old patient with type 1 diabetes for 12 years is reported to have developed background retinopathy. Diabetes control used to be poor but in recent years his HbA1c has averaged 7.5%. His blood pressure is 128/80 mmHg. He has had a screen for microalbuminuria within the last month and this was negative.

This man's blood pressure is in the normal range for the population. He has, however, developed some vascular damage. The main risk factors for retinopathy are duration of diabetes (he has only had diabetes for 12 years), glycaemic control, smoking, higher blood pressure and nephropathy. As part of his assessment, he should be asked about smoking.

There is evidence that treatment of blood pressure in the United Kingdom Prospective Diabetes Study (UKPDS) [8] significantly decreased the progression of retinopathy in people with type 2 diabetes, though the pressures in this study were significantly higher (154/87 mmHg vs. 144/82 mmHg) than those of this patient. In type 1 diabetes, the only well proven strategy to prevent progression of retinopathy is tight glycaemic control [36]. There has been some interest in the potential role of ACEIs or AIIRB therapy to prevent retinopathy progression and there are some ongoing studies [37]. The effect of lisinopril on progression of retinopathy in normotensive (blood pressure 123/81 mmHg) people with type 1 diabetes was studied as part of the EUCLID study [38]. Retinopathy progression was reduced, but methodological concerns have been raised regarding this paper [2]. The authors concluded that large randomised controlled studies are required before changes of clinical practice are advocated.

The approach to this patient would therefore be to encourage improved diabetes control if possible. It would be reasonable to discuss the weak evidence for ACE inhibition with the patient and reach a conclusion with him whether or not to start therapy, based on his preference. This therapy could be introduced on a trial basis and withdrawn if there were any significant side-effects.

Case Scenario 4

A 58-year-old man is referred back to the clinic. Diabetes was diagnosed 5 years ago. He has been treated with metformin and a statin. He has a history of intermittent claudication but continues to smoke 40 cigarettes each day. High blood pressure (168/94 mmHg) was noted by his primary care physician 2 years ago and initially treated with a thiazide diuretic (bendroflumethazide 2.5 mg daily). At this time, his serum potassium was noted to be 3.2 mmol/l. Three months ago, lisinopril 10 mg

Table 9.1 Potentially correctable causes of hypertension

Group	Disorders
Drug ingestion	OCP, NSAIDs, liquorice, glucocorticoids
Renal	Renovascular disease, polycystic kidneys, chronic renal failure (all causes)
Adrenal cortex	Primary hyperaldosteronism, Cushing's syndrome, some adrenal enzyme defects
Adrenal medulla	Phaeochromocytoma
Other endocrine disorders	Acromegaly, hypothyroidism
Miscellaneous	Coarctation of the aorta, sleep apnoea syndrome

NSAIDs = non-steroidal anti-inflammatory drugs; OCP = oral contraceptive pill.

was added to his therapy. His serum creatinine was 110 μmol/l before starting ACEI and increased to 145 μmol/l but remained stable at this concentration. The albumin–creatinine ratio was 21 mg/ mmol. The referral letter suggested investigations for 'secondary causes of hypertension' might be considered.

WHEN AND HOW TO INVESTIGATE FOR A SECONDARY CAUSE OF HYPERTENSION

The true prevalence of secondary hypertension is unknown. Various published estimates are usually based upon selected populations and an oft-quoted figure is <1% of unselected hypertensive patients. Whilst it is intuitively attractive to think that detection and correction of a secondary cause of hypertension is in the best interests of a patient, this has never been established for any of the secondary causes. Although, therefore, there is no evidence that a missed secondary cause in a patient with well controlled BP is a cause for concern, most would hope to recognise the historical and clinical clues of a patient with a phaeochromocytoma and as this is relatively non-controversial, we will discuss it no more here.

The usual causes of hypertension that are considered are outlined in Table 9.1 and, in the assessment of any patient with hypertension, a careful drug history should detect those agents that might cause an increase in BP (e.g. oral contraceptive pill, OCP) and those that may significantly compromise the efficacy of many anti-hypertensive agents (e.g. non-steroidal anti-inflammatory drugs, NSAIDs). It is to be hoped that acromegaly and Cushing's syndrome would be suspected clinically and, as both of these conditions can give rise to diabetes mellitus, it is particularly important that clinic doctors remain vigilant.

The condition to consider in the patient described in case scenario 4, who is already demonstrating vascular disease, is renovascular hypertension.

RENAL ARTERY STENOSIS

Atheromatous disease accounts for more than 90% of all cases of renal artery stenosis (RAS). The true prevalence of this condition is uncertain but it has been noted in 30% of patients with coronary artery disease [39] and 50% of elderly patients or those with diffuse atherosclerotic vascular disease [40]. It seems clear also that the prevalence increases with age and is commoner in patients with diabetes [41]. Finally, up to 14% of patients beginning dialysis in the USA have atherosclerotic renal artery stenosis [42] and, in such situations, this is invariably bilateral in nature (Figure 9.6). Atheromatous renal artery stenosis is thus a common and progressive disorder that may or may not be clinically apparent [43]. As indicated above it remains uncertain as to how important it is that this condition is detected, let alone treated directly.

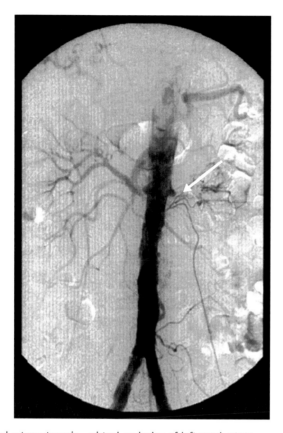

Figure 9.6 Bilateral renal artery stenosis – virtual occlusion of left renal artery.

PATHOGENESIS OF HYPERTENSION IN RAS

Current ideas on how BP increases with RAS are based largely on animal experiments such as those where a clip is placed around the renal artery of a young rat. BP increases almost immediately and this is paralleled by a rise in plasma levels of renin. That the increase in pressure is a direct effect of angiotensin II is supported by the fact that blockade of the production of angiotensin II or its action can abolish the rise in BP, i.e. BP rises as a direct pressor effect of angiotensin II. At the stage where BP and renin are elevated, removal of the clip corrects the hypertension. If the clip is left *in situ* BP remains high while renin falls towards baseline. At this stage, the hypertension is still correctable by removal of the clip and presumably a different mechanism for hypertension must exist (possibly via salt and water retention). This effect can be mimicked by infusion of sub-pressor doses of angiotensin II in either animals or man [44]. Ultimately, a stage is reached in the rat where removal of the clip does not correct the hypertension and, it is hypothesised, irreversible changes in the arterioles of the contralateral kidney or wider vascular bed result in an ongoing elevation of BP due to increases in total peripheral resistance [45]. How all of this relates to the human situation is a matter of conjecture, although it is well known that most patients with RAS and hypertension have normal circulating levels of renin and the renin level is a poor predictor of the BP response to revascularisation.

RENOVASCULAR HYPERTENSION

The term renovascular hypertension is specific and should be reserved for patients in whom correction of RAS reduces or normalises BP. The coexistence of RAS and hypertension does not therefore necessarily indicate causality and this is a major dilemma in managing such patients. RAS may cause hypertension, hypertension may induce atherogenesis and cause RAS, or the two may simply be epiphenomena.

RAS can cause both hypertension and renal failure but whether or not revascularisation is clinically beneficial remains uncertain [46]. The potential for relatively non-invasive correction of RAS with the advent of renal artery angioplasty and stenting has resulted in an explosion of non-controlled studies, and much of what is published in the literature is probably of little value in helping the discerning physician decide whether to look for or treat RAS. The increased frequency of so-called 'drive-by' renal angiography [47] during procedures for coronary imaging has resulted in an increase in renal artery interventions [48]. The authors have recently been very critical of such guidelines [49]. One of us was also part of an early randomised controlled trial of renal artery angioplasty versus medical therapy in hypertensive patients with unilateral or bilateral RAS [50]. The patient numbers were small, but there appeared to be a benefit in terms of BP reduction in patients with bilateral disease. The study was not powered to address changes in renal function. Shortly thereafter, the larger DRASTIC (Dutch Renal Artery Stenosis Intervention Cooperative) study group [51] published negative results, although there was much crossing-over of patients between the medical and intervention groups. A striking observation made during recruitment for this study was that, amongst patients with resistant hypertension (defined as poor BP control on two or more drugs), there was a 20% *prevalence* of significant RAS. We still do not know what to do about RAS, and most guidelines are based upon expert opinion only [52]. A recent issue of the journal *Circulation* published a debate on the pros and cons of intervention [53, 54] and many observers await the outcome of the large prospective, randomised CORAL (Cardiovascular Outcomes in Renal Atherosclerotic Lesions) trial, which, hopefully, will answer the main questions as to whether revascularisation of RAS will control BP and/or prevent the decline in renal function [55].

In the meantime, what advice can we give to the practicing clinician looking after patients with diabetes, a group with a high prevalence of vascular disease?

- Treat blood pressure aggressively with multiple drugs and do not search for RAS if BP is controlled.
- Consider looking for RAS in:
  - Hypertensive patients under 25 years of age (may have the fibromuscular hyperplastic form of RAS).
  - Patients where renal function deteriorates on an ACEI or angiotensin II receptor blockers (ARB).
  - Patients with truly resistant hypertension (three or even four drugs), particularly if they have overt vascular disease elsewhere.
  - Patients with 'flash' pulmonary oedema: these have relatively normal left ventricular systolic function but have repeated attacks of pulmonary oedema.
  - Patients presenting with malignant or accelerated phase hypertension: note that although the prevalence of RAS might be high in this group, it remains arguable whether to look for it if BP is well controlled with drugs.

The patient in case scenario 4 has had an increase of serum creatinine since the introduction of ACEI of around 30%, but this has stabilised and is not continuing to increase. He may well have renovascular disease. So long as his blood pressure remains controlled and renal function is stable we would not investigate further at this stage. He should continue to be prescribed an ACEI. We urge caution in the search for RAS in the absence of good evidence of benefit from intervention.

PRIMARY HYPERALDOSTERONISM

A form of secondary hypertension that has received much attention in recent years is the autonomous secretion of the adrenal mineralocorticoid aldosterone. On 29 October 1954, Jerome Conn gave his presidential address at the 27th Annual Meeting of the Central Society for Clinical Research in the United States of America [56]. He described a female patient with hypertension who was cured by the removal of an adrenal tumour that secreted aldosterone. This condition has since been eponymously named Conn's syndrome. Renin had been known about for over 50 years and as assays became available for the measurement of renin activity in plasma, aldosterone in urine and subsequently plasma, it has become clear that Conn's syndrome of aldosterone excess resulted in sodium retention and suppression of renin. The hallmark of Conn's syndrome was high aldosterone production with a suppressed renin. Initially, all patients investigated had hypokalaemia and it became apparent that not all patients with low renin–aldosterone excess had an adrenal adenoma [57]. In early series, about a quarter of such patients had what came to be called idiopathic hyperplasia or pseudohyperaldosteronism [58]. These patients did not have a discreet tumour but had nodular adrenal glands [59]. Some nodules could be large, being indistinguishable from true tumours when using a variety of imaging techniques [60]. While the removal of an aldosterone-producing adrenal adenoma resulted in cure of hypertension in at least 70% of cases, surgery for nodular hyperplasia did not [61]. There were even examples in the literature of patients who had both adrenal glands removed but who remained hypertensive following replacement therapy. This is not surprising if it is appreciated that the nodules from hyperplastic glands do not make aldosterone whereas tumours do [62]. This observation threw into question the whole notion of what so-called primary hyperaldosteronism meant. Diagnosing primary aldosterone excess has always been difficult because most of the drugs that are used in the treatment of hypertension have an effect on the renin–angiotensin–aldosterone axis. Drugs either stimulate (diuretics, ACEI) or suppress (β-blockers) renin. The observation that no drugs simultaneously suppress renin while stimulating aldosterone led to arguments that the ratio of aldosterone to renin (aldosterone–renin ratio, ARR) might be a good screening test for primary aldosterone excess and this was first demonstrated in 1981 [63]. It is important to remember, however, that primary hyperaldosteronism is not identical with Conn's syndrome and most of the cases diagnosed through the use of ARR turn out to have idiopathic hyperplasia. A recent review highlights current thinking around an apparent explosion of primary hyperaldosteronism such that up to 15% of unselected hypertensive subjects may have this condition [64]. Discovering a high ARR is just the beginning, however, and further confirmatory investigations include saline or fludrocortisone suppression tests (to show that the aldosterone production is autonomous) [65]. This is then followed by imaging such as computed tomography (CT) scanning or the use of radiolabelled cholesterol (Figure 9.7). The limitations of CT scanning have led some to argue that adrenal venous sampling is necessary to determine the presence of unilateral aldosterone production [66]. The cost-effectiveness of this approach has been challenged [67], as most cases do not have a surgically correctable problem. Indeed, Kaplan has suggested that, in the USA, it might cost US$250 000 (at year 2000 prices), to detect one curable case of Conn's syndrome [67]. The way the ARR is used has also changed over time. It is now largely accepted that many drugs can affect the ratio, particularly β-blockers and, because the ratio is largely driven by a low renin, many now advocate the presence of a high aldosterone as well.

Perhaps the most interesting development has been the suggestion that mineralocorticoid antagonists such as spironolactone might have an increasing role to play in the manage-

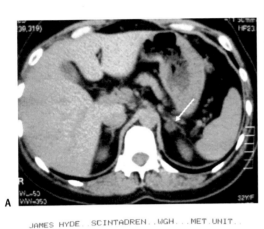
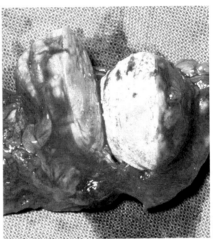
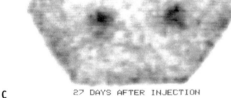

Figure 9.7 Primary hyperaldosteronism. A. CT scan (Conn's tumour, arrowed): B. Surgical specimen (Conn's tumour): C. Seleno-cholesterol scan (hyperplasia).
CT = computed tomography.

ment of patients with resistant hypertension [68], a view supported by the latest publication to come out of the ASCOT (Anglo-Scandavian Cardiac Outcomes Trial) study [69].

It is difficult to be sure how these observations on primary hyperaldosteronism are relevant in the management of the patient with diabetes in case scenario 4. The presence of hypokalaemia, particularly if unprovoked by diuretic therapy, should still raise the spectre of aldosterone excess in patients with diabetes. A pragmatic trial of spironolactone in all patients resistant to three drugs is probably the best management strategy.

Whether we should chase a secondary cause in this or similar patients is moot: the evidence base for reducing cardiovascular events by effective drug treatment in the hypertensive diabetic patient is overwhelming and the cost-effectiveness of a strategy of 'chasing the rainbow' is far from clear. Be wary of evangelists!

ORGANISING CARE

It has been recognised for many years that many people with high blood pressure are not diagnosed and, of those diagnosed, a significant proportion are not treated or do not achieve ideal blood pressures [70]. This is despite the evidence of successful reduction of vascular events with multifactorial intervention [71]. Standard systems to organise care do not seem to be very successful in addressing this. It is possible that new initiatives such as payment-by-results [72] will be of positive influence. There has been recent work describing protocol-driven nurse- or pharmacist-provided care that has shown good improvement in blood pressure control using a more intensive intervention than that usually available and that the decrease of blood pressure is sustained [73, 74]. In one such study, the blood pressure decreased significantly despite the addition of little more antihypertensive therapy, suggesting that the benefit may relate to improved concordance with prescribed therapy. There is strong evidence to support the concern that patients with diabetes may not take all of their prescribed medication [75], particularly when prescribed multiple-dose rather than single-dose therapy. This was shown in diabetes for oral hypoglycaemic agents. It would be surprising if concordance with antihypertensive medication were any different.

Case Scenario 5

An 82-year-old woman presents to the medical assessment area of her local hospital with a 5-day history of diarrhoea and vomiting. She has an 8-year history of diabetes and hypertension. Her current therapy is metformin 500 mg thrice-daily, lisinopril 20 mg daily, bendroflumethiazide 2.5 mg daily and amlodipine 10 mg daily. At a diabetes clinic 1 month ago her HbA1c was noted to be 7.2 %, blood pressure 138/76 mmHg, and serum creatinine 72 µmol/l. There was no microalbuminuria. Assessment on admission revealed a glucose of 12 mmol/l, a serum creatinine of 210 µmol/l and a urea of 24 mmol/l. Her blood pressure was 100/68 mmHg.

As diabetes physicians, we attempt to give good advice regarding the management of glucose control during sick days. This is particularly important in those with type 1 diabetes. We actively encourage these individuals to continue insulin when they are unable to eat to prevent diabetic ketoacidosis. Many older patients are admitted to hospital with dehydration and renal failure due to a dehydrating illness such as gastroenteritis. In this situation, continuing to take ACE inhibitors, diuretics and metformin may be positively harmful. It is difficult to estimate the precise contribution of therapy to the overall condition of the patient in case scenario 5. If she had stopped her medication when becoming dehydrated, it is likely that her renal failure would have been less severe. It is appropriate to advise patients starting such therapy that it might be best to discontinue their antihypertensive treatment during an acute dehydrating illness.

SUMMARY

The measurement, assessment and treatment of blood pressure in diabetes results in some interesting clinical dilemmas. There is a lot of information in the medical literature that can guide a clinician in his or her decision making. Often, many factors have to be considered and a pragmatic solution reached that balances the risks and benefits to the individual patient.

REFERENCES

1. Adler AI, Stratton IM, Neil HA *et al.* Association of systolic blood pressure with the macrovascular and microvascular complications of type 2 diabetes (UKPDS 36). United Kingdom Prospective Diabetes Study Group. *Br Med J* 2000; 321:412–419.
2. SIGN 55 Management of diabetes. Scottish Intercollegiate Guidelines Network. Edinburgh. 2001 (*www.sign.ac.uk*).
3. American Diabetes Association Clinical Practice Recommendations 2006. *Diabetes Care* 2006; 29(Suppl 1): S4–S42.

4. British Cardiac Society, British Hypertension Society, Diabetes UK, HEART UK, Primary Care Cardiovascular Society, The Stroke Association. JBS2: Joint British Societies' guidelines on prevention of cardiovascular disease in clinical practice. *Heart* 2005; 91:1–52(doi:10.1136/hrt.2005.079988).

5. Hansson L, Zanchetti A, Carruthers SG *et al.* Effects of intensive blood-pressure lowering and low-dose aspirin in patients with hypertension: principal results of the Hypertension Optimal Treatment (HOT) randomised trial. HOT Study Group. *Lancet* 1998; 351:1755–1762.

6. Williams B, Poulter NR, Brown MJ *et al.* British Hypertension Society Guidelines. Guidelines for management of hypertension: report of the fourth working party of the British Hypertension Society, 2004 – BHS IV. *J Hum Hypertens* 2004; 18:139–185.

7. Royal College of Physicians of Edinburgh Diabetes Register Group. Predicting vascular risk in type 1 diabetes: stratification in a hospital based population in Scotland. *Diabet Med* 2005; 22:164–171.

8. UK Prospective Diabetes Study Group. Tight blood pressure control and risk of macrovascular and microvascular complications in type 2 diabetes: UKPDS 38. *Br Med J* 1998; 317:703–713.

9. Padfield, Paul L. Self-monitored blood pressure: a role in clinical practice? *Blood Pressure Monitoring* 2002; 7:41–44.

10. O'Brien E, Asmar R, Beilin L *et al.* European Society of Hypertension Working Group on Blood Pressure Monitoring. Practice guidelines of the European Society of Hypertension for clinic, ambulatory and self blood pressure measurement. *J Hypertens* 2005; 4:697–701.

11. Verdecchia P, Staessen JA, White WB *et al.* Properly defining white coat hypertension. *Eur Heart J* 2002; 23:106–109.

12. Messerli FH, Coliga D. Masked hypertension and white coat hypertension: therapeutic navigation between Scylla and Charybdis. *J Am Coll Cardiol* 2005; 546:516–517.

13. Pickering TG, Shimbo D, Haas D. Ambulatory blood pressure monitoring. *N Engl J Med* 2006; 354:2368–2374.

14. Giles TD. Circadian rhythm of blood pressure and the relation to cardiovascular events. *J Hypertens* 2006; 24(Suppl 2):S11-S16.

15. Sega R, Facchetti R, Bombelli M *et al.* Prognostic value of ambulatory and home blood pressures compared with office blood pressure in the general population: follow up results from the PAMELA study. *Circulation* 2005; 111:1777–1783.

16. O'Brien. Unmasking hypertension. *Hypertension* 2005; 45:481–482.

17. Staessen JA, Thijs L, Fagard R *et al*, for the Systolic Hypertension in Europe Trial Investigators. Predicting cardiovascular risk using conventional vs ambulatory blood pressure in older patients with systolic hypertension. *JAMA* 1999; 282:539–546.

18. Clement DL, de Buyzere ML, Bacquer DA *et al.* Prognostic value of ambulatory blood pressure readings in patients with treated hypertension. *N Engl J Med* 2003; 348:2407–2415.

19. Benediktsson R, Padfield PL. Maximizing the benefit of treatment in mild hypertension: three simple steps to improve diagnostic accuracy. *Quart J Med* 2004; 97:15–20.

20. Ramsay LE, Williams B, Johnston GD *et al.* British Hypertension Society Guidelines for Hypertension Management 1999: Summary. *Br Med J* 1999; 319:630–635.

21. Verberk WJ, Kroon AA, Kessels AGH *et al.* Home blood pressure measurement, a systematic review. *J Am Coll Cardiol* 2005; 46:743–751.

22. Strachan MW, Gough K, McKnight JA, Padfield PL. Ambulatory blood pressure monitoring: is it necessary for the routine assessment of hypertension in people with diabetes? *Diabet Med* 2002; 19:787–789.

23. Williams B, Poulter NR, Brown MJ *et al.* Guidelines for management of hypertension: report of the fourth working party of the British Hypertension Society, 2004 – BHS IV. *J Hum Hypertens* 2004; 18:139–185.

24. Hovind P, Rossing P, Tarnow L, Smidt UM, Parving HH. Progression of diabetic nephropathy. *Kidney Int* 2001; 59:702–709.

25. Fuller JH, Stevens LK, Wang SL. Risk factors for cardiovascular mortality and morbidity: the WHO Mutinational Study of Vascular Disease in Diabetes. *Diabetologia* 2001; 44(Suppl 2):S55-S64.

26. Strippoli GFM, Bonifati C, Craig M, Navaneethan SD, Craig JC. Angiotensin converting enzyme inhibitors and angiotensin II receptor antagonists for preventing the progression of diabetic kidney disease. Cochrane Database of Systematic Reviews 2006, Issue 4, Art No.: CD006257.

27. Bakris GL, Weir MR, Secic M, Campbell B, Weis-McNulty A. Differential effects of calcium antagonist subclasses on markers of nephropathy progression. *Kidney Int* 2004: 65:1991–2002.

28. Briggs GG. Drug effects on the fetus and breast-fed infant. *Clin Obstet Gynecol* 2002; 45:6–21.

29. Cooper WO, Hernandez-Diaz S, Arbogast PG *et al*. Major congenital malformations after first-trimester exposure to ACE inhibitors. *N Engl J Med* 2006; 354:2443–2451.
30. Duckitt K, Harrington D. Risk factors for pre-eclampsia at antenatal booking: systematic review of controlled studies. *Br Med J* 2005; 330:565.
31. Evers IM, de Walk, HW, Visser GHA. Risk of complications of pregnancy in women with type 1 diabetes: nationwide prospective study in The Netherlands. *Br Med J* 2004; 323:915.
32. Ekbom P, Damm P, Feldt-Rasmussen B, Feldt-Rasmussen U, Molvig J, Mathiesen ER. Pregnancy outcome in type 1 diabetic women with microalbuminuria. *Diabetes Care* 2001; 24:1739–1744.
33. Collins R, Yusuf S, Petor R. Overview of randomised trials of diuretics in pregnancy. *Br Med J* 1985; 290;17–23.
34. Confidential Enquiry into Maternal and Child Health. Maternity services in 2002 for women with type 1 and type 2 diabetes. *RCOG Press* 2004; London.
35. von Dadelszen P, Ornstein MP, Bull SP, Logan AG, Koren G, Magee LA. Fall in mean arterial pressure and fetal growth restriction in pregnancy hypertension: a meta-analysis. *Lancet* 2000; 355:87–92.
36. Diabetes Control and Complications Trial Research Group. The effect of intensive treatment of diabetes on the development and progression of long-term complications in insulin-dependent diabetes mellitus. *New Engl J Med* 1993; 329:977–986.
37. Sjolie AK, Porta M, Parving HH, Bilous R, Klein R. The DIRECT Programme Study Group The DIabetic REtinopathy Candesartan Trials (DIRECT) Programme: baseline characteristics. *J Renin Angiotensin Aldosterone Syst* 2005; 6:25–32.
38. Chaturvedi N, Sjolie A-K, Stephenson JM, Abrahamian H. Effect of lisinopril on progression of retinopathy in normotensive people with type 1 diabetes. *Lancet* 1998; 351:28–31.
39. Harding MB, Smith LR, Himmelstein SI *et al*. Renal artery stenosis: prevalence and associated risk factors in patients undergoing routine cardiac catheterisation. *J Am Soc Nephrol* 1992; 2:1608–1616.
40. Missouris CG, Buckenham T, Cappuccio FP *et al*. Renal artery stenosis: a common and important problem in patients with peripheral vascular disease. *Am J Med* 1994; 96:10–14.
41. Sawacki PT, Kaiser S, Heinemann I *et al*. Prevalence of renal artery stenosis in diabetes mellitus – an autopsy study. *Ann Int Med* 1991; 229:489–492.
42. United States Renal Data System, 1997 annual data report. NIH, National Institute of diabetes and digestive and kidney diseases, 1997.
43. Safian RD, Textor SC. Renal artery stenosis. *N Engl J Med* 2001; 344:431–442.
44. Lever AF. The fast and slowly developing pressor effect of angiotensin II. In: Robertson JIS, Nichols GM (eds). *The Renin-Angiotensin System*. Gower Medical Publishing, London, 1993, Vol 1; 28: pp 1–9.
45. Robertson JIS, Renin and the pathophysiology of renovascular hypertension In: Robertson JIS, Nichols GM (eds). *The Renin-Angiotensin System*. Gower Medical Publishing, London, 1993, Vol 2; 55: pp 1–34.
46. Balk E, Raman G, Chung M *et al*. Effectiveness of management strategies for renal artery stenosis: a systematic review. *Ann Int Med* 2006; 145:901–912.
47. White CJ, Jaff MR, Haskal ZJ *et al*. Indications for renal arteriography at the time of coronary arteriography: a science advisory from the American Heart Association Committee on Diagnostic and Interventional Cardiac Catheterization, Council on Clinical Cardiology, and the Councils on Cardiovascular Radiology and Intervention and on Kidney in Cardiovascular Disease. *Circulation* 2006; 114:1892–1895.
48. Levin A, Linas S, Luft FC *et al*, on behalf of the ASN HTN Advisory Group, Denver Health Medical Center, Denver, Colo., USA. Controversies in renal artery stenosis: a review by the American Society of Nephrology Advisory Group on Hypertension. *Am J Nephrol* 2007; 27:212–220.
49. Dear JW, Padfield PL, Webb DJ. New guidelines for drive-by renal arteriography may lead to an undesirable increase in percutaneous intervention. *Heart* 2007; 93:1528–1532.
50. Webster J, Marshall F, Abdalla M *et al*. Randomised comparison of percutaneous angioplasty vs continued medical therapy for hypertensive patients with atheromatous renal artery stenosis. Scottish and Newcastle Renal Artery Stenosis Collaborative Group. *J Hum Hypertens* 1998; 12:329–335.
51. van Jaarsveld BC, Krijnen P, Pieterman H *et al*. The effect of balloon angioplasty on hypertension in atherosclerotic renal-artery stenosis. Dutch Renal Artery Stenosis Intervention Cooperative Study Group. *N Engl J Med* 2000; 342:1007–1114.
52. Lerman LO, Chade AR. Atherosclerotic process, renovascular disease and outcomes from bench to bedside. *Curr Opin Nephrol Hypertens* 2006; 15:583–587.
53. Cooper CJ, Murphy TP. The case for renal artery stenting for treatment of renal artery stenosis. *Circulation* 2007; 115:263–270.

54. Dworkin LD, Jamerson KA. Case against angioplasty and stenting of atherosclerotic renal artery stenosis. *Circulation* 2007; 115:271–276.

55. Cooper CJ, Murphy TP, Matsumoto A *et al.* Stent revascularization for the prevention of cardiovascular and renal events among patients with renal artery stenosis and systolic hypertension: rationale and design of the CORAL trial. *Am Heart J* 2006; 152:59–66.

56. Conn JW. Primary aldosteronism, a new clinical syndrome. *J Lab Clin Med* 1955; 45:3–17.

57. Young WF, Hogan MJ, Klee GG, Grant CS, van Heerden JA. Primary aldosteronism: diagnosis and treatment. *Mayo Clin Proc* 1990; 65:96–110.

58. Baer L, Brunner HR, Buhler F, Laragh JA. Pseudo-primary aldosteronism, a variant of low-renin essential hypertension? In: *Hypertension.* Henest J, Loiw E (eds). Springer Verlag, Berlin, 1972, pp 459–472.

59. Padfield PL, Brown JJ, Davies DL *et al.* The myth of idiopathic hyperaldosteronism, *Lancet* 1981; 2:83–84.

60. Radin DR, Manoogian C, Nadicr JL. Diagnosis of primary hyperaldosteronism: importance of correlating CT findings with endocrinologic studies. *Am J Roentgenol* 1992; 158:553–557.

61. Spark RF, Melby JC. Aldosteronism in hypertension: the spironolactone response test. *Ann Intern Med* 1968; 169:685–695.

62. Neville AM, O'Hare MJ, The human adrenal gland: aspects of structure, function and pathology. In: *The Human Adrenal Gland.* James VHT (ed). Academic Press, London, 1979.

63. Hiramatsu K, Yamada T, Jukimura Y *et al.* A screening test to identify aldosterone-producing adenoma by measuring plasma renin activity, *Arch Intern Med* 1981; 141:1589–1594.

64. Young WF. Primary aldosteronism: renaissance of a syndrome. *Clin Endoc* 2007; 66:607–618.

65. Stowasser M, Gordon RD. Monogenic mineralocorticoid hypertension. *Best Pract Res Clin Endocrinol Metab* 2006; 20:401–420.

66. Young WF. Primary aldosteronism: diagnosis. In: Mansoor GA (ed). *Secondary Hypertension: Clinical Presentation, Diagnosis and Treatment.* Humana Press, Totowa, NJ, 2004, pp 119–137.

67. Kaplan NM. Cautions over the current epidemic of primary aldosteronism. *Lancet* 2001; 357:953–954.

68. Lim PO, Jung RT, MacDonald TM. Raised aldosterone to renin ratio predicts antihypertensive efficacy of spironolactone: a prospective cohort follow-up study, *Br J Clin Pharmacol* 1999; 48:756–760.

69. Chapman N, Dobson J, Wilson S *et al*, Anglo-Scandinavian Cardiac Outcomes Trial Investigators. Effect of spironolactone on blood pressure in subjects with resistant hypertension. *Hypertension* 2007; 49:839–845.

70. Eliasson B, Cederholm J, Nilsson P, Gudbjornsdottir S. The gap between guidelines and reality: type 2 diabetes in a national diabetes register 1996–2003. *Diabet Med* 2005; 22:1420–1426.

71. Gaede P, Vedel P, Larsen N, Jensen GV, Parving HH, Pedersen O. Multifactorial intervention and cardiovascular disease in patients with type 2 diabetes. *N Engl J Med* 2003; 348:383–393.

72. Doran T, Fullwood C, Gravelle H *et al.* Pay-for-performance programs in family practices in United Kingdom. *N Engl J Med* 2006; 355:375–384.

73. Cockburn AJ, McKnight JA, Kinnear M, Lannigan NA, Strachan MWJ. Impact of a pharmacist-led cardiovascular risk reduction clinic on cardiovascular risk factor targets in people with diabetes. *Diabet Med* 2005; 22(Suppl 2):62.

74. Woodward A, Wallymahmed M, Wilding J, Gill G. Successful cardiovascular risk reduction in type 2 diabetes by nurse-led care using an open clinical algorithm. *Diabet Med* 2006; 23:780–787.

75. Donnan PT, MacDonald TM, Morris AD. Adherence to prescribed oral hypoglycaemic medication in a population of patients with type 2 diabetes: a retrospective cohort study. *Diabet Med* 2001; 19:279–284.

10

Angiotensin converting enzyme inhibitors and angiotensin receptor blockers

J. Segura, L. M. Ruilope

INTRODUCTION

The prevalence of diabetes mellitus is rising rapidly, especially in the developed countries of the world. Based on current definitions, type 2 diabetes mellitus affects around 12% of those aged 40–74 years and almost 20% of those aged over 74 years in industrialised countries [1]. The current prevalence of 150 million affected subjects worldwide is projected to increase to 220 million by 2010 and to 300 million by 2025 [2].

Diabetes mellitus is characterised by an increased prevalence of cardiovascular and renal disease, which account for the great majority of deaths in this population [3]. Both are facilitated by the same risk factors, which frequently include high blood pressure, dyslipidaemia, obesity and smoking. In order to control cardiovascular and renal risk it is mandatory to attain a strict control of all of the different factors participating in the process [4]. Suppression of the renin–angiotensin system is very important in this respect and can be obtained either by the administration of an angiotensin-converting enzyme inhibitor (ACEI) or an angiotensin receptor blocker (ARB). The aim of this chapter is to review the evidence in favour of both forms of therapy in diabetic patients as well as in those prone to becoming diabetic.

PREVENTION OF CARDIOVASCULAR MORBIDITY AND MORTALITY IN DIABETIC PATIENTS

A recent meta-analysis of data from 61 prospective observational studies on mortality from vascular disease among subjects without previous vascular disease has shown that blood pressure (BP) levels are strongly associated with the age-specific mortality rates from stroke; almost as strongly as with the mortality rates from ischaemic heart disease and with those from other vascular causes [5] (Figures 10.1–10.3). Among people with no previous vascular disease, the usual BP values are positively related to the risks of death from vascular disease, not only among subjects who might be considered hypertensive, but also among those who would usually be considered normotensive (at least down to 'normal' BP levels of 115/75 mmHg) [5]. Taking into account the continuous relationship that is observed between BP

Julián Segura, MD, PhD, Nephrologist, Hypertension Unit, Department of Nephrology, Hospital 12 de Octubre, Madrid, Spain.

Luis M. Ruilope, MD, PhD, Nephrologist, Hypertension Unit, Department of Nephrology, Hospital 12 de Octubre, Madrid, Spain.

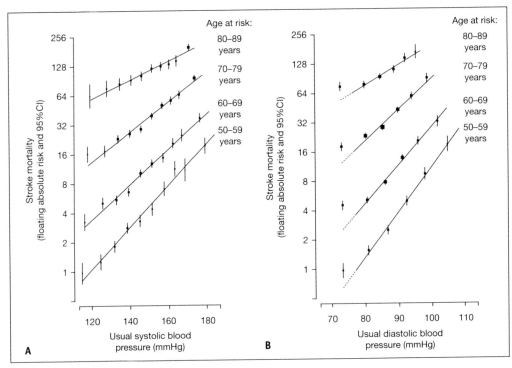

Figure 10.1 Stroke mortality rate in each decade of age versus normal blood pressure at the start of that decade. **A.** Systolic pressure. **B.** Diastolic pressure.
CI = confidence interval.

levels and the risk of death from vascular disease, the absolute benefit of a lower BP level is likely to be greatest for those at greatest absolute risk of vascular disease, in particular diabetic patients, irrespectively of their BP. These results have also confirmed previous data about the relationship between BP levels below the usual diagnostic criteria of arterial hypertension and cardiovascular risk.

In patients with type 2 diabetes, using the cut-off point of 140/90 mmHg, the prevalence of hypertension is up to three times greater than in age- and sex-matched patients without diabetes [6, 7]. Increasing age, obesity and the onset of renal disease are all factors increasing the likelihood of hypertension in diabetic patients [6, 7]. Central obesity is an increasing factor predisposing to the development of diabetes and hypertension [8]. Moreover, people with hypertension have a high prevalence of insulin resistance and, consequently, an increased risk of developing type 2 diabetes mellitus [9]. Major cardiovascular events are more than twice as likely in patients with both diabetes and hypertension than in patients with either disease alone [3, 10]. In a long-term follow-up study comparing the 7-year incidence of myocardial infarction (fatal and non-fatal) among 1373 non-diabetic subjects with the incidence among 1059 diabetic subjects, all from a Finnish population-based study, Haffner and colleagues [11] showed that diabetic patients without coronary heart disease present a similar cardiovascular risk than non-diabetic patients with coronary artery disease (Figure 10.4). These data remain, however, a matter of some debate due to the absence of confirmation from other studies [12].

In recent years, blood glucose levels have been recognised as an independent cardiovascular risk factor. This risk increases continuously, starting well below the current threshold

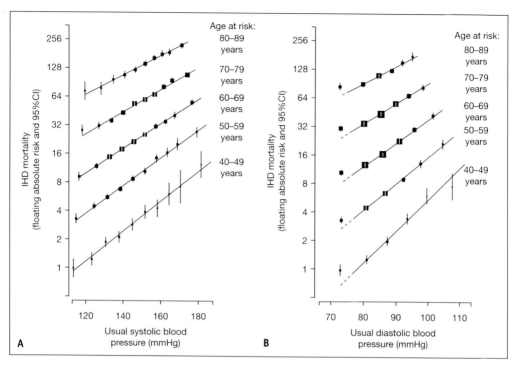

Figure 10.2 Ischaemic heart disease (IHD) mortality rate in each decade of age versus normal blood pressure at the start of that decade. **A.** Systolic pressure. **B.** Diastolic pressure. CI = confidence interval.

for the diagnosis of diabetes mellitus [13, 14]. Accumulating evidence suggests that individuals with non-diabetic ranges of hyperglycaemia are already at risk of cardiovascular diseases [15, 16]. A recent meta-analysis of available prospective studies has reviewed the association between blood glucose levels and cardiovascular risk in the non-diabetic range, confirming their usefulness as risk markers for cardiovascular disease among apparently healthy individuals without diabetes [17]. Individuals with either impaired fasting glucose or impaired glucose tolerance have similar risks of cardiovascular diseases. Those who fulfilled the criteria for both disorders carried a greater risk of developing cardiovascular diseases [18]. More recently, the Risk Factor in Impaired Glucose Tolerance for Atherosclerosis and Diabetes (RIAD) study has shown that all categories of prediabetic hyperglycaemia have a higher cardiovascular risk factor level (more obesity, higher levels of triglycerides, lower high-density lipoprotein [HDL]-cholesterol and elevated blood pressure values) compared to control subjects with normal glucose tolerance [19].

It has recently been described that previously undiagnosed diabetes and impaired glucose tolerance are common in patients presenting with an acute myocardial infarction [20, 21], despite the exclusion of patients with previously diagnosed diabetes or with blood glucose concentrations of >11 mmol/l at hospital admission. Norhammar and colleagues [21] have shown that the true prevalence of diabetes mellitus among people with myocardial infarction might be as high as 45%. Very recently, the Euro Heart Survey has reported the finding that more than two-thirds of patients referred to hospitals with acute ischaemic events showed an impairment of carbohydrate metabolism [22]. Recent data from the Valsartan in Acute Myocardial Infarction Trial (VALIANT) have shown that diabetes mellitus, whether newly diagnosed or previously known, is associated with poorer long-term

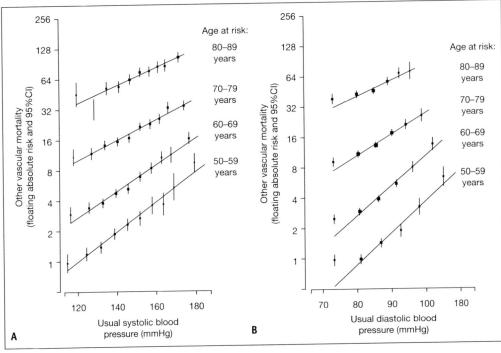

Figure 10.3 Other vascular (not stroke or ischaemic heart disease) mortality rate in each decade of age versus normal blood pressure at the start of that decade. **A.** Systolic pressure. **B.** Diastolic pressure. CI = confidence interval.

outcomes after myocardial infarction in high-risk patients [23]. A similarly increased prevalence of pre-diabetes has been recently described in patients following a transient ischaemic attack or ischaemic stroke [24]. The poor prognosis of patients with newly diagnosed diabetes, despite having baseline characteristics similar to those patients without diabetes, supports the idea that metabolic abnormalities contribute to their adverse outcomes [23].

A growing body of evidence from controlled trials has been reported indicating that rigorous control of blood pressure below the conventional goal of <140/90 mmHg markedly reduces cardiovascular morbidity and mortality in diabetic patients [25]. In consequence, recently published guidelines for the management of arterial hypertension recommended that blood pressure in type 2 diabetic patients must be lowered, whenever possible, to <130/80 mmHg, using effective and well-tolerated antihypertensive agents, generally in combination [4, 26]. Recently, published data from the subgroup of hypertensive type 2 diabetic patients have confirmed the need for lower BP goals during the treatment of these patients [27].

MECHANISMS UNDERLYING DIABETES AND HYPERTENSION

Both insulin resistance and endothelial dysfunction are the initial underlying pathogenetic mechanisms in arterial hypertension and diabetes mellitus that increase cardiovascular and renal risk. Insulin resistance is present in type 2 diabetes, obesity and arterial hypertension, and is frequently accompanied by the features that characterise the metabolic syndrome [28]. This abnormality is accompanied by a compensatory hyperinsulinaemia, but the individual contributions of either of these two conditions remain incompletely understood and continue

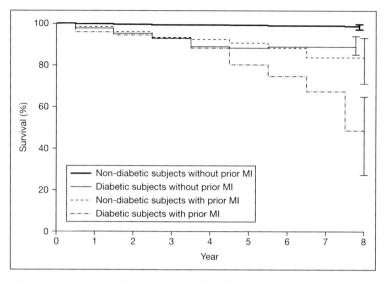

Figure 10.4 Kaplan–Meier estimates of the probability of death from coronary heart disease in 1059 subjects with type 2 diabetes and 1378 non-diabetic subjects with and without prior myocardial infarction.

to be the subject of intense investigation. The effects of compensatory hiperinsulinaemia in the vasculature have been recently summarised and comprise three important aspects:

1. Inability to maintain endothelial nitric oxide synthase (eNOS) activity and nitric oxide (NO) production.
2. Inability to maintain vascular smooth muscle cell (VSMC) quiescence and counteract platelet-derived growth factor (PDGF).
3. Increased ability to promote phenylation of Ras and Rho proteins and to potentiate the action of other growth-promoting agents [28].

In the presence of insulin resistance, hyperinsulinaemia may exert a detrimental influence on the arterial wall and this could potentiate the development of atherosclerosis. This fact suggests that amelioration of insulin resistance with exercise, weight loss, or insulin sensitisers may represent a superior therapeutic approach than simply increasing insulin levels by either administering exogen insulin or insulin secretagogues to patients with insulin resistance [29].

Available data in type 2 diabetes suggest that decreased nitric oxide bioactivity may be the result of nitric oxide breakdown. Type 2 diabetes is associated with increased generation of reactive oxygen species (ROS) [30] and anti-oxidants can improve endothelial dysfunction under experimental conditions [31, 32]. Endothelial dysfunction associated with essential (primary) hypertension is characterised by impaired nitric oxide bioactivity determined by ROS, which scavenges nitric oxide [32]. ROS can be generated by non-enzymatic and enzymatic sources, including nicotinamide adenine dinucleotide phosphate (NAD(P)H) oxidases or xanthine oxidase, cyclo-oxygenase (COX) and nitric oxide synthase (NOS)-induced superoxide production caused by depletion of the cofactor, tetrahydrobiopterin. In the presence of reduced availability of nitric oxide, alternative pathways, including hyperpolarisation, account for endothelium-dependent vasodilatation [33]. In hypertension, endothelial dysfunction can be reversed by both non-pharmacological and pharmacological treatment. Physical exercise can improve endothelium-dependent vasodilatation in the forearm microcirculation [34], whereas antihypertensive drugs show contrasting effects [35]. ACEI were found to improve endothelial function in subcutaneous, epicardial, brachial and renal circu-

Table 10.1 Indications for initial treatment and goals for adult hypertensive diabetic patients

	Systolic	Diastolic
Goal (mmHg)	<130	<80
Behavioral therapy alone (maximum 3 months) then add pharmacological treatment*	130–139	80–89
Behavioral therapy + pharmacologic treatment	≥140	≥90

* Recently published ESH-ESC guidelines recommend lifestyle changes plus drug treatment from the beginning.

lations, whereas they did not enhance the blunted response to acetylcholine in the forearm; similar results are available for angiotensin II receptor antagonists [36].

BLOOD PRESSURE CONTROL IN DIABETIC PATIENTS

High-normal blood pressure and the initial stage of isolated systolic hypertension represent two situations in which doctors are frequently reluctant to begin pharmacological therapy, even though guidelines indicate that this can result in clear benefits [37]. According the American Diabetes Association, Table 10.1 shows the recommendations for initial treatment and goals for adult hypertensive diabetic patients [38]. The attention paid to identifying the antihypertensive agent of first choice for type 2 diabetes may appear rather questionable in view of the need for multiple drugs in order to lower blood pressure to the difficult goal of 130/80 mmHg, as recognised by Kaplan [39] and by an American Consensus Document [40]. Indeed, in the Hypertension Optimal Treatment (HOT) study, the large majority of patients randomised to a diastolic blood pressure (DBP) goal of <80 mmHg were on double- or triple-therapy [41] and in the United Kingdom Prospective Diabetes Study (UKPDS), 29% of patients randomised to tighter blood pressure control were on three drugs and 34% on two drugs [42]. In the two studies on diabetic patients with advanced nephropathy, Irbesartan in Diabetic Nephropathy Trial (IDNT) and Reduction of Endpoints in Non-insulin-dependent diabetes mellitus with the Angiotensin II Antagonist Losartan (RENAAL), an average of 2.5 and 3.0 non-study drugs were required, respectively, in addition to the angiotensin II receptor antagonist [43, 44].

A recent review summarised the results of trials on diabetic patients in which more or less intensive blood pressure lowering was tested, or an active blood pressure lowering regimen was compared with placebo [25]. Ten trials with sufficient power to test the outcomes of greater or smaller lowering of blood pressure were taken into consideration. All ten trials were based on treatment randomisation. Five of them; UKPDS [42], the Appropriate Blood pressure Control in Diabetes study on normotensive patients (ABCD-NT) [45], the ABCD study on hypertensive patients (ABCD-HT) [46], the IDNT [43] and the RENAAL study [44] only included patients with diabetes. The other five: Systolic Hypertension in the Elderly Program (SHEP) [47], Systolic Hypertension in Europe (SystEur) [48], the Perindopril Protection against Recurrent Stroke Study (PROGRESS) [49], HOT study [41] and the Heart Outcomes Prevention Evaluation study (HOPE) [50, 51] included a sizeable number of diabetics within a larger cohort of patients (the larger proportion being non-diabetics) and the evidence they provide derives from subgroup analyses. Figure 10.5 shows data concerning major cardiovascular events, cardiovascular death and total mortality, as these outcomes were primary endpoints in several of the trials, and represent the outcomes with highest numbers in those trials for which the primary endpoint was not a cardiovascular one (renal outcomes were primary endpoints in ACBD-NT, ABCD-HT, IDNT and RENAAL).

Among placebo-treated patients in the two trials on elderly patients with isolated systolic hypertension (SHEP and SystEur), the incidence of major cardiovascular events was, respec-

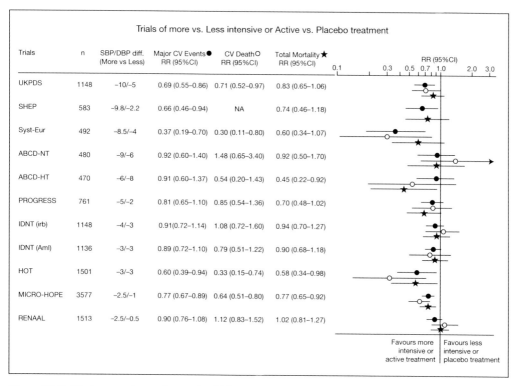

Figure 10.5 Effects on major cardiovascular (CV) events, CV death and total mortality in trials comparing more versus less intensive, or active versus placebo treatment. The first column lists acronyms of the trials (for the Irbesartan in Diabetic Nephropathy Trial (IDNT), the first row is the comparison of irbesartan (Irb) with placebo and the second row is the comparison of amlodipine (Aml) with placebo) and their reference; the second column is the number (n) of diabetic patients; the third column indicates the systolic/diastolic blood pressure difference (SBP/DBP diff) between more intensive (or active) and less intensive (or placebo) treatments. In other columns and in the graphs on the right, the effects are expressed as relative risk (RR) and 95% confidence intervals (95%CI). The trials are ordered by decreasing SBP/DBP differences. ABCD-HT = Appropriate Blood pressure Control in Diabetes on Hypertensive Patients; ABCD-NT = Appropriate Blood pressure Control in Diabetes on Normotensive Patients; HOT = Hypertension Optimal Treatment study; IDNT = Irbesartan in Diabetic Nephropathy Trial; MICRO-HOPE = Heart Outcomes Prevention Evaluation Substudy; PROGRESS = Perindopril Protection against Recurrent Stroke Study; RENAL = Reduction of Endpoints in Noninsulin-dependent diabetes mellitus with the Angiotensin II Antagonist Losartan; SHEP = Systolic Hypertension in the Elderly Program; Syst-Eur = Systolic Hypertension in Europe

tively, 1.71 and 1.90 times higher in the presence of diabetes, and the relative risks (RR) for coronary events were 2.12 and 1.86, those for stroke 1.92 and 2.16, and those for all deaths 1.63 and 2.09. In the HOT study [41], in which all of the patients received intensive blood pressure treatment and 91.5% of the patients had a diastolic blood pressure <90 mmHg, the incidence of major cardiovascular events was 1.71 times higher in diabetics than in non-diabetics, and so was the incidence of myocardial infarction (RR 1.52), stroke (RR 1.65), cardiovascular mortality (RR 2.13) and total mortality (RR 1.45), even after adjusting for the slightly higher systolic blood pressure in treated diabetics [52]. By way of comparison, in the HOT study patients, the relative risk of cardiovascular mortality due to diabetes was only lower than the relative risk due to old age (>65 years) and that due to higher serum creatinine (155 mmol/l or 1.3 mg/dl), and equal to that due to previous coronary heart disease [52]. In the HOPE study only [50], the incidence of major cardiovascular events was just 1.2 times as high in diabetics as in non-diabetics subjects but, in this study, only 46.8% of subjects also had hypertension. However, in HOPE, when diabetes was associated with another powerful predictor of cardiovascular events, such as reduced renal function [52, 53], cardiovascular event incidence among placebo-controlled subjects was approximately twice as frequent as that in non-diabetic subjects with a similar reduction in renal function [54]. However, the high cardiovascular risk found in type 2 diabetics is not only due to the high prevalence of arterial hypertension among these patients. For example, in the normotensive cohort of the ABCD-NT [45], which enrolled patients with a blood pressure of 140/90 mmHg, subjects in the placebo arm (with an average blood pressure of 137/81 mmHg) had an incidence of major cardiovascular events of approximately 16% in 5 years (i.e. approximately three times higher than in the Framingham Heart Study patients with high-normal blood pressure) [55].

As indicated by the data contained in Figure 10.5, trials that showed a statistically significant reduction of cardiovascular events with more intensive blood pressure lowering also showed a statistically significant reduction in cardiovascular death (with the single exception of SHEP, which did not report cardiovascular death among its endpoints), and three trials also showed a significant reduction in total mortality (HOT, MICROHOPE and ABCD-HT). Most trials did not have sufficient statistical power to investigate treatment effects on cause-specific cardiovascular events, but statistically significant reductions were reported, in stroke, by five trials; UKPDS, SHEP, ABCD-NT, PROGRESS, MICROHOPE): in coronary events by three trials (SHEP, MICROHOPE, IDNT-amlodipine arm) and in congestive heart failure by RENAAL).

A recent meta-analysis published by the Blood Pressure Lowering Treatment Trialists' has shown that treatment with any commonly used regimen reduces the risk of total major cardiovascular events, and that larger reductions in blood pressure produce larger reductions in risk [56]. Mean blood pressure differences between randomised groups seemed to be directly associated with differences in risks of stroke, coronary heart disease, major cardiovascular events, cardiovascular death, and total mortality. By contrast, blood pressure differences did not seem to be associated with risk of heart failure [56].

On the whole, evidence that more intensive blood pressure lowering is beneficial in reducing the aggregate of major cardiovascular events in type 2 diabetic patients, although not entirely uncontroversial, appears overwhelming. However, the more specific question on the blood pressure level that should be reached by therapy for cardiovascular prevention in diabetes is more difficult to answer precisely. Even in the five trials showing the most significant reduction in cardiovascular events, blood pressure, particularly systolic blood pressure, remained at relatively high levels as recently reviewed by Mancia and Grassi [57]. Blood pressure values achieved in more intensively treated groups averaged 142/82 mmHg in UKPDS, 148/68 mmHg in SHEP, 153/78 mmHg in SystEur, 143/81 mmHg in HOT and 140/77 mmHg in MICROHOPE. Therefore, diastolic blood pressure values between 77 and 82 mmHg could be achieved, even in trials not exclusively including patients with isolated systolic hypertension. On the other hand, in most positive trials, systolic blood pressure values remained higher than the conventional hypertension threshold of 140 mmHg. Only the two ABCD studies were able to reach quite low blood pressure values (132/78 mmHg in ABCD-HT and 128/75 mmHg in ABCD-NT) but, unfortunately, both of these studies were unsuccessful in convincingly demonstrating a consistent reduction in cardiovascular events with more intensive treatment (only total mortality in ABCD-HT and stroke in ABCD-NT were significantly reduced). However, it should be remarked that no trial suggests an increased cardiovascular risk at the lowest blood pressure achieved.

Nevertheless, in trials including high-risk patients with lower initial blood pressure values, the beneficial cardiovascular effects of ACEI have been observed independently of blood pressure control. The combined analysis of HOPE, the European Trial on Reduction of Cardiac Events with Perindopril in Stable Coronary Artery Disease (EUROPA) and the Prevention of Events with Angiotension Converting Enzyme inhibition (PEACE) trials shows that ACEI reduce serious vascular events in patients with atherosclerosis [58]. In fact, ACEI significantly reduced all-cause mortality (7.8 vs. 8.9%; P = 0.0004), cardiovascular mortality (4.3 vs. 5.2%; P = 0.0002), non-fatal myocardial infarction (5.3 vs. 6.4%; P = 0·0001), all stroke (2.2 vs. 2.8%; P = 0.0004), heart failure (2.1 vs. 2.7%; P = 0.0007), and coronary-artery bypass surgery (6.0 vs. 6.9%; P = 0.0036) [58]. In patients with heart failure and myocardial infarction, ARBs have beneficial effects in patients with heart failure who are intolerant to ACEI and who are on optimal ACEI therapy [59]. In patients with acute high-risk myocardial infarction, the ARB was as effective as an ACEI following myocardial infarction [23, 59]. The addition of an ARB to ACEI and other treatment leads to a further clinically important reduction in relevant cardiovascular events in patients with chronic heart failure and reduced left ventricular ejection fraction [60].

PREVENTION OF RENAL DISEASE IN DIABETICS

PRIMARY PREVENTION OF DIABETIC NEPHROPATHY

Recent clinical trials suggested that inhibition of the renin–angiotensin system may actually prevent nephropathy. The *post hoc* analyses of the reduction in hypertension in the HOPE study [51] and in the Losartan Intervention For Endpoint Reduction in Hypertension (LIFE) study [61] found a lower incidence of overt nephropathy in subjects with type 2 diabetes who received therapy that inhibited the rennin–angiotensin system than in controls. However, these studies were not designed to assess the incidence of microalbuminuria, because patients with microalbuminuria were included in them. The multicentre double-blind, randomised Bergamo Nephrologic Diabetes Complications Trial (BENEDICT) was designed to assess whether angiotensin-converting enzyme inhibitors and non-dihydro-pyridine calcium-channel blockers, alone or in combination, prevented microalbuminuria in subjects with hypertension, type 2 diabetes mellitus and normal urinary albumin excretion [62]. A total of 1204 subjects were randomly assigned to receive at least three years of treatment with trandolapril (at a dose of 2 mg/day) plus verapamil (sustained-release formulation, 180 mg/day), trandolapril alone (2 mg/day), verapamil alone (sustained-release formulation, 240 mg/day), or placebo. The primary endpoint was the development of persistent microalbuminuria (overnight albumin excretion, ≥20 μg/min at two consecutive visits), and it was reached in 5.7% of the subjects receiving trandolapril plus verapamil, 6.0% of the subjects receiving trandolapril, 11.9% of the subjects receiving verapamil and 10.0% of control subjects receiving placebo. In conclusion, in subjects with type 2 diabetes and arterial hypertension, normoalbuminuria and normal renal function, ACE inhibitor therapy with trandolapril plus verapamil or trandolapril alone prevented the onset of microalbuminuria. The renoprotective effect of ACE inhibition did not appear to be enhanced by the addition of a non-dihydropyridine calcium channel blocker. These findings suggest that in hypertensive patients with type 2 diabetes and normal renal function, an ACE inhibitor may be the medication of choice for controlling blood pressure [62]. In the same way, the Randomised Olmesartan and Diabetes Microalbuminuria Prevention (ROADMAP) trial is a large scale European, multicentre, multinational, double-blind, randomised, placebo-controlled, parallel-group study in patients with type 2 diabetes, normoalbuminuria and one or more cardiovascular risk factors. It will randomise 4400 patients to receive an angiotensin receptor blocker, olmesartan, 40 mg once daily, or a placebo. The primary objective is to determine in the study population whether olmesartan, compared with a placebo, prevents or delays the onset of microalbuminuria. The study started in 2004 and will end in 2012 [63].

PREVENTION/DELAY OF OVERT DIABETIC NEPHROPATHY

Diabetic nephropathy has become the leading cause of end-stage renal disease (ESRD) in the United States [6]. Approximately 35% of persons with diabetes will develop diabetic nephropathy, characterised by proteinuria, decreased glomerular filtration rate and increased blood pressure [6]. In fact, development of diabetic nephropathy often pre-dates or occurs simultaneously with the evolution of hypertension in patients with diabetes [7]. In patients with type 2 diabetes, the incidence of nephropathy is approximately 20%. The prevalence and incidence of ESRD are approximately twice what they were 10 years ago [6]. If the trends of the past two decades persist, approximately 175 000 new cases of ESRD will be diagnosed in 2010 [64]. This is due in part to the expectation that the incidence of type 2 diabetes will double within the next 10–15 years and the fact that patients with diabetes are living longer and are thus more likely to develop chronic problems, including ESRD. Recent studies have addressed renal protection in type 2 diabetes. The IDNT evaluated the effects of irbesartan in 1715 patients with hypertension, type 2 diabetes and proteinuria, with urinary protein excretion of ≥900 mg/day [43]. These patients were randomised to irbesartan, placebo or amlodipine groups, with an average follow-up of 2.6 years. The time event for the composite endpoint of a doubling of serum creatinine level, ESRD, or death was 28% in the control group versus 19.8% in the irbesartan group (20% reduction; $P = 0.02$). In another trial, the RENAAL study, losartan (50–100 mg) plus conventional hypertensive therapy was compared with placebo plus conventional hypertensive therapy in 1513 patients [44]. Serum creatinine levels were required to be between 114.9–265.2 pmol/l (1.3–3.0 mg/dl) and urine albumin–creatinine ratio had to be greater than 300 mg/g or 25 mg/mmol. Losartan therapy was associated with a 28% reduction in the risk of ESRD and a 25% reduction in doubling of serum creatinine level. The Irbesartan in Patients with Type 2 Diabetes and Microalbuminuria (IRMA-2) trial examined the possibility that irbesartan could delay or prevent the development of clinical proteinuria in patients with type 2 diabetes, microalbuminuria and a normal serum creatinine [65]. Patients with type 2 diabetes were randomised to receive placebo or irbesartan, 150–300 mg/day. The primary endpoint of the trial was defined as the occurrence of a urinary albumin excretion rate (UAER) >200 µg/min and/or at least 30% higher than baseline on two consecutive measurements. Average blood pressure values were slightly lower in the two groups treated with irbesartan than in the placebo group during the first six months of the study, but this small difference disappeared during the last 12 months of the study. In the irbesartan (150 mg/day) group versus placebo, there was a 39% reduction ($P = 0.08$) in the rate of development of clinical proteinuria, while in the irbesartan (200 mg/day) group there was a 70% reduction in the primary endpoint. Return to a normal UAER (<20 µg/min) was 34% more frequent among patients treated with irbesartan 300 mg/day than among patients in the placebo group. The results of this study demonstrated that irbesartan 300 mg/day could delay progression of microalbuminuria to clinical proteinuria in patients with type 2 diabetes [65]. Microalbuminuria Reduction with Valsartan (MARVAL) [66] was a multicentre, double-blind, randomised parallel study of 332 patients with type 2 diabetes aged 35–75 years with microalbuminuria and normal or high blood pressure. Subjects were randomised to receive valsartan 80 mg/day or amlodipine 5 mg/day over 24 weeks. The reduction of UAER from baseline to the end of the study was greater for the valsartan group than for the amlodipine group. In addition, more patients returned to normal albuminuria status after 24 weeks with valsartan versus amlodipine therapy. These differences were observed in association with equivalent blood pressure-lowering effects of the two agents, again emphasising the unique beneficial effects of ARBs on the diabetic kidney. The results of the Diabetics Exposed to Telmisartan and Enalapril (DETAIL) study showed a similar capacity of enalapril and telmisartan for long-term protection (5 years) of glomerular filtration rate in microalbuminuric type 2 hypertensive diabetic patients [67].

There have also been trials examining the impact of combination of an ACE inhibitor and an ARB on diabetic nephropathy [68, 69]. The Candesartan and Lisinopril Microalbuminuria (CALM) trial [69], a randomised study examining the effect of combining candesartan and lisinopril on microalbuminuria, was conducted in 199 patients with type 2 diabetes. This was a 12-week combination therapy trial, with 12 weeks of prior monotherapy with either candesartan or lisinopril. In this study, the reduction in the urinary albumin–creatinine ratio in those receiving candesartan 16 mg/day and lisinopril 20 mg/day was significantly greater (50% reduction) than that observed with either agent alone (24% for candesartan and 39% for lisinopril). As is often the case with combination therapy, blood pressure values were lower compared with therapy with the individual agent, which makes interpretation of the findings difficult. After 24 weeks of therapy, diastolic blood pressure was reduced to a greater degree with combination therapy (-16.3 mmHg) than with either candesartan (-10.4 mmHg) or lisinopril (-10.7 mmHg) alone.

PREVENTION OF NEW-ONSET DIABETES

Preventing or postponing type 2 diabetes is vital for public healthcare systems, given that diabetic patients have increased cardiovascular morbidity and mortality rates. It should be noted that the relationship between glycaemia and the incidence of diabetes is non-linear [70]. The Hoorn study showed that the risk for conversion to diabetes during 6.5 years of follow-up was more than ten times higher in people with impaired glucose tolerance or impaired fasting glucose in comparison with normoglycaemic subjects [71]. The risk of developing type 2 diabetes is equivalent for impaired glucose tolerance and impaired fasting glucose, but these two abnormalities overlap by only 20–25% [71].

All of this evidence has been considered by the American Diabetes Association in defining pre-diabetes as the presence of either impaired glucose tolerance or impaired fasting glucose [72]. Given that the cut-off point for impaired fasting glucose has been recently reduced to 100 mg/dl [73], the relevance of the pre-diabetes state is clearly reinforced.

Recent data have confirmed this predisposition to develop type 2 diabetes of those subjects presenting pre-diabetes: among 872 participants in the Insulin Resistance Atherosclerosis study (IRAS), those presenting normal glucose tolerance showed an incidence of new-onset diabetes of 8% after 5 years, whereas 33% of individuals with impaired glucose tolerance developed type 2 diabetes during the same time period [74]. These metabolic disturbances have also been described in non-diabetic, first-degree relatives of African-American type 2 diabetic patients who progressed to impaired glucose tolerance and type 2 diabetes [75], and in hypertensive patients presenting with metabolic syndrome [76].

Among overweight American adults aged 45–74 years included in National Health and Nutrition Examination Survey (NHANES) III survey, 12.5% had self-reported diabetes, 10.8% had undiagnosed diabetes, 22.6% had pre-diabetes and 54.1% had normal glucose metabolism [77]. Recent data show that two-thirds of the hypertensive population followed in hospital-located hypertension units exhibited alterations in carbohydrate metabolism [78].

New-onset diabetes commonly appears in the hypertensive population during follow-up. Data from controlled trials clearly show that hypertensive patients under treatment with diuretics or β-blockers exhibited a greater incidence of new-onset diabetes than hypertensive patients under treatment with 'newer' drugs [79]. A recent review indicated that, whereas diuretic therapy increased the risk of new-onset diabetes in comparison to placebo, other antihypertensive drug classes such as ARB, ACEI and calcium channel blockers all reduced such risk (Figure 10.6) [80].

SUMMARY

Arterial hypertension is highly prevalent in type 2 diabetic patients. An early start to antihypertensive therapy, including appropriate lifestyle changes and pharmacological therapy, will contribute to the attainment of the expected goal blood pressure, which is <130/80 mmHg. The use of an angiotensin-converting enzyme inhibitor or an angiotensin receptor blocker, in combination with the antihypertensive drugs frequently required, enhances car-

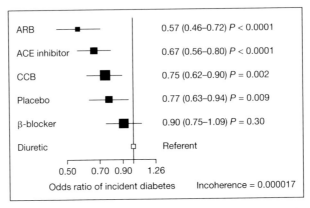

Figure 10.6 Results of the network meta-analysis with the diuretic as the standard of comparison.

diovascular and renal protection. Antidiabetic drugs and the integral management of global cardiovascular risk with a statin (and possibly antiplatelet therapy) are also required.

REFERENCES

1. Harris MI, Flegal KM, Cowie CC et al. Prevalence of diabetes, impaired fasting glucose and impaired glucose tolerance in U.S. adults. The Third National Health and Nutrition Examination Survey, 1998–1994. *Diabetes Care* 1998; 21:518–524.
2. King H, Aubert RE, Herman WH. Global burden of diabetes, 1995–2025. *Diabetes Care* 1998; 21:1414–1431.
3. Stamler J, Vaccaro O, Neaton JD et al. Diabetes, other risk factors, and 12-yr cardiovascular mortality for men screened in the Multiple Risk Factor Intervention Trial. *Diabetes Care* 1993; 16:434–444.
4. The Task Force for the Management of Arterial Hypertension of the European Society of Hypertension and of the European Society of Cardiology. 2007 Guidelines for the management of arterial hypertension. *J Hypertens* 2007; 25:1105–1187.
5. Prospective Studies Collaboration. Age-specific relevance of usual blood pressure to vascular mortality: a meta-analysis of individual data for one million adults in 61 prospective studies. *Lancet* 2002; 360:1903–1913.
6. Bakris GL, Willians M, Dworkin L et al. National Kidney Foundation Hypertension and Diabetes Executive Committees Working Group. Preserving renal function in adults with hypertension and diabetes: a consensus approach. *Am J Kidney Dis* 2000; 36:646–661.
7. Sowers JR, Epstein M, Frohlich ED. Diabetes, hypertension, and cardiovascular disease: an update. *Hypertension* 2001; 37:1053–1059.
8. The Diabetes Control and Complications Trial. Epidemiology of diabetes interventions and complications research group. *N Engl J Med* 2003; 348:2294–2303.
9. Griess TW, Nieto FJ, Shahar E et al. Hypertension and antihypertensive therapy as risk factors for type 2 diabetes mellitus: Atherosclerosis Risk in Communities Study. *N Engl J Med* 2000; 342:905–912.
10. Grundy SM, Benjamin IJ, Burke GL et al. Diabetes and cardiovascular disease. A statement for healthcare professionals from the American Heart Association. *Circulation* 1999; 100:1134–1146.
11. Haffner SM, Lehto S, Ronnemaa T et al. Mortality from coronary heart disease in subjects with type 2 diabetes and in nondiabetic subjects with and without prior myocardial infarction. *N Engl J Med* 1998; 339:229–234.
12. Lee CD, Folsom AR, Pankow JS et al. Atherosclerosis Risk in Communities (ARIC) Study Investigators. Cardiovascular events in diabetic and nondiabetic adults with or without history of myocardial infarction. *Circulation* 2004; 109:855–860.
13. Björnholt J, Erikssen G, Aaser E et al. Fasting blood glucose: an underestimated risk factor for cardiovascular death. Results from a 22-year follow-up of healthy nondiabetic men. *Diabetes Care* 1999; 22:45–49.

14. The DECODE study group on behalf of the European Diabetes Epidemiology Group. Is the current definition for diabetes relevant to mortality risk from all causes and cardiovascular and noncardiovascular diseases? *Diabetes Care* 2003; 26:688–696.

15. DECODE study group on behalf of the European Diabetes Epidemiology group. Glucose tolerance and mortality: comparison of WHO and American Diabetes Association diagnostic criteria. *Lancet* 1999; 354:617–621.

16. Meigs JB, Nathan DM, Wilson PW *et al.* Metabolic risk factors worsen continuously across the spectrum of nondiabetic glucose tolerance. The Framingham Offspring Study. *Ann Intern Med* 1998; 128:524–533.

17. Levitan EB, Song Y, Ford ES *et al.* Is nondiabetic hyperglycemia a risk factor for cardiovascular disease? A meta-analysis of prospective studies. *Arch Intern Med* 2004; 164:2147–2155.

18. Lim SC, Tai ES, Tan BY *et al.* Cardiovascular risk profile in individuals with borderline glycemia: the effect of the 1997 American Diabetes Association diagnostic criteria and the 1998 World Health Organization Provisional Report. *Diabetes Care* 2000; 23:278–282.

19. Hanefeld M, Koehler C, Fuecker K *et al.* Insulin secretion and insulin sensitivity pattern is different in isolated impaired glucose tolerance and impaired fasting glucose: the risk factor in Impaired Glucose Tolerance for Atherosclerosis and Diabetes study. *Diabetes Care* 2003; 26:868–874.

20. Bartnik M, Malmberg K, Norhammar A *et al.* Newly detected abnormal glucose tolerance: an important predictor of long-term outcome after myocardial infarction. *Eur Heart J* 2004; 25:1990–1997.

21. Norhammar A, Tenerz A, Nilsson G *et al.* Glucose metabolism in patients with acute myocardial infarction and no previous diagnosis of diabetes mellitus: a prospective study. *Lancet* 2002; 359:2140–2144.

22. Bartnik M, Ryden L, Ferrari R *et al.* The prevalence of abnormal glucose regulation in patients with coronary artery disease across Europe. The Euro Heart Survey on diabetes and the heart. *Eur Heart J* 2004; 25:1880–1890.

23. Aguilar D, Solomon SD, Kober L *et al.* Newly diagnosed and previously known diabetes mellitus and 1-year outcomes of acute myocardial infarction: the VALsartan In Acute myocardial iNfarcTion (VALIANT) trial. *Circulation* 2004; 110:1572–1578.

24. Kernan WN, Viscoli CM, Inzucchi SE *et al.* Prevalence of abnormal glucose tolerance following a transient ischemic attack or ischemic stroke. *Arch Intern Med* 2005; 165:227–233.

25. Zanchetti A, Ruilope LM. Antihypertensive treatment in patients with type-2 diabetes mellitus: what guidance from recent controlled randomized trials? *J Hypertens* 2002; 20:2099–2110.

26. Chobanian AV, Bakris GL, Black HR *et al.* The Seventh Report of the Joint National Committee on Prevention, Detection, Evaluation, and Treatment of High Blood Pressure. The JNC 7 Report. *JAMA* 2003; 289:2560–2571.

27. Fox JC, Leight K, Sutradhar SC *et al.* The JNC 7 approach compared to conventional treatment in diabetic patients with hypertension: a double-blind trial of initial monotherapy vs. combination therapy. *J Clin Hypertens (Greenwich)* 2004; 6:437–442.

28. Wang CC, Goalstone ML, Draznin B. Molecular mechanisms of insulin resistance that impact cardiovascular biology. *Diabetes* 2004; 53:2735–2740.

29. Dandona P, Aljada A, Mohanty P. The anti-inflammatory and potential anti-atherogenic effect of insulin: a new paradigm. *Diabetologia* 2002; 45:924–930.

30. Chowienczyk PJ, Brett SE, Gopaul NK *et al.* Oral treatment with an antioxidant (raxofelast) reduces oxidative stress and improves endothelial function in men with type II diabetes. *Diabetologia* 2000; 43:974–977.

31. Ting HH, Timimi FK, Boles KS *et al.* Vitamin C improves endothelium-dependent vasodilation in patients with non-insulin-dependent diabetes mellitus. *J Clin Invest* 1996; 97:22–28.

32. Taddei S, Virdis A, Ghiadoni L *et al.* Vitamin C improves endothelium-dependent vasodilation by restoring nitric oxide activity in essential hypertension. *Circulation* 1998; 97:2222–2229.

33. Taddei S, Ghiadoni L, Virdis A *et al.* Vasodilation to bradykinin is mediated by an ouabain-sensitive pathway as a compensatory mechanism for impaired nitric oxide availability in essential hypertensive patients. *Circulation* 1999; 100:1400–1405.

34. Higashi Y, Sasaki S, Kurisu S *et al.* Regular aerobic exercise augments endothelium-dependent vascular relaxation in normotensive as well as hypertensive subjects: role of endothelium-derived nitric oxide. *Circulation* 1999; 100:1194–1202.

35. Taddei S, Virdis A, Ghiadoni L *et al.* Effects of antihypertensive drugs on endothelial dysfunction: clinical implications. *Drugs* 2002; 62:265–284.

36. Brunner H, Cockcroft JR, Deanfield J et al. Endothelial function and dysfunction. Part II: Association with cardiovascular risk factors and diseases. A statement by the Working Group on Endothelins and Endothelial Factors of the European Society of Hypertension. J Hypertens 2005; 23:233–246.

37. Ruilope LM, Usan L, Segura J et al. Intervention at lower blood pressure levels to achieve target goals in type 2 diabetes: PRADID (PResión Arterial en DIabéticos tipo DOS) study. J Hypertens 2004; 22:217–222.

38. American Diabetes Association. Treatment of hypertension in adults with diabetes. Diabetes Care 2003; 26(Suppl 1):S80–S82.

39. Kaplan NM. Management of hypertension in patients with type 2 diabetes mellitus: guidelines based on current evidence. Ann Intern Med 2001; 135:1079–1083.

40. Bakris GL, Williams M, Dworkin L et al. Preserving renal function in adults with hypertension and diabetes: a consensus approach. National Kidney Foundation Hypertension and Diabetes Executive Committees Working Group. Am J Kidney Dis 2000; 36:646–661.

41. Hansson L, Zanchetti A, Carruthers SG et al. Effects of intensive blood-pressure lowering and low-dose aspirin in patients with hypertension: principal results of the Hypertension Optimal Treatment (HOT) randomised trial. Lancet 1998; 351:1755–1762.

42. UK Prospective Diabetes Study Group. Tight blood pressure control and risk of macrovascular and microvascular complications in type 2 diabetes. UKPDS 38. Br Med J 1998; 317:703–713.

43. Lewis EJ, Hunsicker LG, Clarke WR et al. Renoprotective effect of the angiotensin-receptor antagonist irbesartan in patients with nephropathy due to type 2 diabetes. N Engl J Med 2001; 345:851–860.

44. Brenner BM, Cooper ME, de Zeeuw D et al. Effects of losartan on renal and cardiovascular outcomes in patients with type 2 diabetes and nephropathy. N Engl J Med 2001; 345:861–869.

45. Schrier RW, Estacio RO, Esler A et al. Effects of aggressive blood pressure control in normotensive type 2 diabetic patients on albuminuria, retinopathy and strokes. Kidney Int 2002; 61:1086–1097.

46. Estacio RO, Jeffers BW, Hiatt WR et al. The effect of nisoldipine as compared with enalapril on cardiovascular outcomes in patients with non-insulin-dependent diabetes and hypertension. N Engl J Med 1998; 338:645–652.

47. Curb JD, Pressel SL, Cutler JA et al. Effect of diuretic-based antihypertensive treatment on cardiovascular disease risk in older diabetic patients with isolated systolic hypertension. Systolic Hypertension in the Elderly Program Cooperative Research Group. JAMA 1996; 276:1886–1892.

48. Tuomilehto J, Rastenyte D, Birkenhäger WH et al. Effects of calcium-channel blockade in older patients with diabetes and systolic hypertension. N Engl J Med 1999; 340:677–684.

49. PROGRESS Collaborative Study Group. Randomised trial of perindopril-based blood pressure-lowering regimen among 6108 individuals with previous stroke or transient ischaemic attack. Lancet 2001; 358:1033–1041.

50. The Heart Outcomes Prevention Evaluation Study Investigators. Effects of an angiotensin-converting–enzyme inhibitor, ramipril, on cardiovascular events in high-risk patients. N Engl J Med 2000; 342:145–153.

51. Heart Outcomes Prevention Evaluation (HOPE) Study investigators. Effects of ramipril on cardiovascular and microvascular outcomes in people with diabetes mellitus: results of the HOPE study and MICRO-HOPE substudy. Lancet 2000; 355:253–259.

52. Zanchetti A, Hansson L, Dahlöf B et al. Effects of individual risk factors on the incidence of cardiovascular events in the treated hypertensive patients of the Hypertension Optimal Treatment Study. J Hypertens 2001; 19:1149–1159.

53. Ruilope LM, Salvetti A, Jamerson K et al. Renal function and intensive lowering of blood pressure in hypertensive participants of the hypertension optimal treatment (HOT) study. J Am Soc Nephrol 2001; 12:218–225.

54. Mann JFE, Gerstein HC, Pogue J et al, for the HOPE Investigators. Renal insufficiency as a predictor of cardiovascular outcomes and the impact of ramipril: the HOPE randomized trial. Ann Intern Med 2001; 134:629–636.

55. Vasan RS, Larson MG, Leip EP et al. Impact of high-normal blood pressure on the risk of cardiovascular disease. Framingham Heart Study. N Eng J Med 2001; 345:1291–1297.

56. Turnbull F. Blood Pressure Lowering Treatment Trialists' Collaboration. Effects of different blood-pressure-lowering regimens on major cardiovascular events: results of prospectively-designed overviews of randomised trials. Lancet 2003; 362:1527–1535.

57. Mancia G, Grassi G. Systolic and diastolic blood pressure control in antihypertensive drug trials. J Hypertens 2002; 20:1461–1464.

58. Dagenais GR, Pogue J, Fox K *et al*. Angiotensin-converting-enzyme inhibitors in stable vascular disease without left ventricular systolic dysfunction or heart failure: a combined analysis of three trials. *Lancet* 2006; 368:581–588.

59. Tokmakova M, Solomon SD. Inhibiting the renin-angiotensin system in myocardial infarction and heart failure: lessons from SAVE, VALIANT and CHARM, and other clinical trials. *Curr Opin Cardiol* 2006; 21:268–272.

60. McMurray JJ, Ostergren J, Swedberg K *et al*. CHARM Investigators and Committees. Effects of candesartan in patients with chronic heart failure and reduced left-ventricular systolic function taking angiotensin-converting-enzyme inhibitors: the CHARM-Added trial. *Lancet* 2003; 362:767–771.

61. Lindholm LH, Ibsen H, Dahlof B *et al*. Cardiovascular morbidity and mortality in patients with diabetes in the Losartan Intervention For Endpoint reduction in hypertension study (LIFE): a randomized trial against atenolol. *Lancet* 2002; 359:1004–1010.

62. Ruggenenti P, Fassi A, Ilieva AP *et al*, for the Bergamo Nephrologic Diabetes Complications Trial (BENEDICT) Investigators. Preventing microalbuminuria in type 2 diabetes. *N Engl J Med* 2004; 351:1941–1951.

63. Haller H, Viberti GC, Mimran A *et al*. Preventing microalbuminuria in patients with diabetes: rationale and design of the Randomised Olmesartan and Diabetes Microalbuminuria Prevention (ROADMAP) study. *J Hypertens* 2006; 24:403–408.

64. Ruddy M. Angiotensin II receptor blockade in diabetic nephropathy. *Am J Hypertens* 2002; 15:468–469.

65. Parving HH, Lehnert H, Brochner-Mortensen J *et al*. The effect of irbesartan on the development of diabetic nephropathy in patients with type 2 diabetes. *N Engl J Med* 2001; 345:870–878.

66. Viberti G, Wheeldon NM; MicroAlbuminuria Reduction With VALsartan (MARVAL) Study Investigators. Microalbuminuria reduction with valsartan in patients with type 2 diabetes mellitus: a blood pressure-independent effect. *Circulation* 2002; 106:672–678.

67. Barnett AH, Bain SC, Bouter P *et al*. Diabetics Exposed to Telmisartan and Enalapril Study Group. Angiotensin-receptor blockade versus converting-enzyme inhibition in type 2 diabetes and nephropathy. *N Engl J Med* 2004; 351:1952–1961.

68. Agarwal R. Add-on angiotensin receptor blockade with maximized ACE inhibition. *Kidney Int* 2001; 59:2282–2289.

69. Mogensen CE, Neldam S, Tikkanen I *et al*. Randomized controlled trial of dual blockade of reninanglotensin system in patients with hypertension, microalbuminuria, and non-insulin dependent diabetes: the Candesartan and Lisinopril Microalbuminuria (CALM) study. *Br Med J* 2000; 321:1440–1444.

70. Narayan KM, Imperatore G, Benjamin SM *et al*. Targeting people with pre-diabetes. *Br Med J* 2002; 325:403–404.

71. de Vegt F, Dekker JM, Jager A *et al*. Relation of impaired fasting and postload glucose with incident type 2 diabetes in a Dutch population: the Hoorn study. *JAMA* 2001; 285:2109–2113.

72. American Diabetes Association and National Institute of Diabetes, Digestive and Kidney Diseases. The prevention or delay of type 2 diabetes. *Diabetes Care* 2002; 25:1–8.

73. Genuth S, Alberti KG, Bennett P *et al*. Expert Committee on the Diagnosis and Classification of Diabetes Mellitus. Follow-up report on the diagnosis of diabetes mellitus. *Diabetes Care* 2003; 26:3160–3167.

74. D'Agostino RB Jr, Hamman RF, Karter AJ *et al*. Cardiovascular disease risk factors predict the development of type 2 diabetes: the insulin resistance atherosclerosis study. *Diabetes Care* 2004; 27:2234–2240.

75. Osei K, Rhinesmith S, Gaillard T *et al*. Impaired insulin sensitivity, insulin secretion, and glucose effectiveness predict future development of impaired glucose tolerance and type 2 diabetes in pre-diabetic African Americans: implications for primary diabetes prevention. *Diabetes Care* 2004; 27:1439–1446.

76. Segura J, Banegas JR, García-Donaire JA *et al*. Should hypertension guidelines be changed for hypertensive patients with the metabolic syndrome? *J Clin Hypertens (Greenwich)* 2007; 9:595–600.

77. Benjamin SM, Valdez R, Geiss LS *et al*. Estimated number of adults with prediabetes in the US in 2000: opportunities for prevention. *Diabetes Care* 2003; 26:645–649.

78. Garcia-Puig J, Ruilope LM, Luque M *et al*; AVANT Study Group Investigators. Glucose metabolism in patients with essential hypertension. *Am J Med* 2006; 119:318–326.

79. Mancia G, Grassi G, Zanchetti A. New-onset diabetes and antihypertensive drugs. *J Hypertens* 2006; 24:3–10.

80. Elliott WJ, Meyer PM. Incident diabetes in clinical trials of antihypertensive drugs: a network meta-analysis. *Lancet* 2007; 369:201–207.

11

Antiplatelet therapy in diabetes

J. A. Colwell

INTRODUCTION

The risk for coronary heart disease (CHD) events is increased two to four-fold in people with type 2 diabetes [1]. In women with type 2 diabetes, the risk is even greater, when compared to non-diabetic women. In one study, individuals with type 2 diabetes had the same increased risk for CHD death as did non-diabetic patients who had a history of prior myocardial infarction (MI) [2]. In an 18-year follow-up of this population, the investigators found that diabetes without any prior evidence of CHD indicated an even higher risk for CHD death than prior evidence of CHD in non-diabetic subjects [3]. Diabetes has been declared a 'CHD equivalent' by the third Adult Treatment Panel of the National Cholesterol Education Program (NCEP ATPIII) in the United States [4].

Platelets play a critical role in the process of atherothrombosis. Many studies have established that altered platelet function exists in diabetes. Effective antiplatelet agents, including aspirin and clopidogrel have been developed, and have been found to be effective in preventing cardiovascular events in people with diabetes. This chapter will review the evidence in this regard from large-scale prospective randomised trials and will discuss position statements from national and international organisations on antiplatelet therapy. We will also consider the estimation of cardiovascular risk in diabetes, as well as the risks of antiplatelet therapy. Finally, we will briefly review the issues of 'aspirin resistance' as well as the utilisation of aspirin therapy in diabetes, and suggest prospective randomised trials for the future. The goal is to present a balanced view on indications and expectations for the use of antiplatelet therapy in people with diabetes.

RATIONALE FOR ANTIPLATELET THERAPY IN DIABETES

PLATELETS AND ATHEROTHROMBOSIS

Platelets play an important role in atherothrombosis [5], particularly at the site of plaque rupture in the coronary artery. Platelet adherence occurs at sites of endothelial damage, and platelet–endothelial interaction is promoted by activation of platelet and endothelial adhesive receptors [6]. These receptors are activated in diabetes [7]. Collagen fibrils in the subendothelial layer trigger platelet aggregation and release of intraplatelet constituents. Platelet–platelet binding occurs via fibrinogen bridging at glycoprotein (GP) IIb/IIIa receptor sites on platelets. Thrombin cleavage of fibrinogen results in a cross-linked fibrin throm-

John A. Colwell, MD, PhD, Emeritus Professor of Medicine, Division of Endocrinology, Diabetes and Medical Genetics, Medical University of South Carolina, Charleston, South Carolina, USA.

bus. Serotonin, vascular growth factors, adenosine diphosphate (ADP), thromboxane A2 (TXA2) and/or plasminogen activator inhibitor-1 (PAI-1) are released by the aggregating platelets. Some of these factors promote further platelet recruitment, aggregation and release at the site of injury. Clot lysis is suppressed. Smooth muscle cell migration is stimulated and lipoproteins contribute lipids, which are taken up by macrophages and result in foam cells in the atherosclerotic lesion [6, 8–11].

Within the coronary artery, a critical event is plaque rupture, platelet adherence, aggregation, release and thrombus formation. The process occurs at the site of an unstable plaque [12–14]. Here, a thin fibrous cap overlies a lipid core, which also contains smooth muscle cells and activated monocytes. The cap may rupture, resulting in further platelet activation and thrombus formation. Thus, platelets play a key role in atherosclerosis and thrombosis, particularly in the coronary arteries. Inhibition of platelet function, therefore, is a logical strategy to forestall or prevent coronary occlusion [15].

ALTERED PLATELET FUNCTION IN DIABETES

Early observations

Altered platelet function in diabetes has been recognised for over 30 years [16, 17]. A summary of key studies is given in Table 11.1. Increased platelet adhesiveness *in vitro*, primarily mediated by increased von Willebrand factor (vWf) activity, was an early finding in diabetes [18]. Increased platelet sensitivity to a variety of agonists (ADP, epinephrine, collagen, arachidonic acid) occurs when platelets are suspended in citrated plama [17, 19]. Concentrations of agonists, which are relatively inactive when added to platelets from non-diabetic controls, cause the release of platelet constituents from diabetic donors. These observations have been reported in individuals with impaired glucose tolerance [17], type 1 or type 2 diabetes [6, 10, 11], and in animal models of diabetes [20–22]. There are multiple platelet plasma interactions that are operational [16]. These can be demonstrated in washed platelets or platelet-rich plasma from diabetic subjects. One of the first observations was that a minute amount of plasma from an individual with diabetes would potentiate ADP-induced aggregation at low concentrations of ADP [16]. This was called 'plasma factor', and was found in excess in diabetic individuals with microvascular and cardiovascular disease [16, 19]. Some of the contributing 'plasma factors' that have been identified are vWf [18], fibrinogen [23], immune complexes [24], and glycated low-density lipoproteins (LDL) [25]. Platelet–plasma interactions contribute not only in an increase in platelet aggregation and release in diabetes, but also to platelet–platelet and/or platelet–endothelial interactions.

Many findings were reproduced in platelet-rich plasma from animal models of diabetes. They were also seen in washed platelets from animal models [20, 21] or from diabetic subjects [6, 7, 11, 17, 19, 26]. Other findings included decreased platelet membrane fluidity [21], probably from protein glycation, and decreased platelet stores of the anti-oxidant Vitamin C [27]. Increased release of thromboxane from arachidonic acid was demonstrated in platelets from diabetic subjects [28]. Platelet turnover was found to be increased in diabetes and platelet survival was shortened [19, 22]. These findings are seen particularly in those diabetic individuals with established vascular disease. Increased platelet turnover and consequent production of young platelets (megathrombocytes) contribute to platelet hyperaggregability [22]. Indicators of *in vivo* platelet activation include increased plasma levels of β-thromboglobulin (BTG), platelet factor-4 (PF-4), platelet-derived growth factors (PDGF), and increased urinary excretion of 11-dehydro-thromboxane in type 2 diabetic individuals [6, 11, 26]. Further *in vivo* evidence is provided by the findings of platelet micro-thrombi in the vessels of patients with diabetes [29, 30], and in animal models [31]. Thus, there was ample evidence from older studies that antiplatelet therapy had a pathophysiological rationale in the prevention of vascular events in diabetes mellitus.

Table 11.1 Early observations of altered platelet function in diabetes mellitus

In vitro	In vivo
↑ Adhesiveness ↑ Aggregability ↑ Thromboxane synthesis ↑ Sensitivity to prostacyclin	↑ Turnover ↓ Survival
Platelet–plasma interactions[a] ↓ Membrane fluidity ↑ Storage and release of PAI-1 ↓ Vitamin C levels	↑ Megathrombocytes ↑ Plasma BTG, PF-4, PDGF ↑ Urinary thromboxane ↑ Platelet microthrombi

↓ and ↑ indicate decrease and increase, respectively.
a = 'Plasma factor', von Willebrand factor, fibrinogen, immune complexes, glycated LDL; BTG = β-thromboglobulin; LDL = low-density lipoprotein; PAI-1 = plasminogen activator inhibitor-1; PDGF = platelet-derived growth factor; PF-4 = platelet factor-4.

Recent observations

In more recent years, the story of altered platelet function in diabetes has been amplified. The results of some of these studies are given in Table 11.2. In particular, there have been advances in the understanding of platelet metabolism and of surface receptors. In some recent reviews [32–35], both appear to contribute to the alterations of platelet behaviour in diabetes.

Nitric oxide (NO) is an important modulator of platelet adherence, aggregation and release [32]. Platelet NO production is decreased in type 1 and type 2 diabetes [33]. Decreased uptake of the NO precursor l-arginine, and decreased production of NO by platelets from diabetic subjects have been found. Since NO is an inhibitor of platelet adhesion and aggregation, these findings may relate to heightened *in vitro* sensitivity of platelets from patients with diabetes. Further, hyperglycaemia decreases NO release and advanced glycation products are scavengers of NO [33]. Platelet activation is associated with increased protein tyrosine phosphorylation and protein kinase C (PKC) stimulation in diabetes [34]. Increased platelet intracellular calcium stores have been found in diabetes and accelerated calcium mobilisation contributes to platelet activation [35]. Increased phosphoinositide turnover in type 2 diabetes may be linked to the high intracellular calcium content and to PKC activation [34].

After platelet activation, there is an increased expression of GP surface receptors in both type 1 and type 2 diabetes [36–42]. The GPIIb/IIIa receptor binds fibrinogen, leading to platelet aggregation. GPIb-V-IX acts as a receptor for vWf and is a substrate for thrombin. P-selectin is an alpha granule protein that is expressed on the platelet surface with degranulation. P-selectin glycoprotein ligand (PSGL-1) is a ligand on white blood cells for P-selectin. P-selectin mediates the interaction of activated platelets with neutrophils and monocytes. Increased adhesiveness and/or aggregation of erythrocytes, leucocytes and platelets has been found in the peripheral blood of people with diabetes [43, 44]. Leucocyte–platelet aggregates produce procoagulant and mitogenic materials that may play a role in thrombosis. Interaction of activated platelets with monocytes, mediated by P-selectin, can activate tissue factor and the blood coagulation cascade.

Thus, alterations of the intensive coagulation system, the fibrinolytic system, and platelet function are frequently present in diabetes. Accordingly, several pharmaceutical modulators of platelet function have been developed and their effect in primary and secondary prevention of cardiovascular events has been studied in people with diabetes.

Table 11.2 Recent observations of altered platelet function in diabetes mellitus

Intracellular metabolism	
↓ NO sensitivity and production	↓ L-arginine uptake ↑ Homocysteine and ↓ NO release ↑ Glucose and ↓ NO release
↑ Protein tyrosine phosphorylation ↑ PKC stimulation ↑ Intracellular calcium content ↑ or ↓ Phosphoinositide turnover	
Surface receptors ↑ Expression of adhesive receptors	GP IIb/IIIa: fibrinogen GPIb-V-IX: von Willebrand factor PSGL-1: P-selectin (on white blood cells) CD36: thrombospondin
↑ Platelet-erythrocyte-leukocyte adhesion ADP receptor activation	

↑ and ↓ indicate increase and decrease, respectively.
ADP = adenosine diphosphate; GP = glycoprotein; NO = nitric oxide; PKC = protein kinase C;
PSGL-1 = P-selectin glycoprotein ligand-1

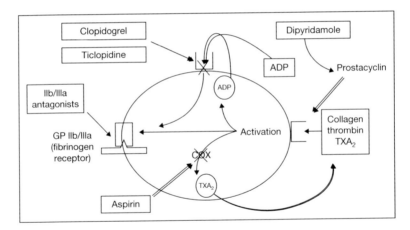

Figure 11.1 Mechanism of action of antiplatelet agents.
ADP = adenosine diphosphate; GP = glycoprotein; TXA2 = thromboxane A2.

MAJOR ANTIPLATELET DRUGS

Aspirin

Aspirin produces an irreversible loss of the enzymatic activity of thromboxane synthase, the cyclo-oxygenase enzyme that catalyses the conversion of prostanoid precursors to thromboxane (TXA2, Figure 11.1) [45]. Its effect is rapid after oral ingestion, resulting in an immediate action on platelets in the portal circulation. Inhibition of thromboxane production lasts for the 8–10 day lifespan of these platelets, since platelets cannot synthesise new enzymatic protein. The system is very sensitive to low doses of aspirin, with 70–100 mg orally virtually completely suppressing thromboxane synthesis. The inhibiting effect is cumulative, and daily doses of 30–50 mg in normal subjects provide almost complete suppression of thromboxane synthesis after 7–10 days of administration [45]. Theoretically, it is advisable to use an aspirin dosage that will not inactivate endothelial cyclo-oxygenase. This should allow for the production of prostacyclin, a potent platelet anti-aggregant. Low-dose preparations of aspirin appear to yield persistent suppression of platelet thromboxane synthesis. However, accelerated platelet turnover may occur in diabetes and require controlled release aspirin, higher doses or multiple daily dosing [46]. Aspirin has been the first-choice antiplatelet agent in the majority of controlled clinical trials.

Clopidogrel

This drug acts by inhibiting the binding of ADP to its low affinity platelet receptor (Figure 11.1) [47, 48]. This will inhibit platelet aggregation and it is not dependent upon thromboxane inhibition. Thus, clopidogrel may be effective in the absence of aspirin or may be additive to aspirin's inhibition of thromboxane synthesis. Activation of low affinity purigenic platelet receptors leads to calcium mobilisation and a platelet conformational change [47, 48]. This, in turn, activates the platelet GPIIb/IIIa receptor complex, which increases fibrinogen binding and platelet aggregation. Inhibition of ADP binding with clopidogrel is concentration-dependent, with significant inhibition after 2–3 days of 75 mg of clopidogrel orally. This persists for 7–10 days after therapy is stopped, as new platelets enter the circulation. As would be predicted from the mechanism described, clopidogrel will act synergistically with aspirin and/or GPIIb/IIIa receptor antagonists to inhibit platelet aggression.

GPIIb/IIIa receptor antagonists

Monoclonal antibodies to GPIIb/IIIa and arginine–glycine aspartic acid compounds have been developed that inhibit fibrinogen binding to these GP receptors [49, 50]. Abciximab binds to the GPIIb/IIIa receptor, prevents fibrinogen and vWf binding, and inhibits platelet aggregation. Other antagonists of this receptor complex are eptifibatide and tirofiban. These are given intravenously and inhibit platelet aggregation in a concentration-dependent manner. This is reversible 4–8 hours after cessation of the infusion. Oral agents are under study. In diabetes, the major use of these agents has been in patients with acute coronary syndromes.

Picotamide

Picotamide is a drug that has dual antiplatelet actions. It inhibits thromboxane synthesis and also antagonises TXA2 receptors at equivalent concentrations. It enhances endothelial formation of prostacyclin. This should result in inhibition of platelet aggregation and increased activity of anti-aggregetory prostaglandins. The drug is a derivative of methoxy-isophthalic acid, and is given in divided oral doses of 900–1200 mg daily. Preliminary studies in type 2 diabetic subjects with peripheral arterial disease have been reported from Europe [51], and are considered below.

PROSPECTIVE RANDOMISED TRIALS OF ANTIPLATELET AGENTS IN DIABETES

SECONDARY PREVENTION

Meta-analyses by the Antiplatelet Trialists' Collaboration

There have been two major meta-analyses of antiplatelet trials in high-risk patients, usually with a previous myocardial infarction or stroke. In 1994, 145 randomised trials in 70 000 high-risk patients were reviewed [52]. In 2002, the analysis was updated by including the results of 287 studies in 135 000 patients [53]. Overall, allocation to antiplatelet therapy (usually aspirin) reduced the combined outcome of any serious vascular event in high-risk patients by 25%, non-fatal myocardial infarction by 33%, non-fatal stroke by 25% and cardiovascular mortality by 16%.

Only nine of the 287 studies (3%) were undertaken solely in diabetic subjects, and in only two was aspirin the chosen antiplatelet agent. Results were clearly dominated by the large Early Treatment in Diabetic Retinopathy Study (ETDRS) [54]. Overall, the results of these trials in high-risk diabetic subjects were similar to those in the entire patient group. Antiplatelet therapy is now accepted as the appropriate approach in patients who have had a previous cardiovascular event (secondary prevention).

Peripheral arterial disease in diabetes

Veterans Affairs (VA) Cooperative Study
One of the first studies of antiplatelet agents in type 2 diabetic subjects was in patients who had already had an amputation for gangrene [55]. In this study, 325 mg of aspirin plus 75 mg of dipyridamideamole or matching placebos were given three times daily for 3 years to 231 VA patients. No effect on the primary combined endpoint of amputation of the opposite extremity plus vascular death was seen. There was a significant reduction in stroke and transient ischaemic attack (TIA), a predefined secondary combined endpoint.

Drug Evaluation in Artherosclerotic Vascular Disease in Diabetes (DAVID) study
In the DAVID study, 1209 patients with type 2 diabetes and peripheral arterial disease (PAD) were randomised to receive either picotamide (600 mg bid) or aspirin (320 mg daily) for 2 years [51]. Overall mortality was the primary endpoint and was significantly lower in those who received picotamide (3.0%) compared to those given aspirin (5.5%) ($P = 0.0474$). Relative risk ratio for mortality (picotamide vs. aspirin) was 0.55 (95% confidence interval [CI] 0.31–0.98). The secondary study endpoint, mortality plus non-fatal vascular events, was slightly (but not significantly) reduced in the picotamide group.

Acute coronary syndrome

This issue has been explored in detail in a recent review article [48]. In brief, studies have indicated that aspirin, in combination with clopidogrel, and/or with a platelet GPIIb/IIIa inhibitor, will lower the risk of adverse cardiovascular events in patients with acute coronary syndromes (ACS). The majority of these studies have been of short duration and were undertaken in populations with limited numbers of diabetic subjects. Generally, beneficial effects have been seen in the entire population, with non-significant trends in the same direction in diabetic subgroups.

There has been one meta-analysis of 30-day mortality in diabetic patients with ACS who received platelet GPIIb/IIIa inhibitor or placebo [56]. There was a significant reduction in 30-day mortality from 6.2% to 4.6% ($P = 0.007$) in this meta-analysis.

RANDOMISED TRIALS OF ASPIRIN IN DIABETIC SUBJECTS AT HIGH VASCULAR RISK

There are two key studies of aspirin therapy in large numbers of diabetic subjects who were at high vascular risk. In one, the ETDRS study, all of the patients had diabetic retinopathy, the majority had hypertension, and many had suffered a previous cardiovascular event [54]. In the Hypertension Optimal Treatment (HOT) study, all patients had hypertension [57]. Thus, cardiovascular risk was high in the diabetic patients in both studies.

Early Treatment of Diabetic Retinopathy Study (ETDRS)
This is the largest study of aspirin therapy in a diabetic population. It was primarily designed to explore photocoagulation approaches for pre-proliferative retinopathy and/or maculopathy in 3711 type 1 and type 2 diabetic patients. The design compared the effects of 650 mg of aspirin daily versus placebo on the progression of retinopathy, retinal or vitreous bleeding, maculopathy and cardiovascular events. In the first 5 years of follow-up, the relative

risk for myocardial infarction was 0.72 (99% CI 0.55–0.95; $P \leq 0.01$) for the aspirin versus placebo comparison. Over the full 7 years of the trial, relative risk for MI was 0.83 (95% CI 0.66–1.04; $P \leq 0.05$). The change in relative risk was attributed to decreased adherence late in the study, particularly the use of antiplatelet agents in the placebo group. There was no effect of aspirin on retinopathy, and there was no increase in gastrointestinal, retinal or vitreous bleeding with aspirin [58].

HOT trial

This was designed as a study of antihypertensive therapy in 18 790 hypertensive men and women. Diabetes was present in 1501 subjects. In the antihypertensive therapy study, there was a 51% reduction in vascular events in the diabetic subgroup, which was targeted to a diastolic blood pressure of ≤ 80 mmHg versus the group targeted to ≤ 90 mmHg. In this study, patients were randomised to 75 mg of aspirin daily or placebo and cardiovascular events were followed. Overall, there was a 36% reduction in the risk for myocardial infarction in the group randomised to aspirin ($P = 0.002$). The results in the diabetic subgroup were not reported separately. However, the investigators stated that the relative benefit on major cardiovascular events on myocardial infarction were *'about the same'* in the diabetic subjects. There was no increase in hemorrhagic stroke or in fatal bleeding in the aspirin group in the entire cohort.

RANDOMISED TRIALS OF ASPIRIN IN SUBJECTS AT LOW VASCULAR RISK

Primary Prevention Project (PPP)

This was a randomised trial designed to test whether treatment with 100 mg aspirin and/or 300 mg of Vitamin E would reduce frequency of major cardiovascular events in 4495 diabetic and non-diabetic patients with one or more cardiovascular risk factors [59]. After a mean follow-up of 3.6 years, the relative risk for the aspirin versus non-aspirin comparison for the combined endpoint of cardiovascular death, stroke or myocardial infarction was 0.59 (95%CI 0.37–0.94). The prospective design included a study of 4000 subjects with diabetes. However, recruitment was stopped after only 1031 patients were entered, due to the benefit seen in the entire trial. In the diabetic group, there were fewer myocardial infarctions with aspirin therapy (5 vs. 10, or 1% vs. 2%), but CHD event rates were very low (<1% per year), and the findings did not reach statistical significance [60].

US Physicians' Health Study (USPHS)

This was a primary prevention study in 22 071 American male physicians in which 325 mg of aspirin was given every other day and compared to placebo [61]. Average follow-up was 5 years, and there was a 44% reduction in the risk of myocardial infarction in the aspirin group. In the small subgroup of diabetic men in the study, 26 of 258 (10.8%) of those randomised to placebo, versus 11 of 258 randomised to aspirin (4.3%) had a myocardial infarction. No statistical analysis was reported. A simple Chi square analysis yields a P value of <0.01.

Women's Health Study

This was a trial that compared 100 mg of aspirin to Vitamin E 600 IU every other day in 39 876 initially healthy women [62]. They were followed for 10 years, with a combined primary endpoint of non-fatal myocardial infarction, non-fatal stroke and cardiovascular death. In the aspirin group, there was a non-significant reduction in risk for this primary cardiovascular endpoint of 9% ($P = 0.13$). There was a significant 17% reduction in risk of stroke in the aspirin group, primarily related to a 24% decrease in the risk of ischaemic stroke. Subgroup analysis showed a significant reduction in major cardiovascular events (ischaemic stroke, myocardial infarction) with aspirin in women 65 years of age or older.

There were 1027 women who had diabetes at baseline in this study. The aspirin group had a significant 19% reduction in ischaemic stroke ($P = 0.05$), but had no significant reduction in myocardial infarction. The event rate for myocardial infarction was low, at approximately 0.6% per year. No breakdown of diabetic women over age 65 was given.

The study shows that very low-dose aspirin (100 mg every other day) will prevent ischaemic stroke in diabetic women.

The Prevention of Progression of Arterial Disease and Diabetes (POPADAD) trial

This was a study to determine if aspirin (100 mg) and anti-oxidant therapy, combined or alone, would reduce the development of cardiovascular events in people with diabetes and peripheral vascular disease [63]. 1276 adults with type 1 or 2 diabetes and ankle brachial pressure index of 0.99 or less, but no symptomatic cardiovascular disease, were followed for 6.7 years (median). Two hierarchical composite endpoints were used:

1. Death from coronary heart disease or stroke, non-fatal myocardial infarction or stroke, or above ankle amputation for critical limb ischemia.
2. Death from coronary heart disease or stroke. No difference was seen between aspirin vs. no aspirin in either primary endpoint.

This study had a slower than expected recruitment rate and lower event rates than predicted. This reduced the power of the study to detect a difference in cardiovascular events between the aspirin vs. no aspirin groups.

Low-Dose Aspirin for Primary Prevention of Atherosclerotic Events in Patients with type 2 Diabetes: A Randomized Controlled Trial (JPAD).

This was a prospective randomised trial of aspirin (81 or 100 mg per day) vs. no aspirin in 2539 Japanese type 2 diabetic patients without a history of atherosclerotic disease [64]. They had a median follow-up of 4.37 years. Primary endpoints were fatal and non-fatal ischemic heart disease or stroke and peripheral vascular disease.

There were 68 atherosclerotic events in the aspirin group (13.6 per 1000 person-years) and 86 in the non aspirin group (17.0 per 1000 person-years). This yielded a hazard ratio (HR) of 0.80, with 95% confidence interval (CI) of 0.58–1.10 ($P = 0.16$). Fatal coronary and cardiovascular events occurred in 1 patient (aspirin group) vs. 10 patients (non-aspirin group; HR 0.10; 95%CI, 0.01–0.79, $P = 0037$.) In 1363 patients aged 65 years or older, the incidence of atherosclerotic events was significantly lower in the aspirin group (45 events = 6.3%) than in the non-aspirin group (59 events = 9.2%; HR=0.68; 95%CI, 0.46–0.99, $P = 0.047$).

Thus, there were a non-signifcant trend favouring a beneficial effect of aspirin on the primary endpoint, and significant effects of aspirin on the secondary endpoint of fatal coronary and cerebrovascular events. Futher, a subgroup analysis in those patients aged 65 years or older showed a significant benefit of aspirin on the incidence of atherosclerotic events. This study was also underpowered for the primary endpoint due to an event rate that was one-third of the rate used in sample size calculations. Collectively, the results are encouraging, and indicate that larger studies in low-risk diabetic subjects are needed.

Results from these eight studies in diabetic subjects are shown in Table 11.3. It is clear that more studies are indicated in people with diabetes, particularly those at low CHD risk.

Meta-analyses of primary prevention trials

In addition to the USPHS, HOT and PPP trials, there are two other published primary prevention trials of aspirin vs. placebo in low-risk individuals. In one meta-analysis (which did not include the PPP trial), aspirin was associated with a significant 30% reduction in myo-

Table 11.3 Trials of aspirin versus placebo in diabetes mellitus: effect on myocardial infarction (MI) or ischaemic stroke

Trial	n	%F	Years	Endpoint	Aspirin (mg/day)	Relative risk	P
USPHS [61]	533	0	5	MI	325 (q.o.d.)	0.39	0.01*
ETDRS [54]	3711	44	5	MI	650	0.72	0.01$^\Delta$
HOT [57]	1501	47	3.8	MI	75	0.64	0.002+
PPP [60]	1031	58	3.7	MI	100	NS	NS
WHS [62]	1027	100	10	Ischaemic Stroke	100 (q.o.d.)	0.81	0.05
POPADAD [63]	1276	57	6.7	composite**	100	0.98	0.86
JPAD [64]	2539	45	4.37	composite**	81 or 100	0.80	0.16

* = Chi Square analysis; $^\Delta$ = 1st 5 years; + = Entire cohort, including diabetes; %F = percentage of females in study; ** See text
ETDRS = Early Treatment Diabetic Retinopathy Study; HOT = Hypertension Optimal Treatment; JPAD = Japanese Primary Prevention of Atherosclerosis with Aspirin for Diabetes; NS = not significant; POPADAD = Prevention of Progression of Arterial Disease and Diabetes; PPP = Primary Prevention Project; USPHS = US Physicians' Health Study; WHS = Women's Health Study.

cardial infarction and a 15% reduction in all cardiovascular events [65]. However, risk of major bleeding with aspirin did not outweigh benefit when the CHD event rate was ≤0.6% per year. These authors concluded that aspirin treatment for primary prevention is safe and worthwhile at a coronary event risk ≥1.5% per year, safe but of limited value at a coronary risk of ≥1.0% per year, and unsafe at a coronary risk of ≤0.5% per year. When results from the PPP trial were included in a separate meta-analysis of five primary prevention trials, similar significant risk reductions were found: 32% for the first MI and 15% for all cardiovascular events [66].

There were approximately 3000 low-risk diabetic patients out of a total of 55 580 (5.4%) randomised participants in these five trials. A preliminary analysis has indicated a nonsignificant 25% reduction in coronary events among those diabetic patients randomised to aspirin therapy [67]: 3.9% of aspirin-allocated patients and 4.9% of placebo-allocated patients had coronary events (P = 0.1), during a mean follow-up of 5 years. These findings provide additional support for new randomised trials of aspirin versus placebo in diabetic patients at low cardiovascular risk.

POSITION STATEMENTS ON ASPIRIN USE TO PREVENT CARDIOVASCULAR EVENTS

Position statements on aspirin therapy for patients at high risk for CHD events have been released by four organisations.

AMERICAN DIABETES ASSOCIATION (ADA)

After the results of the ETDRS were released, the ADA issued a Technical Review [68] and a Position Statement [69]. This has been reissued yearly, with minor modifications. The current recommendations are summarised as follows:

■ Use aspirin therapy (75–162 mg/day) as a secondary prevention strategy in those individuals with diabetes with a history of myocardial infarction, vascular bypass procedure,

stroke or transient ischaemic attack, peripheral vascular disease, claudication and/or angina.
- Use aspirin therapy (75–162 mg/day) as a primary prevention strategy in those with type 1 or type 2 diabetes at increased cardiovascular risk, including those who are >40 years of age and who have one or more risk factors (family history of cardiovascular disease [CVD], hypertension, smoking, dyslipidaemia or albuminuria).
- People with aspirin allergy, bleeding tendency, receiving anticoagulant therapy, recent gastrointestinal bleeding or clinically active hepatic disease are *not* candidates for aspirin therapy. Other antiplatelet agents may be a reasonable alternative for patients with high risk.

AMERICAN HEART ASSOCIATION (AHA)

Guidelines issued by the AHA emphasize the estimation of cardiovascular risk in choosing candidates for aspirin therapy [70]. The AHA recommends that 75–160 mg/day be used in people at high risk for coronary heart disease (CHD). This was defined as ≥10% in 10 years.

US PREVENTIVE SERVICES TASK FORCE (USPSTF)

The USPSTF, after a thorough review of available evidence, issued guidelines that were more aggressive [71]. The task force recommended that physicians discuss the use of aspirin to prevent CHD in patients at a 5-year risk of CHD of >3% (10 year risk ≥6%).

EUROPEAN SOCIETY OF CARDIOLOGY (ESC)

A task force of ESC has issued more conservative guidelines [72]. They concluded that the available evidence supports the daily use of aspirin (75–100 mg) for the long-term prevention of serious vascular events in individuals with a CHD risk ≥3% per year.

In low-risk individuals, the ESC stated that the benefit/risk profile is uncertain. The task force noted, however, that a meta-analysis of four primary prevention trials suggested that aspirin treatment is *'safe and worthwhile'* at a coronary event risk ≥1.5% per year.

A summary of these recommendations is given in Table 11.4.

ESTIMATION OF CARDIOVASCULAR RISK IN DIABETES

Diabetes is viewed by the ATP III report as a *'cardiovascular risk equivalent'* [4]. Yet, there are many variables among diabetic individuals, including type 1 or 2 diabetes, age, duration of diabetes, gender, blood pressure, cigarette smoking, as well as biochemical cardiovascular risk variables such as HbA1c, lipids and microalbuminuria.

The Framingham estimation of risk [73, 74] is valuable for non-diabetic individuals, but has limitations for people with diabetes. The model is drawn from a small sample size of 337 diabetic patients and includes no measure of glycaemia or duration of diabetes. Recently, Stevens and colleagues have developed the UKPDS risk engine, which is designed to predict CHD in type 2 diabetes [75]. The model is derived from the results of the UKPDS, where 4540 men and women with recently diagnosed type 2 diabetes were followed in the trial for a mean of 10.5 years. This model, in contrast to the Framingham system, is diabetes-specific. It takes into account age at diagnosis and duration of diabetes, glycosylated haemoglobin (HbA1c), systolic hypertension, cholesterol–HDL cholesterol ratio, cigarette smoking, gender and ethnicity. In diabetes, it is the preferred model to estimate CHD risk, which is defined as fatal or non-fatal myocardial infarction or sudden death.

Table 11.4 Summary of recommendations for aspirin therapy

Organisation	Year	Recommendation	Aspirin dosage (mg/day)
ADA [68, 69]	1998	Diabetes (≥40 yrs of age) + 1 or more CV risk factors	75–162
AHA [70]	2002	10 year risk of first CHD event ≥10%	75–150
USPSTF [71]	2002	5 year risk of CHD ≥3%	75
ESC [72]	2003	1 year risk of CHD ≥3% 'Safe and worthwhile' at 1 year Risk of CHD ≥1.5%	75–100

ADA = American Diabetes Association; AHA = American Heart Association; CHD = coronary heart disease; ESC = European Society of Cardiology; USPSTF = US Preventive Services Task Force.

Table 11.5 Estimates of diabetic individuals eligible for aspirin therapy

CHD cut-off point (%/yr)	Organisation	% of diabetes ≥ cut-off point
≥0.6	USPSTF [71]	94%
≥1.0	AHA [70]	85%
≥1.5	ESC [72]	73%, 65%
High CHD risk	ADA [68, 69]	98%

ADA = American Diabetes Association; AHA = American Heart Association; CHD = coronary heart disease; ESC = European Society of Cardiology; USPSTF = US Preventive Services Task Force.

Since this model is based upon follow-up of recently diagnosed diabetic individuals and excludes those with recent myocardial infarction or stroke, it will underestimate CHD risk in a general adult diabetic population. By this system, the majority of people with diabetes would exceed the guidelines for aspirin therapy from the USPSTF and the AHA (Table 11.5).

There are two recent population studies in the United Kingdom in newly diagnosed type 2 diabetic subjects who were free from vascular disease. Estimations of CHD risk were done using the UKPDS risk engine [75, 76]. In one study, 700 male and female diabetic subjects without arterial complications were evaluated from nine general practices [77]. Overall, the 10-year CHD risk was 21.5% (2.15% per year). If a ≥1.5% per year CHD risk were used, about 65% of these diabetic individuals would have been eligible for aspirin therapy. A higher percentage would have been eligible if USPSTF, ADA or AHA recommendations were followed. In a second study of 428 newly diagnosed diabetic patients in Southampton, UK [76], 73–94% of these type 2 diabetic subjects would be eligible for aspirin therapy, depending on the cut-off point used (Table 11.5). If recommendations from the ADA were followed, Rolka and colleagues found that 98% of 1503 adult diabetic individuals in the Third National Health and Nutrition Examination Survey in the USA would be eligible for aspirin therapy [78]: 27% of these were secondary prevention and 71% primary prevention patients. Calculation of projected CHD risk using the UKPDS risk engine (or comparable systems to be developed for diabetic populations) provides the best quantitative tool to guide the decision about aspirin therapy in type 2 diabetic individuals.

RISKS OF ANTIPLATELET THERAPY

In non-diabetic individuals, long-term therapy with low dose aspirin approximately doubles the risk of major gastrointestinal (GI) tract bleeding [79]. This translates into an estimated excess of one or two major bleeding episodes per 1000 adults treated with low-dose aspirin for one year. Whether this applies to diabetic subjects is unclear. It is of interest that major GI bleeding was rarely reported in the ETDRS, in spite of a relatively high aspirin dosage of 650 mg/day. It is estimated that there is an absolute excess of haemorrhagic strokes of about 1–2 per 10 000 patients with aspirin therapy. Risk of serious bleeding rises with increased doses of aspirin and with age [80]. The risk is particularly high in subjects with acute coronary syndrome, where combined antiplatelet therapy is often given, and dosages usually exceed the low doses recommended for chronic therapy.

In the ETDRS, serial retinal photographs revealed that there was no increased risk of retinal or vitreous bleeding in diabetic subjects, even with aspirin doses of 650 mg/day. Further, in the HOT study, there was no increase in major haemorrhagic stroke in this large cohort of hypertensive individuals who were under intensive therapy for hypertension, when aspirin was prescribed at a dose of 100 mg/day.

There may be gastric irritation with aspirin, usually manifested by heartburn. Use of enteric-coated aspirin may be helpful. Occasionally, allergy to aspirin may occur, and desensitisation or switching to another antiplatelet agent is indicated. A past history of ulcer is a relative contraindication to aspirin therapy because of the potential for GI bleeding. Proton pump inhibitors have been shown to decrease the risk of GI bleeding with aspirin in one study [80].

'ASPIRIN RESISTANCE'

A concept of 'aspirin resistance' has arisen [81, 82] and may be recognised clinically as an individual who suffers a cardiovascular event while on aspirin therapy. One study indicated that the baseline level of a urinary thromboxane metabolite (11 dehydrothromboxane B_2) in individuals on aspirin therapy (by history) was associated with an increased risk of cardiovascular death and of myocardial infarction [83]. There have been a number of attempts to define 'aspirin resistance' by *in vitro* responsiveness of platelets to various agonists [81]. However, in one recent study, only one of 143 patients who were taking 325 mg aspirin daily was found to be 'aspirin resistant' when the thromboxane substrate, arachidonic acid, was used as the agonist [84]. It is apparent that this issue remains a research question. While 'aspirin resistance' (manifested as treatment failure) is present in some patients with diabetes mellitus, more studies are needed to define accurate and sensitive predictive tests as well as therapeutic approaches to address this issue.

There are a number of theoretical reasons to expect that aspirin would not be 100% effective in preventing cardiovascular events in diabetic subjects. As already noted, platelet function is quite complicated in the diabetic state (Tables 12.1 and 12.2). One of the first alterations of platelet aggregation that was described in diabetes was an interaction of normal platelets with 'platelet aggregation enhancing factor(s)' found in people with diabetes, especially those with vascular disease [16]. Candidates for this activity include immune complexes, lipoproteins, glycosylated proteins, fibrinogen and von Willebrand factor [6]. These interactions are demonstrated using ADP-induced platelet aggregation, and may not necessarily involve the thromboxane system. Thus, plasma–platelet interaction in diabetes is one theoretical explanation for treatment failure with aspirin therapy. Other candidates for 'aspirin resistance' include erythrocyte-induced platelet activation, cigarette smoking, poor patient compliance, aspirin-insensitive thromboxane biosynthesis from macrophages or endothelial cells and mutations of the cyclo-oxygenase-1 (COX-1) gene in platelets [81]. A clinical cause of 'aspirin resistance' is the interference by ibuprofen for COX-1 binding sites for aspirin

Table 11.6 Prevalence of aspirin use in patients with diabetes mellitus

Study	Years	Aspirin use		Comments
		Primary prevention (% pts)	Secondary prevention (% pts)	
NHANES III [78]	1988–94	13	37	US survey (NHANES)
Wood et al [87]	1999		63	Outpatients with cardiovascular disease
Krein et al [88]	2000	59	79	25 VA Medical Centers
Krumholz et al [89]	2001		62	Medicare recipients
Cull et al [90]	1997	20	76	Longitudinal study
	2001	35	82	

NHANES = National Health and Nutrition Examination Survey; pts = patients; VA = Veterans Affairs.

[85]. Recent studies have indicated that enteric-coated aspirin may not adequately suppress thromboxane production in some patients with stable cardiovascular disease [86].

If recurrent vascular events occur despite the chronic use of aspirin, a consensus view is that this be defined as treatment failure, rather than 'aspirin resistance'. The therapeutic strategy in such diabetic patients must await the results of properly designed prospective trials.

ASPIRIN UTILISATION IN DIABETES

In spite of guidelines for aspirin use in patients at high risk for CHD events, utilisation appears to be less than optimal. A summary of aspirin use in patients with diabetes is given in Table 11.6. Usage is highest in patients who have already had a cardiovascular event (>60% in recent studies). As a primary prevention strategy, aspirin use ranges from 20–59% in recent studies. Counselling of staff and patients in the Veterans Affairs system has led to an increase in aspirin use.

As previously noted, the Antiplatelet Trialists' Collaboration reviewed 287 antiplatelet trials in 135 000 patients [52]. Aspirin was the antiplatelet agent in diabetic subjects in only two of these trials. As noted in Table 11.3, only ~7800 diabetic subjects have been randomised to aspirin (in doses ranging from 100 mg every other day to 650 mg/day) versus placebo. Furthermore, only one study (ETDRS) has solely enrolled diabetic subjects. This study accounts for 48% of diabetic patients studied in randomised trials of aspirin versus placebo. Thus, the database is badly in need of expansion. Accordingly, one major prospective trial is now in the planning stage and another is ongoing. As we have noted, evidence for aspirin therapy in diabetic individuals who are at relatively low risk for a cardiovascular event are limited. A Study of Cardiovascular Events in Diabetes (ASCEND), will compare 75 mg of aspirin versus 1 g/day of omega-3 fatty acids in 10 000 newly-diagnosed type 1 or 2 diabetic volunteers over age 40 years, without clinical vascular disease [67, 91]. A 2×2 factorial design will be used. Primary endpoints are non-fatal myocardial infarction, non-fatal stroke and cardiovascular death. The event rate is estimated to be 2% per year. This study will give valuable information on the efficacy and safety of low-dose aspirin therapy in those type 2 diabetic subjects who are at relatively low cardiovascular risk for fatal or non-fatal MI and stroke.

There is one ongoing trial (Clopidogrel for High Atherothrombotic Risk and Ischemic Stabilization, Management and Avoidance, CHARISMA) that is evaluating safety and efficacy of 75–162 mg of aspirin plus 75 mg of clopidogrel versus aspirin alone in high-risk patients [92]. A total of 15 602 adult patients with established coronary, cerebral or peripheral arterial disease are enrolled. The primary endpoint is the composite of vascular death, myocardial infarction, or stroke. The entry criteria and the large sample size indicate that the diabetic subgroup will be substantial in number. Thus, the trial should provide useful new information on the benefits and risks of dual antiplatelet therapy for people with diabetes. It will be viewed as a mixed secondary and high-risk primary prevention trial.

The best evidence for efficacy of aspirin therapy comes from the ETDRS, where a large dose (650 mg of aspirin daily) was compared to placebo therapy in type 1 and type 2 diabetic patients with retinopathy. This was a mixed primary and secondary trial, since some of these patients had cardiovascular events before entry. Thus, there is evidence in support of high-dose aspirin therapy in diabetic patients who are at high cardiovascular risk. Increased severe GI bleeding was not seen. A prospective trial in type 2 diabetic patients with a cardiovascular risk of >2% per year, which compares low versus high-dose aspirin, would be a useful study. If techniques to clearly identify 'aspirin resistant' diabetic subjects at baseline are developed and agreed upon, one would also like to explore combinations of aspirin and clopidogrel versus aspirin alone in these individuals.

Information on aspirin therapy in women with diabetes has been reported in the Women's Health Study [62] and the ETDRS [58]. Low-dose aspirin in the former trial reduced the risk for ischaemic stroke among diabetic women and reduced cardiovascular events in women over age 65 (many of whom may have had diabetes). The effects of a high aspirin dose on CHD in the ETDRS were less successful in women than in men. A recent meta-analysis of aspirin therapy for primary prevention of cardiovascular events in large, randomised trials indicated that aspirin was effective in reducing MI in men and ischaemic stroke in women [93]. Small numbers of diabetic subjects precluded an analysis of a diabetic subgroup. Additional trials are needed in women with diabetes who are at a CHD risk of ≥1% per year. Results from the ASCEND Trial [67, 91] will provide useful information on this issue, as will findings from the CHARISMA Trial [92].

SUMMARY

In the United States, there are approximately 20 million people with diabetes mellitus. There are at least as many additional individuals who can be classified, on the basis of fasting plasma glucose levels between 100 and 126 mg/dl, as having 'pre-diabetes'. Others are at high cardiovascular risk from the metabolic syndrome. Cardiovascular disease is often manifested clinically by myocardial infarction and is the major cause of death in diabetic and pre-diabetic individuals and in those with the metabolic syndrome. Prior to the last decade, while significant advances were made in reducing cardiovascular mortality in the non-diabetic population, there was only a minimal decrease among men, and an actual increase in women with diabetes between 1971–1975 and 1982–1984 [94]. More recently, and presumably related to more intensive management of lipids, blood pressure, glycaemia and other CHD risk factors in people with diabetes, an encouraging drop in cardiovascular complications has been reported among the small cohort of diabetic individuals in the Framingham Study (1950–1966 vs. 1977–1995) [95].

It is unclear what role aspirin therapy has played in these trends. Aspirin therapy is underutilised in diabetes, particularly as a primary prevention strategy (Table 11.6). After a coronary event, recent studies indicate that 63–82% of people with diabetes in the USA and the UK are placed on aspirin therapy. However, <35% of adults with diabetes are currently taking aspirin regularly, in spite of guidelines from the ADA, AHA, USPSTF and ESC. In part, this may reflect the need for more data on primary prevention and/or the lack of recognition that diabetes should be viewed as a *'cardiovascular risk equivalent'* [4]. In this context, data from secondary prevention trials [56, 57] and studies of diabetic subjects at high CHD risk [53, 56] would support the use of aspirin in the majority of people with diabetes [69–71].

Perhaps the most useful guidelines for clinical decision-making are those issued yearly by the ADA since 1998 [69]. Low dose aspirin (75–162 mg/day) is recommended. Here, diabetic individuals who are clearly at high cardiovascular risk are defined. In addition to those who have already had a cardiovascular event, the guidelines required an adult (>40 years old) with a diagnosis of type 1 or type 2 diabetes, and at least one additional risk factor: hypertension, lipid abnormality, cigarette smoking and albuminuria. This virtually assures a predicted coronary heart disease event rate of ≥1.5% per year. This rate is greater that that proposed by the AHA [70] or USPSTF [71], and is supported by the ESC [72]. Until newer studies are completed, this strategy for aspirin therapy should provide clear benefit in the prevention of myocardial infarction in these individuals with diabetes.

These predicted benefits must be balanced against projected risks. Aspirin should not be used in individuals with a bleeding disorder, or anticoagulant therapy. It must be used with caution, if at all, in patients with a history of ulcer disease. Here, concomitant therapy with a proton pump inhibitor such as omeprazole is an option [80]. Future studies should clarify indications for the long-term use of combined antiplatelet therapy and/or higher doses of aspirin in cases of treatment failure.

In conclusion:

1. There is a pathophysiological rationale for aspirin therapy in diabetes.
2. There is support from controlled clinical trials that aspirin therapy is effective in reducing the risk of myocardial infarction in diabetic patients.
3. People with diabetes have a high risk for coronary heart disease events, and this risk can be quantified accurately.
4. Four major professional societies have issued position statements in support of aspirin therapy in patients with high CHD risk ranging from 0.6–1.5% per year. The majority of type 2 diabetic patients are at or exceed the threshold of 1% per year.
5. 75–162 mg of aspirin/day should be prescribed for adult diabetic subjects at high CHD risk (≥1% per year, or with ≥1 CHD risk factor).
6. There is a need for prospective randomised trials of low versus high-dose aspirin, clopidogrel + aspirin versus aspirin alone, etc. in low- and high-risk diabetic populations.
7. Additional studies of antiplatelet therapy in women with diabetes are needed.

REFERENCES

1. Stamler JM, Vaccaro O, Neaton JD et al. Diabetes, other risk factors, and 12-yr cardiovascular mortality for men screened in the Multiple Risk Factor Intervention Trial. Diabetes Care 1993; 16:434–444.
2. Haffner SM, Lehto S, Ronnemaa T et al. Mortality from coronary heart disease in subjects with type 2 diabetes and in nondiabetic subjects with and without prior myocardial infarction. N Engl J Med 1998; 339:229–234.
3. Juutilainen A, Lehto S, Ronnemaa T et al. Type 2 diabetes as a 'Coronary Heart Desease Equivalent'. Diabetes Care 2005; 28:2901–2907.
4. Expert Panel on Detection, Evaluation, and Treatment of High Blood Cholesterol in Adults. (Adult Treatment Panel III). JAMA 2001; 285:2486–2497.
5. Ross R. Atherosclerosis: an inflammatory disease. N Engl J Med 1999; 340:115–126.
6. Colwell JA, Jokl R. Vascular thrombosis in diabetes. In: Porte D, Sherwin R, Rifkin H (eds). Diabetes Mellitus: Theory and Practice, 6th edition. Appleton & Lange, Norwalk, CT, 1996, pp 207–216.
7. Tschoepe D, Driesch E, Schwippert B et al. Exposure of adhesion molecules on activated platelets in patients with newly diagnosed IDDM is not normalized by near-normoglycaemia. Diabetes 1995; 44:890–894.
8. Jokl R, Colwell JA. Clotting disorders in diabetes. In: Alberti KGMM, Zimmet P, DeFronzo RA, et al. (eds). International Textbook of Diabetes Mellitus, 2nd edition. John Wiley & Sons Ltd, Chichester, UK, 1997, pp 1543–1557.

9. Ceriello A. Coagulation activation in diabetes mellitus: the role of hyperglycaemia and therapeutic prospects. *Diabetalogia* 1993; 36:1119–1125.
10. Sobol AB, Watala C. The role of platelets in diabetes-related vascular complications. *Diabetes Res Clin Pract* 2000; 50:1–16.
11. Ostermann H, van de Loo J. Factors of the hemostatic system in diabetic patients: a survey of controlled studies. *Haemostasis* 1986; 16:386–416.
12. Fuster V, Badimon J, Chesebro JH. Plaque rupture, thrombosis, and therapeutic implications. *Haemostasis* 1996; 26(4 suppl):269S–284S.
13. Davies MJ. Stability and instability: two faces of coronary atherosclerosis: The Paul Dudley White Lecture 1995. *Circulation* 1996; 94:2013–2020.
14. Falk E, Ahah PK, Fuster V. Coronary plaque disruption. *Circulation* 1995; 92:657–671.
15. Schafer AI. Antiplatelet therapy. *Am J Med* 1996; 101:199–209.
16. Kwaan HC, Colwell JA, Cruz S *et al*. Increased platelet aggregation in diabetes mellitus. *J Lab Clin Med* 1972; 80:236–246.
17. Sagel J, Colwell JA, Crook L *et al*. Increased platelet aggregation in early diabetes mellitus. *Ann Intern Med* 1975; 82:733–738.
18. Sarji KE, Schraibman HB, Chambers A *et al*. Quantitative studies of von Willebrand factor (vWf in normal and diabetic subjects: role of vWf in second-phase platelet aggregation). *Microcirculation* 1976; II:296–297.
19. Colwell JA, Nair RM, Halushka PV *et al*. Platelet adhesion and aggregation in diabetes mellitus. *Metabolism* 1979; 28:394–400.
20. Winocour PD, Lopes-Virella M, Laimins M *et al*. Effect of insulin treatment in streptozotocin-induced diabetic rats on *in vitro* platelet function and plasma von Willebrand factor activity and factor VIII-related antigen. *J Lab Clin Med* 1985; 6:319–325.
21. Winocour PD, Watala C, Kinlough-Rathbone RL. Membrane fluidity is related to the extent of glycation of proteins, but not to alterations in the cholesterol to phospholipids ratio in isolated platelet membranes from diabetic and control subjects. *Thromb Haemost* 1992; 67:575–581.
22. Winocour PD, Laimins M, Colwell JA. Platelet survival in streptozotocin-induced diabetic rats. *Thromb Haemost* 1984; 51:307–312.
23. Ceriello A. Fibrinogen and diabetes mellitus: is it time for intervention trials? *Diabetologia* 1997; 33:731–734.
24. VanZile J, Kilpatrick M, Laimins M *et al*. Platelet aggregation and release of ATP after incubation with soluble immune complexes purified from the serum of diabetic patients. *Diabetes* 1981; 30:575–582.
25. Watanabe J, Wohltmann HJ, Klein RL *et al*. Enhancement of platelet aggregation by low-density lipoproteins from IDDM patients. *Diabetes* 1988; 37:1652–1657.
26. Davi G, Belvedere M, Vigneri S *et al*. Influence of metabolic control on thromboxane biosynthesis and plasma plasminogen activator inhibitor type 1 in non-insulin-dependent diabetes mellitus. *Thromb Haemost* 1996; 76:34–37.
27. Sarji KE, Kleinfelder J, Brewington P *et al*. Decreased platelet Vitamin C in diabetes mellitus: possible role in hyperaggregation. *Thromb Res* 1979; 15:639–650.
28. Halushka PV, Rogers RC, Loadholdt CB. Increased platelet thromboxane synthesis in diabetes mellitus. *J Lab Clin Med* 1981; 97:87–96.
29. Kwaan HC, Colwell JA, Suwanwela N. Disseminated intravascular coagulation in diabetes mellitus, with reference to the role of increased platelet aggregation. *Diabetes* 1972; 21:108–113.
30. Boeri D, Maiello M, Lorenzi M. Increased prevalence of microthromboses in retinal capillaries of diabetic individuals. *Diabetes* 2001; 50:1432–1439.
31. Ishibashi T, Tanaka K, Taniguchi Y. Platelet aggregation and coagulation in the pathogenesis of diabetic retinopathy in rats. *Diabetes* 1981; 30:601–606.
32. Loscalzo J. Nitric oxide insufficiency, platelet activation and arterial thrombosis. *Circ Res* 2001; 88:756–762.
33. Trovati M, Anfossi G. Mechanisms involved in platelet hyperactivation and platelet-endothelium interrelationships in diabetes mellitus. *Curr Diab Rep* 2002; 2:316–322.
34. Vinik AI, Erbas T, Park TS *et al*. Platelet dysfunction in type 2 diabetes. *Diabetes Care* 2001; 24:1476–1485.
35. Li Y, Woo V, Bose R. Platelet hyperactivity and abnormal Ca2+ homeostasis in diabetes mellitus. *Am J Physiol Heart Circ Physiol* 2001; 280:H1480–H1489.

36. Tschoepe D, Driesch E, Schwippert B *et al*. Exposure of adhesion molecules on activated platelets in patients with newly diagnosed IDDM is not normalized by near-normoglycaemia. *Diabetes* 1995; 44:890–894.

37. Tschoepe D, Rosen P, Schwippert B *et al*. Platelets in diabetes: the role in haemostatic regulation in atherosclerosis. *Semin Thromb Hemost* 1993; 19:122–128.

38. Tschoepe D, Rauch R, Schwippert B. Platelet-leukocyte-cross-talk in diabetes mellitus. *Horm Metab Res* 1997; 29:631–635.

39. Tschoepe P, Oresen L, Kaufmann S *et al*. Evidence for abnormal glycoprotein receptor expression on diabetic platelets. *Eur J Clin Invest* 1990; 20:166–170.

40. Tschoepe D, Schwippert G, Schettler B *et al*. Increased GPIIb/IIIa expression and altered DNA-ploidy pattern in megakaryocytes of diabetic BB rats. *Eur J Clin Invest* 1992; 22:591–598.

41. Tschoepe D, Roesen P, Esser J *et al*. Large platelets circulate in an activated state in diabetes mellitus. *Semin Thromb Hemost* 1991; 17:433–438.

42. Tschoepe D. The activated megakaryocyte-platelet-system in vascular disease: focus on diabetes. *Semin Thromb Hemost* 1995; 21:152–160.

43. Fusman R, Rotstein R, Elishkewich K *et al*. Image analysis for the detection of increased erythrocyte, leukocyte and platelet adhesiveness/aggregation in the peripheral blood of patients with diabetes mellitus. *Acta Diabetol* 2001; 38:129–134.

44. Kaplar M, Keppelmayer J, Veszpremi A *et al*. The possible association of *in vivo* leukocyte-platelet heterophylic aggregate formation and the development of diabetic angiopathy. *Platelets* 2001; 12:419–422.

45. Patrono C. Aspirin as an antiplatelet drug. *N Engl J Med* 1994; 330:1287–1294

46. DiMinno G, Silver MJ, Cerbone AM *et al*. Trial of repeated low-dose aspirin in diabetic angiopathy. *Blood* 1986; 68:886–891.

47. Mills CDB, Puri R, Hu C-J *et al*. Clopidogrel inhibits the binding of ADP analogues to the receptor mediating inhibition of platelet adenylate cyclase. *Arterioscler Thromb* 1992; 12:430–436.

48. Colwell JA, Nesto RW. The platelet in diabetes. Focus on prevention of ischemic events. *Diabetes Care* 2003; 26:2181–2188.

49. Coller BS. A new murine monoclonal antibody reports an activation-dependent change in the conformation and/or microenvironment of the platelet glycoprotein IIb/IIIa complex. *J Clin Invest* 1985; 76:101–108.

50. Coutre S, Leung L. Novel antithrombotic therapeutics targeted against platelet glycoprotein IIb/IIIa. *Annu Rev Med* 1995; 46:257–265.

51. Nerisezneri GG, Coccheri S, Marubini E, Violi F, for the committees and the investigators of the Drug Evaluation in Atherosclerotic Vascular Disease in Diabetes (DAVID) Study Group. Picotamide, a combined inhibitor of thromboxane A2 synthase and receptor, reduces 2-year mortality in diabetics with peripheral arterial disease: the DAVID Study. *Eur Heart J* 2004; 25:1845–1852.

52. Antiplatelet Trialists' Collaboration. Collaborative overview of randomized trials of antiplatelet therapy: I. Prevention of death, myocardial infarction, and stroke by prolonged antiplatelet therapy in various categories of patients. *Br Med J* 1994; 308:81–106.

53. Antithrombotic Trialists' Collaboration. Collaborative meta-analysis of randomized trials of antiplatelet therapy for prevention of death, myocardial infarction, and stroke in high risk patients. *Br Med J* 2002; 324:71–86.

54. ETDRS Investigators. Aspirin effects on mortality and morbidity in patients with diabetes mellitus. *JAMA* 1992; 268:1292–1300.

55. Colwell JA, Bingham SF, Abraira C *et al*. Veterans administration cooperative study on antiplatelet agents in diabetic patients after amputation for gangrene: II. Effects of aspirin and dipyridamole on atherosclerotic vascular disease rates. *Diabetes Care* 1986; 9:140–148.

56. Roffi M, Chew DP, Mukherjee D *et al*. Platelet glycoprotein IIb/IIIa inhibitors reduce mortality in diabetic patients with non-ST-segment-elevation acute coronary syndromes. *Circulation* 2001; 104:2767–2771.

57. Hansson L, Zanchetti A, Carruthers SG *et al*. Effects of intensive blood-pressure lowering and low-dose aspirin in patients with hypertension: principal results of the hypertension optimal treatment (HOT) randomized trial. *Lancet* 1998; 351:1755–1762.

58. Early Treatment Diabetic Retinopathy Study Research Group. Effects of aspirin treatment on diabetic retinopathy: ETDRS report number 8. *Ophthalmology* 1991; 98:757–765.

59. Collaborative Group of the Primary Prevention Project. Low-dose aspirin and Vitamin E in people at cardiovascular risk: a randomized trial in general practice. *Lancet* 2001; 357:89–95.

60. Sacco M, Pellegrini R, Roncaglioni MC et al. Primary prevention of cardiovascular events with low-dose aspirin and Vitamin E in type 2 diabetic patients. Diabetes Care 2003; 26:3264–3272.

61. Steering Committee of the Physicians' Health Study Research Group. Final report on the aspirin component of the ongoing Physicians Health Study. N Engl J Med 1989; 321:129–135.

62. Ridker PM, Cook NR, Lee IM et al. A randomized trial of low-dose aspirin in the primary prevention of cardiovascular disease in women. N Engl J Med 2005; 352:1293–1304.

63. Belch J, MacCuish A, Campbell I et al. The prevention of progression of arterial disease and diabetes (POPADAD) trial: factorial randomized placebo controlled trial of aspirin and anti-oxidants in patients with diabetes and asymptomatic peripheral arterial disease. BMJ 2008; 337:a1840.

64. Ogawa H, Nakagama M, Morimoto T et al. Low-dose aspirin for primary prevention of atherosclerotic events in patients with type 2 diabetes. JAMA 2008; 300:2134–2141.

65. Sanmuganathan PS, Ghahramani P, Jackson PR et al. Aspirin for primary prevention of coronary heart disease: safety and absolute benefit related to coronary risk derived from meta-analysis of randomized trials. Heart 2001; 85:265–271.

66. Eidelman RS, Hebert PR, Weisman SM, Hennekens CH. An update on aspirin for the primary prevention of cardiovascular disease. Arch Int Med 2003; 163:2006–2010.

67. ASCEND protocol. 2005; pp1–20. Available by email: ascend@ctsu.ox.ac.uk

68. Colwell JA. Aspirin therapy in diabetes. Diabetes 1997; 20:1767–1771.

69. American Diabetes Association. Clinical practice recommendations. Diabetes Care 2002; 24:S62–S63.

70. AHA Scientific Statement. AHA guidelines for primary prevention of cardiovascular disease and stroke: 2002 up date. Circulation 2002; 106:388–391.

71. US Preventive Services Task Force. Aspirin for the primary prevention of cardiovascular events: summary of the evidence. Ann Intern Med 2002; 136:161–172.

72. Patrono C, Backmann F, Beigent C et al. Expert consensus document on the use of antiplatelet agents. Eur Heart J 2004; 25:166–181.

73. Anderson KM, Wilson PW, Odell PM, Kannel WB. An updated coronary risk profile. A statement for health professionals. Circulation 1991; 83:356–362.

74. Anderson KM, Odell PM, Wilson PW, Kannel WB. Cardiovascular disease risk profiles. Am Heart J 1991; 121:293–298.

75. Stevens RJ, Kothari V, Adler A et al. The UKPDS risk engine: a model for the risk of coronary heart disease in type II diabetes (UKPDS 56). Clinical Science 2001; 101:671–679.

76. Guzder RN, Gutling WK, Muller MA et al. Prognostic value of the Framingham cardiovascular risk equation and the UKPDS risk engine for coronary heart disease in newly diagnosed type 2 diabetes: results from a United Kingdom Study. Diabetes Med 2005; 22:554–562.

77. Song SH, Brown PM. Coronary heart disease risk assessment in diabetes mellitus: comparison of UKPDS risk engine with Framingham risk assessment function and its clinical implications. Diabet Med 2004; 21:238–245.

78. Rolka DB, Fagot-Campagna A, Narayan KM. Aspirin use among adults with diabetes: estimates from the Third National Health and Nutrition Examination Survey. Diabetes Care 2001; 24:197–201.

79. Garcia Rodriguez LA, Hernandes-Diaz S, de Abajo FJ. Association between aspirin and upper gastrointestinal complications: systematic review of epidemiologic studies. Br J Clin Pharmacol 2001; 52:563–571.

80. Chan FKL, Ching JYL, Hung LCT et al. Clopidogrel versus aspirin and esomeprazole to prevent recurrent ulcer bleeding. N Engl J Med 2005; 352:238–244.

81. Mason PJ, Freedman JE, Jacobs AK. Aspirin resistance: current concepts. Reviews in Cardiovasc Med 2004; 5:156–163.

82. Gum PA, Kottke-Marchant K, Poggio ED et al. Profile and prevalence of aspirin resistance in patients with cardiovascular disease. Am J Cardiol 2001; 88:230–235.

83. Eikelboom JW, Hirsch J, Weitz JI et al. Aspirin-resistant thromboxane biosynthesis and the risk of myocardial infarction, stroke, or cardiovascular death in patients at high risk for cardiovascular events. Circulation 2002; 105:1650–1655.

84. Tantry U, Bliden K, Hayes K et al. Overestimation of aspirin resistance. JACC 2005; 45(suppl A).

85. Catella-Lawson F, Reilly MP, Kapoor SC et al. Cyclooxygenase inhibitors and the antiplatelet effects of aspirin. N Engl J Med 2001; 345:1809–1817.

86. Maree AO, Curtin RJ, Dooley M et al. Platelet response to low-dose enteric-coated aspirin in patients with stable cardiovascular disease. J Am Coll Cardiol 2005; 47:1258–1263.

87. Wood DM, Plehwe WE, Coloman PG. Aspirin usage in a large teaching hospital diabetes clinic setting. *Diabet Med* 1999; 16:605–608.

88. Krein SL, Vijan S, Pogach LM *et al*. Aspirin use and counseling about aspirin among patients with diabetes. *Diabetes Care* 2002; 25:965–970.

89. Krumholz HM, Chen YT, Want Y *et al*. Aspirin and angiotensin-converting enzyme inhibitors among elderly survivors of hospitalization for an acute myocardial infarction. *Arch Intern Med* 2001; 161:538–544.

90. Cull CA, Neil A, Holman RR. Changing aspirin use in UK patients with type 2 diabetes. *Diabetes* 2002; 51(suppl 2):A156.

91. Hennekens CH, Knatterud GL, Pfeffer MA. Use of aspirin to reduce risks of cardiovascular disease in patients with diabetes. *Diabetes Care* 2004; 27:2752–2754.

92. Bhatt DL, Topol EJ. Clopidogrel added to aspirin versus aspirin alone in secondary prevention and high-risk primary prevention: rationale and design of the clopidogrel for high atherothrombotic risk and ischemic stabilization, management, and avoidances (CHARISMA) Trial. *Am Heart J* 2004; 148:264–268.

93. Berger JS, Roncaglioni MC, Avanzini F *et al*. Aspirin for the primary prevention of cardiovascular events in women and men. *JAMA* 2006; 295:306–313.

94. Gu K, Cowie CC, Harris MI. Diabetes and decline in heart disease mortality in US adults. *JAMA* 1999; 281:1291–1297.

95. Fox CS, Coady S, Sorlie PD *et al*. Trends in cardiovascular complications of diabetes. *JAMA* 2004; 292:2495–2499.

12

Diabetes and folic acid

C. van Guldener, Y. M. Smulders

INTRODUCTION

Patients with type 1 or type 2 diabetes mellitus have an increased risk of cardiovascular events. Macrovascular disease involves atherothrombotic changes in the aorta and the coronary, carotid, renal and iliac arteries, while microangiopathic changes contribute to nephropathy, retinopathy and possibly also to neuropathy. In type 1 diabetes mellitus, microvascular complications are more common than large vessel abnormalities, but coronary heart disease has a high occurrence in these patients, especially when diabetes is long-standing and/or when nephropathy is present. In patients with type 2 diabetes mellitus, the risk of cardiovascular events is 2- to 4-fold higher than individuals without diabetes. Given that type 2 diabetes mellitus is the most common form of diabetes (~90–95% of all cases) and that its incidence is rapidly increasing, management of cardiovascular disease and their risk factors is extremely important in these patients.

Apart from diabetes-related risk factors (hyperglycaemia, hyperinsulinaemia, obesity, hypertension, hypertriglyceridaemia), traditional risk factors (hypercholesterolaemia, smoking) are known to increase the risk of cardiovascular disease in patients with diabetes. However, the atherothrombotic process in diabetes is complex and alternative risk factors, such as alterations in folate–homocysteine metabolism, may be involved.

Folate is a B Vitamin, which plays an important role in deoxyribonucleic acid (DNA) synthesis and in the methionine–homocysteine methylation cycle. In terms of cardiovascular disease, homocysteine is the most extensively studied parameter of folate metabolism. As folate and homocysteine are biochemically linked (see below), plasma homocysteine level is modulated by the folate status. A reduction in folate status leads to an increase in plasma homocysteine level, both of which have been linked to the development of cardiovascular disease [1–3].

In this chapter, the role of folate with emphasis on homocysteine in the development and occurrence of arterial vascular disease in diabetes mellitus is discussed. In addition, the therapeutic potential of folate supplementation for primary and secondary prevention of cardiovascular disease in patients with diabetes mellitus is addressed.

Coen van Guldener, MD, PhD, Internist, Department of Internal Medicine, Amphia Hospital, Breda, The Netherlands.

Yvo M. Smulders, MD, PhD, Internist, Department of Internal Medicine, VU University Medical Center, Amsterdam, The Netherlands.

FOLATE AND HOMOCYSTEINE METABOLISM

FOLATE

In 1941, Mitchell and co-workers [4] isolated a nutritional growth factor for *Streptococcus faecalis* from spinach leaves, which they called folic acid (*folium* is Latin for 'leaf'). At present, the term folic acid is reserved for pteroylglutamic acid, which is actually a synthetic compound, whereas the term folate is used to indicate the group of naturally occurring vitamins that are biochemically related to pteroylglutamic acid.

Folate, also named Vitamin B_9, is a water-soluble vitamin that plays an essential role in many different biochemical processes. Its main function is to enable enzymes to pass on one-carbon groups to a variety of target molecules. To fulfil this role, folate appears in various different biochemical forms, which are referred to as folate vitamers. Different folate vitamers pass on different one-carbon groups, such as methyl (CH_3), formyl (CHO), and methylene (CH_2) groups.

Humans cannot synthesise folate, and thus rely on food absorption and effective cellular retention of folates. The minimal daily requirement for folate is 50 µg, but a daily intake of 200 µg is recommended, whereas the intake in pregnant women should be at least 400 µg.

Folates in natural, non-enriched foods are predominantly present in the reduced forms 5-methyltetrahydrofolate (5-MTHF) and formyltetrahydrofolate. Attached to these are polyglutamyl chains of various lengths (usually <9 glutamyl residues). After stomach passage, the ingested food folates are joined by folate monoglutamates originating from biliary secretion. Subsequently, the polyglutamyl chain is deconjugated by the intestinal brush border enzyme conjugase, leaving folate monoglutamates, which are absorbed into the enterocytes. Folate monoglutamates that are not already in the form of 5-MTHF are transformed to 5-MTHF during passage through the intestinal cells and are subsequently transported to the circulation. 5-MTHF is the thus predominant form of circulating folate.

Folate is eliminated from the body by excretion via urine and faeces (mostly via biliary excretion) and by conversion to p-aminobenzoylglutamate. The latter pathway may account for the loss of more than 50% of normal daily folate intake.

Intracellular folate metabolism is complex, and important pathways are displayed in Figure 12.1. After cell entry, 5-MTHF-monoglutamate is available primarily for homocysteine remethylation, catalysed by methionine synthase and resulting in the formation of tetrahydrofolate. The next step in intracellular folate metabolism is for tetrahydrofolate to acquire a new one-carbon unit. The 3-carbon of serine is the predominant source for one-carbon donation in this reaction, in which methylenetetrahydrofolate is formed. Methylenetetrahydrofolate has three possible metabolic fates. In the first, it can directly donate its methylene (CH_2) group in the thymidylate synthase reaction for the biosynthesis of pyrimidines for DNA synthesis. Alternatively, methylenetetrahydrofolate can be converted to 5-10-methenyltetrahydrofolate, which undergoes rapid subsequent conversion to 10-formyltetrahydrofolate, which donates its formyl (CHO) group for purine synthesis, another essential step in DNA synthesis. The third fate for methylenetetrahydrofolate is irreversible conversion to 5-MTHF in a reaction catalysed by methylenetetrahydrofolate reductase (MTHFR), which has riboflavin (Vitamin B_2) as a cofactor. The function of 5-MTHF is to donate its methyl (CH_3) group to homocysteine, reconverting it to methionine in a reaction catalysed by the enzyme methionine synthase, with Vitamin B_{12} (methylcobalamin) as an essential cofactor.

FOLIC ACID

Folic acid is the oxidised form of folate and does not occur in nature. It can be generated from natural folates by chemical oxidation. A main advantage of folic acid is that it is more

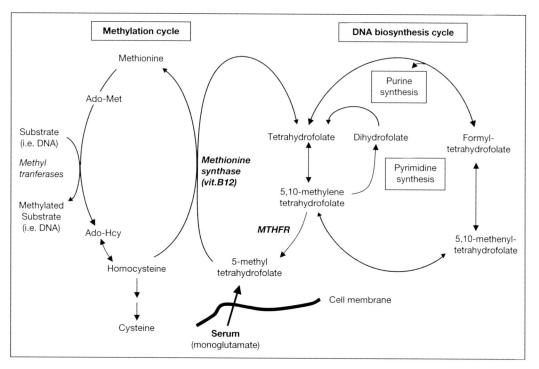

Figure 12.1 Important pathways in folate–homocysteine metabolism. For explanation, see text. AdoMet = S-adenosylmethionine; AdoHcy = S-adenosylhomocysteine; DNA = deoxyribonucleic acid; MTHFR = methylenetetrahydrofolatereductase.

stable during long-term (months to several years) storage and food processing and, as such, is more suitable for effective food enrichment. Because folic acid occurs only in the mono-glutamate form, its bioavailability after ingestion is not limited by intestinal deconjugation of the polyglutamyl chain. As a result of these advantages, and because its industrial pro-duction is relatively cheap, folic acid is the main folate vitamer used for pharmacological treatment. Folic acid itself, however, is not biologically active, as it cannot bind and pass on one-carbon groups. Low-dose folic acid is absorbed by the enterocyte and, during absorp-tion and hepatic passage, converted via dihydrofolate, to tetrahydrofolate by the enzyme dihydrofolate reductase. Single high-doses of folic acid exceeding 200 μg, however, saturate intestinal and hepatic dihydrofolate reductase capacity, and thus result in the appearance of unmetabolised, oxidised folic acid in the systemic circulation [5]. Much of this folic acid is rapidly excreted via the urine, and the remainder is reduced to tetrahydrofolate in the course of several hours.

HOMOCYSTEINE

Homocysteine is the transmethylation product of its sole precursor, methionine (Figure 12.1). Methionine is an essential amino acid derived from dietary or endogenous proteins, or from homocysteine. In the transmethylation pathway, methionine is converted to S-adenosylmethionine (AdoMet), which donates its activated methyl group to a variety of acceptors including DNA, ribonucleic acid (RNA), hormones, neurotransmitters, lipids, small molecules, myelin basic protein, and many other proteins/enzymes, to form

S-adenosylhomocysteine (AdoHcy). The enzymes catalysing these methylation reactions are called methyltransferases. AdoHcy is subsequently hydrolysed to homocysteine. Homocysteine can either be remethylated to methionine or be transsulphurated to cysteine. There are two remethylation pathways. The first was described above and requires 5-methyltetrahydrofolate as a methyl donor. The second remethylation reaction uses betaine as the methyl donor and is catalysed by betaine–homocysteine methyltransferase. The transsulphuration pathway is irreversible and comprises two reactions: from homocysteine to cystathionine (catalysed by cystathionine β-synthase) and from cystathionine to cysteine (by γ-cystathionase). Both enzymes require pyridoxal phosphate (vitamin B_6) as a cofactor. Cysteine can be incorporated into protein, used for the synthesis of compounds such as taurine and glutathione, or be metabolised with its sulphur atom excreted as sulphate. Key regulators of the homocysteine–methionine metabolism are AdoMet, which activates homocysteine transsulphuration and inhibits its remethylation, and AdoHcy, which inhibits methionine transmethylation.

DETERMINANTS OF PLASMA HOMOCYSTEINE CONCENTRATION

GENERAL POPULATION

In the general population, determinants of plasma homocysteine level are age, sex, menopausal state, the 677 C-to-T polymorphism of the methylenetetrahydrofolate reductase gene, plasma Vitamin B_6 and B_{12} levels, smoking and coffee consumption [6–8]. The two strongest determinants of plasma homocysteine concentration, however, are folate status (measured as serum or erythrocyte folate level) and renal function, measured as serum creatinine level or any other method to estimate the glomerular filtration rate. The inverse relationship between renal function and plasma homocysteine level remains largely unexplained, but may relate to uraemic inhibition of homocysteine turnover [9]. Renal dysfunction probably also at least partly explains the higher homocysteine levels that are found with increasing age, in hypothyroidism and during fibrate therapy.

DIABETES MELLITUS

In subjects with diabetes mellitus, plasma homocysteine levels have also been shown to be associated with folate status, renal function, gender, post-menopausal state and smoking [10–18]. Renal function in particular is an important determinant of plasma homocysteine concentration in subjects with diabetes. Not only has it been demonstrated that plasma homocysteine levels are high when renal function is impaired in diabetics, but also that plasma homocysteine is decreased in subjects with glomerular hyperfiltration, often the first stage of diabetes-associated nephropathy [19, 20].

Whether the diabetic state itself, or related metabolic abnormalities, influence plasma homocysteine level is uncertain. There is no obvious direct biochemical link between methionine–homocysteine metabolism and glucose/carbohydrate metabolism, other than insulin-induced protein synthesis, which may decrease plasma methionine level [21]. In a type 1 diabetic animal model, it was shown that plasma homocysteine levels were lower in rats with untreated, streptozotocin-induced diabetes than in diabetic animals treated with insulin or in control animals [22]. As the activity of hepatic betaine–homocysteine methyltransferase and transsulphuration enzymes was increased in the untreated diabetic rats, it was speculated that insulin deficiency leads to enhanced homocysteine catabolism in the liver, a phenomenon that is reversible upon insulin administration [22, 23]. A low plasma homocysteine was also found in Zucker fatty diabetes rats (a type 2 diabetes animal model), which again was accompanied by increased hepatic activity and expression of betaine–homocysteine methyltransferase and transsulphuration enzymes [24]. In humans, somewhat contrasting observations have been reported. In patients with type 2 diabetes, plasma homocysteine does not change during a hyperinsulinaemic–euglycaemic clamp, although homocysteine transsulphuration is decreased during hyperinsulinaemia [25, 26]. From these studies, the precise mode of action of insulin on homocysteine metabolism remains unclear. Other studies, which have examined the relationship between insulin resistance and plasma homocysteine level, have also yielded conflicting results. A positive relation between plasma homocysteine and insulin resistance, as assessed by hyperinsulinaemic–euglycaemic clamping, was found in healthy non-obese subjects [27] and in type 2 diabetics [15]. On the other hand, larger studies using the steady-state plasma glucose concentration during an insulin suppression test [28] and the intravenous glucose tolerance test with minimal model analysis of glucose disappearance [29] have not confirmed this relation in healthy subjects. Insulin resistance (as estimated by the homeostasis model assessment) was similar in hyper- and normohomocysteinaemic type 2 diabetes patients [30]. Another study in patients with type 2 diabetes showed that aggressive intravenous insulin therapy improved metabolic control and insulin sensitivity, but did not lower plasma homocysteine [31]. Fasting insulin levels, another index of insulin resistance, have been shown to relate positively with plasma homocysteine in obese children and adolescents [32], but in non-diabetic adults a weak, negative association was found [33], while no significant relation was found in adult type 2 diabetics [15]. In a mixed group of healthy subjects, glucose-intolerant subjects and type 2 diabetes patients, there was only a weak positive relation [34]. Taken together, no consistent pattern emerges from these studies and the relationship between plasma homocysteine level and insulin resistance, if any, seems marginal. Other diabetes-related factors such as glycosylated haemoglobin (HbA1c) level, duration of diabetes and insulin dependency do not have a significant influence on plasma homocysteine level [10, 13, 17, 18, 30]. Some drugs commonly used in diabetes may influence homocysteine levels. Metformin, for example, may impair cobalamin and possibly folate absorption, and may increase plasma homocysteine level by 4% [35]. In contrast to statins, which have a neutral effect, fibrates increase plasma homocysteine concentration, possibly by a renal mechanism [36, 37].

Whether these factors lead to differences in plasma homocysteine level between patients with diabetes and healthy subjects is unclear. Studies that have adjusted for renal function and vitamin status suggest that diabetic patients and healthy controls have similar plasma homocysteine levels [38–40]. In addition, there are no consistent differences in plasma homocysteine levels between patients with type 1 and 2 diabetes mellitus [19].

MICROVASCULAR DISEASE

MICROALBUMINURIA

Microalbuminuria is a strong predictor of cardiovascular events in diabetes, especially in type 2 diabetes, while in type 1 diabetes, microalbuminuria mainly predicts progression to overt nephropathy. The cause of microalbuminuria is unknown, but the most accepted view is that microalbuminuria reflects systemic vascular, possibly endothelial, dysfunction. As homocysteine is thought to induce endothelial dysfunction, hyperhomocysteinaemia could contribute to microalbuminuria.

A summary of studies on the association between plasma homocysteine and microalbuminuria is given in Table 12.1.

In both type 1 and type 2 diabetes, there are considerable differences in outcomes, with some studies finding a significant association between urinary albumin excretion and plasma homocysteine level [34, 38, 39, 41–46], while others did not observe such a relationship [10, 18, 30, 40, 47–49]. The discrepancies between these studies may relate to the cross-sectional design of most studies, with limited numbers of patients of different ethnic backgrounds, comorbidity, renal function and vitamin status. Importantly, most studies that did find a significant association did not adjust for renal function. In the largest study of

Table 12.1 Studies on the association between homocysteine and microalbuminuria in diabetes mellitus

Study	Design	Type 1 / Type 2 diabetes (n/n)	Outcome
Agardh [47]	Cross-sectional	76 / 0	No significant association
Cronin [40]	Cross-sectional	119 / 0	No significant association**
Hofmann [41]	Cross-sectional	75 / 0	Significant association**
Chico [38]	Cross-sectional	75 / 90	Significant association**
Chiarelli [43]	Cross-sectional	61 / 0	Significant association**
Vaccaro [39]	Cross-sectional	66 / 0	Significant association**
Soedamah-Muthu [18]	Cross-sectional	533 / 0	No significant association*
Hoogeveen [34]	Cross-sectional	0 / 164	Significant association*
Lanfredini [42]	Cross-sectional	0 / 33	Significant association**
Smulders [10]	Cross-sectional	0 / 85	No significant association**
Buysschaert [30]	Cross-sectional	0 / 122	No significant association**
Davies [48]	Cross-sectional	0 / 260	No significant association*
Abdella [49]	Cross-sectional	0 / 358	No significant association**
Ozmen [45]	Cross-sectional	0 / 75	Significant association**
de Luis [46]	Cross-sectional	0 / 155	Significant association**
Jager [44]	Prospective, 6.1 yr	0 / 66 + 250 non-diabetic subjects	Significant association*

*adjusted for renal function; **not adjusted for renal function.

type 1 diabetics (n = 533), there was no significant relationship between homocysteine and microalbuminuria [18]. The only prospective study examining the link between hyperhomocysteinaemia and microalbuminuria is the follow-up part of the Hoorn Study, a population-based cohort study [44]. During a mean follow-up of 6.1 years of 316 normoalbuminuric subjects (of whom 66 had type 2 diabetes), the cumulative incidence of microalbuminuria was 14% (95% confidence interval [CI] 9.7–18.3) in non-diabetic subjects, and 22.7% (95%CI 12.9–32.5) among type 2 diabetics. In subjects with a baseline homocysteine level of >19.0 µmol/l, the odds ratio for developing microalbuminuria was 5.1 (1.1–23.0) compared to those with a plasma homocysteine of <9.1 µmol/l (Figure 12.2). In the subgroup of patients with type 2 diabetes, the association could not be reliably estimated due to the fact that there were an insufficient number of diabetic subjects with hyperhomocysteinaemia. Taken together, these studies suggest that homocysteine may be involved in the development of microalbuminuria in type 2 diabetes, but it remains to be established whether this association is causal, e.g. by inducing endothelial or mesangial abnormalities in the kidney, or that both have a common, yet unidentified origin.

NEPHROPATHY

A summary of studies addressing the association between plasma homocysteine and diabetic nephropathy is given in Table 12.2.

In patients with chronic kidney disease, whether diabetic or non-diabetic in origin, it is generally assumed that renal insufficiency is the cause of the rise in plasma homocysteine. There are, however, only a few studies that have prospectively examined the relationship between plasma homocysteine and renal function. The only study in diabetic patients found that plasma homocysteine was significantly associated with the rate of decline in glomerular filtration rate (GFR) in 157 type 1 diabetic patients with diabetic nephropathy (GFR 80 ml/

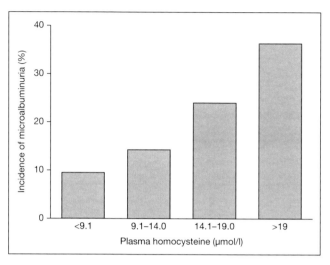

Figure 12.2 Cumulative incidence of (micro)albuminuria per category of homocysteine level. Estimated by age-adjusted, sex-adjusted and glucose tolerance-adjusted logistic regression analyses (with permission from [44]).

Table 12.2 Studies on the association between homocysteine and nephropathy in diabetes mellitus

Study	Design	Type 1 / Type 2 diabetes (n/n)	Outcome
Hovind [50]	Prospective, 7 yr	157 / 0	No significant association with decline in GFR**
Looker [17]	Prospective, 8.6 yr	0 / 229	No significant association with occurence of macroalbuminuria*
Soedamah-Muthu [18]	Cross-sectional	533 / 0	Significant association with macroalbuminuria*

*adjusted for renal function; **not adjusted for renal function.

min; range 23–143 ml/min), which were followed for a median of 7 years [50]. This relationship, however, was no longer significant after adjustment for other risk factors, such as blood pressure and albuminuria.

The relation between homocysteine and macroalbuminuria, another feature of diabetic nephropathy, has been examined in two studies [17, 18]. In a cross-sectional study of 533 patients with type 1 diabetes, plasma homocysteine was significantly related to macroalbuminuria, also after adjustment for renal function [18]. In a prospective study of 229 type 2 diabetics followed for 8.6 years, plasma homocysteine was not associated with the development of macroalbuminuria [17].

RETINOPATHY

A summary of studies on the association between plasma homocysteine and diabetic retinopathy is given in Table 12.3.

Table 12.3 Studies on the association between homocysteine and retinopathy in diabetes mellitus

Study	Design	Type 1 / Type 2 diabetes (n/n)	Outcome
Hultberg [51]	Cross-sectional	79 / 0	No significant association**
Agardh [47]	Cross-sectional	76 / 0	No significant association
Hofmann [41]	Cross-sectional	75 / 0	Significant association**
Cronin [40]	Cross-sectional	119 / 0	No significant association**
Agardh [52]	Cross-sectional	49 / 0	No significant association*
Vaccaro [39]	Cross-sectional	64 / 0	Significant association*
Buysschaert [53]	Cross-sectional	71 / 0	No significant association*
Soedamah-Muthu [18]	Cross-sectional	533 / 0	No significant association*
Smulders [10]	Cross-sectional	0 / 85	No significant association
Stabler [11]	Cross-sectional	0 / 452	No significant association
Buysschaert [30]	Cross-sectional	0 / 122	No significant association**
Hoogeveen [54]	Cross-sectional	0 / 171	Significant association*
Abdella [49]	Cross-sectional	0 / 358	No significant association*
de Luis [46]	Cross-sectional	0 / 155	No significant association**
Looker [17]	Prospective, 8.9 yr	0 / 266	Significant association with proliferative retinopathy*

*adjusted for renal function; **not adjusted for renal function.

In type 1 diabetes, most studies find no significant association between hyperhomocysteinaemia and retinopathy [10, 11, 18, 30, 40, 46, 47, 49, 51–53]. In contrast, in a study by Hofmann and colleagues [41], it appeared that type 1 diabetics with retinopathy had higher homocysteine levels, but these subjects also had a higher prevalence of nephropathy, which was not adjusted for. In another small cross-sectional study of 66 patients with type 1 diabetes, plasma homocysteine was higher in patients with proliferative retinopathy (9.5 ± 2.6 µmol/l) compared to those with background retinopathy (8.1 ± 2.6 µmol/l) and to those without retinopathy (7.3 ± 3.0 µmol/l), without apparent differences in renal function [39]. In the Hoorn study, no significant association between the presence of retinopathy and hyperhomocysteinaemia was detected in 454 non-diabetic subjects (odds ratio [OR] 1.01 [0.44–2.33]) after adjustment for age, sex, HbA1c, hypertension and serum creatinine [54]. In patients with diabetes (n = 171), however, the association was much stronger (OR 3.33 [0.99–11.19]). In the only prospective study, Looker and colleagues [17] found that a 5 µmol/l increase in plasma homocysteine was associated with an increased incidence of proliferative retinopathy among 212 subjects with type 2 diabetes (incident rate ratio 1.62 [1.16–2.28]). Although not all studies concur, it seems that hyperhomocysteinaemia may be involved, although to a small extent, in the occurrence of proliferative retinopathy in patients with diabetes.

NEUROPATHY

Studies addressing the relationship between plasma homocysteine and diabetic neuropathy are summarised in Table 12.4.

The pathobiological mechanism leading to peripheral and/or autonomic neuropathy in diabetes mellitus is complex and not completely understood. Factors that are proposed to be involved include hyperglycaemia, autoimmunity and neurotrophic or vascular insufficiency. Homocysteine could contribute to neuropathy by acting as a direct neurotoxic agent or by causing neurovascular impairment.

Table 14.4 Studies on the association between homocysteine and neuropathy in diabetes mellitus

Study	Design	Type 1 / Type 2 diabetes (n/n)	Outcome
Cronin [40]	Cross-sectional	119 / 0	Significant association only for autonomic neuropathy in males**
Hofmann [41]	Cross-sectional	75 / 0	No significant association**
Buysschaert [53]	Cross-sectional	71 / 0	No significant association*
Stabler [11]	Cross-sectional	0 / 452	No significant association**
Hoogeveen [57]	Cross-sectional	0 / 162	No significant association**
Buysschaert [30]	Cross-sectional	0 / 122	No significant association**
Ambrosch [55]	Cross-sectional	0 / 65	Significant association*
Cohen [56]	Cross-sectional	0 / 448	Significant association only for autonomic neuropathy
Abdella [49]	Cross-sectional	0 / 358	No significant association*
de Luis [46]	Cross-sectional	0 / 155	No significant association**
Spoelstra-de Man [58]	Cross-sectional	0 / 184	No significant association with cardiovascular autonomic function*

*adjusted for renal function; **not adjusted for renal function.

Although in some studies, a significant relation was found between plasma homocysteine level and the presence of autonomic or peripheral neuropathy [40, 55, 56], most studies concluded that no such association is present [11, 30, 41, 46, 49, 53, 57, 58]. As no prospective studies have examined the relationship between homocysteine and diabetic neuropathy, the role of hyperhomocysteinaemia in the development of diabetic neuropathy remains unclear, but, if it does exist, would appear to be small.

MACROVASCULAR DISEASE

Studies on the association between plasma homocysteine and macrovascular disease, defined as coronary, carotid–cerebrovascular or peripheral arterial disease, are summarised in Table 12.5.

In type 1 diabetes patients, no significant relationship between plasma homocysteine concentration and total macrovascular disease was found in two cross-sectional studies [18, 53]. Most studies in type 2 diabetes, however, showed a significant relation between plasma homocysteine and the presence of vascular disease [11, 30, 59–62]. In a cross-sectional study among 631 participants in the Hoorn study, it was found that the odds ratio for any cardiovascular disease for an increase of 5 μmol/l in plasma homocysteine was 1.38 (1.03–1.85) for non-diabetics, 1.55 (1.01–2.38) for subjects with an impaired glucose tolerance and 2.33 (1.11–4.90) for subjects with diabetes [60] (Figure 12.3). There were no significant differences in risk for coronary, cerebrovascular or peripheral vascular disease. Prospective studies in type 2 diabetes have shown mixed results. Plasma homocysteine was not associated with overall cardiovascular events in 1575 subjects with diabetic nephropathy who were followed for 2.6 years in the Irbesartan in Diabetic Nephropathy (IDNT) trial [62].

Cross-sectional [10, 16, 63–65] and prospective [66, 67] studies that have focused on coronary artery disease as a manifestation of macrovascular disease in type 2 diabetes, found that plasma homocysteine was an independent predictor of coronary heart disease (Figure 12.4). There are relatively few studies of the relationship between homocysteine and carotid, cerebral or peripheral artery disease separately in diabetes mellitus [12, 16, 68–70], which precludes definite conclusions.

Table 12.5 Studies on the association between homocysteine and macrovascular disease in diabetes mellitus

Study	Design	Type 1 / Type 2 diabetes (n/n)	Outcome
All macrovascular diseases			
Buysschaert [53]	Cross-sectional	71 / 0	No significant association*
Soedamah-Muthu [18]	Cross-sectional	533 / 0	No significant association*
Araki [59]	Cross-sectional	0 / 136	Significant association*
Hoogeveen [60]	Cross-sectional	0 / 173	Significant association*
Stabler [11]	Cross-sectional	0 / 452	No significant association
Buysschaert [30]	Cross-sectional	0 / 122	Significant association*
Tan [61]	Cross-sectional	0 / 123	Significant association
Friedman [62]	Prospective, 2.6 yr	0 / 1575[#]	No significant association*
Coronary artery disease			
Kaye [16]	Cross-sectional	354 / 392	No significant association*
Smulders [10]	Cross-sectional	0 / 85	Significant association
Okada [63]	Cross-sectional	0 / 46	Significant association**
Passaro [64]	Cross-sectional	0 / 318	Significant association**
Al-Nozah [65]	Cross-sectional	0 / 209	No significant association**
Becker [66]	Prospective, 10 yr	0 / 140	Significant association**
Soinio [67]	Prospective, 7 yr	0 / 830	Significant association*
Stroke			
Kaye [16]	Cross-sectional	354 / 392	No significant association*
Carotid artery disease			
Mazza [12]	Cross-sectional	0 / 130	No significant association**
Scaglione [68]	Cross-sectional	0 / 124	No significant association*
Becker [69]	Cross-sectional	0 / 140	Significant association
Peripheral artery disease			
Ciccarone [70]	Cross-sectional	0 / 354	Significant association*

*adjusted for renal function; **not adjusted for renal function; [#]all with nephropathy.

MORTALITY

Studies on the relationship between plasma homocysteine and mortality are given in Table 12.6.

There are four prospective studies that have investigated whether elevated plasma homocysteine levels are associated with increased mortality in diabetes. Firstly, Stehouwer and colleagues [71] reported data from 211 patients with type 2 diabetes less than 70 years old who were followed for a median of 6.4 years. The 6-year cumulative all-cause mortality hazard in the upper plasma homocysteine tertile (≥8.2 µmol/l) was significantly higher (44%) compared to the middle (6.2–8.1 µmol/l) and the lower tertile (≤6.1 µmol/l), in which the mortality hazards were 14% and 15%, respectively. Secondly, in an Israeli study of 239 subjects with diabetes followed for 9–11 years, an adjusted hazard ratio for all-cause mortality of 2.1 (0.9–4.9) was found in subjects in the highest quartile (non-fasting plasma homocysteine >13.0 µmol/l) compared to those in the lowest quartile (plasma homocysteine <8.2 µmol/l) [72]. Thirdly, Hoogeveen and co-workers [73] performed a nested case-control analysis using data from the Hoorn study. The fasting homocysteine levels of 171 subjects who died during a 5-year follow-up were compared with those of 640 survivors. For subjects with hyperhomocysteinaemia (plasma homocysteine >14 µmol/l), the 5-year odds ratio for

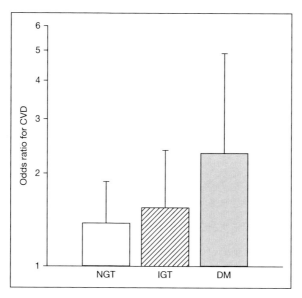

Figure 12.3 Odds ratio for cardiovascular disease after stratification by glucose tolerance category. The error bars represent the upper half of the 95%CI. Odds ratios are calculated per 5 µmol/l increment of serum total homocysteine, adjusted for age, sex, hypertension, ever smoking, hypercholesterolaemia and serum creatinine. $P <0.05$; $P = 0.07$ for interaction (with permission from [60]).
CI = confidence interval; CVD = cardiovascular disease; DM = diabetes mellitus; IGT = impaired glucose tolerance; NGT = normal glucose tolerance.

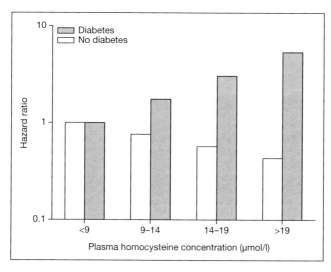

Figure 12.4 Adjusted hazard ratios for coronary events among diabetics and non-diabetics per category increment of serum homocysteine (with permission from [66]).

Table 12.6 Studies on the asociation between homocysteine and mortality in diabetes mellitus

Study	Design	Type 1 / Type 2 diabetes (n/n)	Outcome
All-cause mortality			
Stehouwer [71]	Prospective, 6.4 yr	0 / 211	Significant association*
Kark [72]	Prospective, 9–11 yr	0 / 139	Significant association*
Hoogeveen [73]	Prospective, 5 yr	0 / 184	Significant association**
Cardiovascular mortality			
Stehouwer [71]	Prospective, 6.4 yr	0 / 211	No significant association*
Soinio [67]	Prospective, 7 yr	0 / 830	Significant association*

*adjusted for renal function; **not adjusted for renal function.

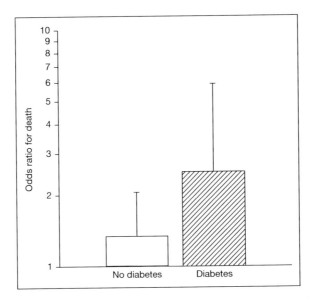

Figure 12.5 Odds ratios for 5-year overall death associated with hyperhomocysteinaemia (>14 μmol/l) after stratification by diabetes (yes/no). Error bars represent upper half of 95%CI. Odds ratios are adjusted for age, sex, hypertension, hypercholesterolaemia, current smoking and serum albumin (P <0.05, P = 0.08 for interaction) (with permission from [73]).
CI = confidence interval.

mortality was 1.6 (1.1–2.3). When diabetic and non-diabetic subjects were analysed separately, the odds ratio for mortality remained significant at 2.5 (1.1–5.9) in patients with diabetes only. This study not only shows, therefore, that hyperhomocysteinaemia is an independent mortality risk factor, but also that the associated risk is about twice as high in diabetics compared to non-diabetics (Figure 12.5). Finally, Soinio and colleagues [67] examined a large cohort of 830 patients with type 2 diabetes. After a follow-up of 7 years, coronary heart disease mortality was 26.1% in patients with a plasma homocysteine ≥15 μmol/l, compared to 13.5% in subjects with a plasma homocysteine <15 μmol/l (relative risk, RR 2.94 [1.72–5.01]) (Figure 12.6).

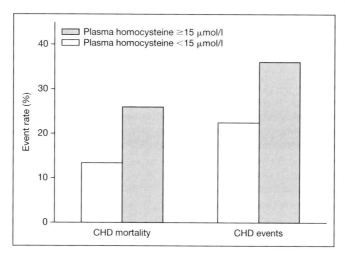

Figure 12.6 Coronary events by plasma homocysteine concentration in individuals with type 2 diabetes (with permission from [67]).
CHD = coronary heart disease.

Taken together, there is strong evidence that plasma homocysteine is an independent predictor of (cardiovascular) mortality in patients with diabetes mellitus.

PATHOPHYSIOLOGICAL CONSIDERATIONS

ENDOTHELIAL DYSFUNCTION

Homocysteine is thought to mediate its vasculotoxic effects by several mechanisms, most of which relate to the impairment of endothelial regulatory functions [74]. Endothelial cell damage, decreased nitric oxide availability, oxidative stress, smooth muscle cell proliferation, increased leukocyte adhesion, enhanced platelet aggregation, impaired fibrinolysis and induction of a chronic inflammatory state have all been implicated in homocysteine-induced vascular disease. To what extent these mechanisms are operative in diabetes is unknown. In patients with type 1 diabetes, Hofmann and colleagues [41] found a positive correlation between serum soluble thrombomodulin, a putative marker for endothelial damage, and plasma homocysteine concentration. Several other biochemical markers of endothelial dysfunction, leukocyte adhesion and inflammation have been investigated in diabetic patients in the Hoorn study [75, 76]. Becker and colleagues [75] found weak but significant associations between plasma homocysteine and von Willebrand factor and soluble vascular cell adhesion molecule-1 in a population of 170 subjects with diabetes and 440 non-diabetics. These relationships were independent of the presence of diabetes. In another study, plasma homocysteine did not materially affect the strength of the relative risk of soluble vascular cell adhesion molecule-1 level as a risk marker for cardiovascular mortality in type 2 diabetics [76]. The relationship between compounds from homocysteine–folate metabolism on the one hand and endothelium-dependent vasodilation on the other hand was studied *in vivo* by the reactive hyperaemia model of the brachial artery in a group consisting of 236 type 2 diabetics, 133 subjects with impaired glucose tolerance and 232 subjects with normal glucose tolerance [77]. The main finding was that 5-MTHF and AdoMet levels, but not homocysteine levels, were positively associated with endothelium-dependent vasodilation, independently of the glucose tolerance status.

The negative effects of disturbances in homocysteine metabolism on endothelial function have been ascribed to the reduced bioavailability of nitric oxide due to auto-oxidation of homocysteine in plasma, which leads to oxidative inactivation of nitric oxide. A recent study supported this concept by demonstrating, in aortic rings from diabetic rats, that reduced endothelium-dependent vasodilation upon exposure to homocysteine can be reversed by co-administration of superoxide dismutase [78]. Alternatively, by inhibiting dimethylarginine dimethylaminohydrolase, an enzyme that catabolises asymmetric dimethylarginine (ADMA), homocysteine may lead to accumulation of this endogenous inhibitor of nitric oxide synthase.

Taken together, these studies suggest that the link between hyperhomocysteinaemia and atherothrombotic disease in diabetes cannot readily be explained by endothelial dysfunction (as reflected by plasma von Willebrand factor concentration or flow-mediated vasodilatation). Alternatively, mechanisms as yet unknown may also be in operation.

HYPOMETHYLATION

Because a key function of folate metabolism is to provide sufficient one-carbon substrate for methylation, disturbances of folate metabolism are likely to be induce alterations in methylation status. From a biochemical perspective, a low folate status would lead to a decreased supply of (S-adenosyl)methionine and an accumulation of (S-adenosyl)homocysteine, which in turn would inhibit AdoMet-dependent methyltransferases. There is no reliable assessment of the adequacy of whole body methylation, but a potentially useful marker for methylation status is global DNA methylation.

In humans, it has been shown that higher plasma homocysteine is indeed independently related to high AdoHcy and lower lymphocyte DNA methylation [79]. The effect has been shown to occur with homocysteine close to physiological concentrations (10–50 µmol/l) in vascular endothelial cells [80]. Vascular endothelial cells in particular may be susceptible to this effect of homocysteine because they lack the homocysteine-metabolising enzymes cystathionine β-synthase and betaine hydroxymethyltransferase activity, and thus cannot dispose of homocysteine via the transsulphuration route.

An increasing number of studies indicate that DNA damage and altered gene expression play a role in cardiovascular disease. In part, this may be the result of DNA alterations, particularly hypomethylation, caused by disturbed folate metabolism. For example, the micronucleus index, a measure of genetic instability, correlates with hyperhomocysteinaemia and the MTHFR (methylenetetrahydrofolate reductase) 677 TT genotype, and is associated with the severity of coronary artery disease [81]. In addition, leukocyte DNA methylation is lower in patients with cardiovascular disease than in healthy controls [82]. DNA hypomethylation has also been shown in human atherosclerotic lesions [83]. As methylation of the promotor regions of genes is an important mechanism of regulation of gene expression (i.e. 'epigenetic regulation'), one possibility that links hypomethylation to vascular disease is that DNA hypomethylation hallmarks altered expression of specific (but as yet unknown) genes involved in atherothrombosis. Alternatively, DNA hypomethylation may reflect hypomethylation of other molecules (particularly proteins) that are involved in the pathogenesis of cardiovascular disease.

In view of the possible causal role of hypomethylation in the pathogenesis of atherosclerosis, and in view of the association between hyperhomocysteinaemia and hypomethylation, the possibility that the predictive effect of homocysteine for cardiovascular disease is, in fact, at least partly explained by hypomethylation deserves investigation.

DNA BIOSYNTHESIS

Assessment of the DNA synthesis cycle, another part of folate metabolism, may also be of interest. The best-known clinical manifestation of impairment of this cycle, megaloblastic anaemia, occurs relatively late and is thus an insensitive marker. A more suitable method is assessment of the degree of uracil misincorporation in DNA. When the availability of methylenetetrahydrofolate is limited, uracil may be misincorporated into DNA, which has mutagenic effects. In addition, in the attempt to repair itself, the DNA molecule is broken to remove the uracil molecule, eventually resulting in DNA double-strand breaks and chromosomal damage. The role of a low folate state in causing uracil misincorporation has been well established. Although there is some literature on the adverse vascular effects of anticancer drugs that inhibit the thymidylate synthase pathway [84], there are no data specifically addressing the role of uracil misincorporation in the pathogenesis of atherothrombosis. However, in view of the diversity of the effects of disturbed DNA synthesis on cell proliferation, mutagenesis and gene expression, such a role cannot be excluded.

TREATMENT

Although hyperhomocysteinaemia can be treated with folic acid, Vitamin B_6, Vitamin B_{12} and betaine, folate treatment is the cornerstone of any homocysteine lowering therapy. Exceptions are patients who are deficient for Vitamin B_{12} or the enzyme cystathionine β-synthase, who should primarily be treated with Vitamin B_{12} and Vitamin B_6, respectively. Because virtually all homocysteine lowering regimens contain folate, it is less relevant from a therapeutic point of view whether it is a high homocysteine or a low folate that is causing cardiovascular disease.

Folic acid lowers lower fasting plasma homocysteine levels by about 25% in doses of 0.5–5 mg/day [85]. The reduction is greater at higher pre-treatment plasma homocysteine concentrations. The most effective dose appears to be 0.8 mg/day, with little or no additional homocysteine lowering effect of higher doses [86]. Vitamin B_{12} has a marginal additive effect of about 7%, while Vitamin B_6 provides no extra effect [85].

Folic acid can improve endothelium-dependent vasodilatation in subjects with hyperhomocysteinaemia, hypercholesterolaemia and coronary artery disease [87–89]. In patients with chronic kidney disease, no improvement in flow-mediated dilatation was seen after folic acid therapy [90]. Folic acid(-containing) therapy has no significant effects on plasma markers of endothelial function, inflammation and oxidative stress[(91, 92].

The vascular effects of folic acid in diabetes have been studied to a limited extent. In streptozotocin-induced diabetic rats, 5-methyltetrahydrofolate restored the impaired hyperpolarising factor-mediated vasodilation in the renal microcirculation, indicating that folic acid may improve endothelial dysfunction in diabetes [93]. Studies in humans with diabetes have indeed indicated that endothelium-dependent vasodilatation may be improved by folic acid. In young type 1-diabetes patients, flow-mediated dilatation in the brachial artery was significantly improved after 8 weeks treatment with 5 mg folic acid [94], and in patients with type 2-diabetes, intra-arterial administration of 5-methyltetrahydrofolate led to an improvement of serotonin-induced vasodilatation [95]. On the other hand, in a placebo-controlled trial of 41 type 2 diabetes patients, treatment with 5 mg folic acid for 6 months did not improve plasma markers of endothelial dysfunction and inflammation [96].

Surrogate endpoint trials, mostly with non-diabetic subjects, have shown heterogeneous effects of homocysteine lowering therapy. In one study, a reduction was found in the incidence of abnormal exercise electrocardiogram (ECG) [97] and, in another study, fewer restenoses were reported after coronary angioplasty [98]. However, in a study in which coronary stenting was performed, homocysteine lowering therapy appeared to have the opposite effect [99].

Some clinical endpoint studies have recently been completed and have, surprisingly, shown overall neutral effects of homocysteine lowering therapy. In an open-label trial among 593 patients with stable coronary artery disease, no beneficial effect was found of folic acid treatment on mortality and a composite vascular endpoint [100]. There was also no benefit of folic acid treatment on recurrent stroke or other vascular endpoints in the Vitamin Intervention for Stroke Prevention (VISP) trial, which included 3680 stroke patients [101]. In a secondary prevention study among 3749 patients with myocardial infarction, homocysteine lowering treatment was not associated with a lower risk of new cardiovascular events [102]. The percentage of patients with diabetes was too small in this study (10%) to perform a subgroup analysis for these patients. In the Heart Outcomes Prevention Evaluation (HOPE) 2 study, 5522 patients with vascular disease and/or diabetes were randomised to multivitamin treatment (2.5 mg folic acid, 50 mg Vitamin B_6 and 1 mg Vitamin B_{12}) or placebo [103]. Active treatment lowered plasma homocysteine by 2.4 μmol/l, but did not significantly reduce the primary endpoint, i.e. the composite of death from cardiovascular causes, myocardial infarction and stroke (RR 0.95; 95%CI 0.84–1.07; $P = 0.41$). There was no difference in effect between diabetics ($n = 2209$) and non-diabetics ($n = 3313$) (P for interaction = 0.64).

Other randomised trials in women at high risk of cardiovascular disease [104], individuals undergoing coronary angiography [105], and patients with advanced chronic kidney disease [106] neither showed beneficial effects of folate-based homocysteine-lowering treatment on cardiovascular events. A recent meta-analysis, however, indicated that folic acid supplementation may lower the risk of stroke by 18% (RR 0.82; 95%CI 0.68–1.00; $P = 0.045$) [107].

To date, no endpoint studies have been carried out in subjects with diabetes only.

The apparent discrepancies between the epidemiological studies and the intervention studies are interesting. Accepting the strong evidence implicating homocysteine as an independent risk factor for cardiovascular disease, several explanations for the results of the intervention trials merit consideration. Firstly, it is possible that homocysteine lowering requires a longer period to demonstrate a favourable effect than the duration of follow-up in the intervention trials. Secondly, it may not be homocysteine, but an associated compound or biochemical process (which may be less susceptible to homocysteine lowering therapy) that is responsible for the vasculotoxic effects ascribed to homocysteine itself. In this respect, potential candidates are Ado-Hcy, ADMA and global hypomethylation. Finally, it is possible that the strategy that is used to lower plasma homocysteine is not appropriate. As outlined at the beginning of this chapter, high-dose folic acid therapy results in the presence of unmetabolised folic acid in the systemic circulation, the effects of which have never been properly addressed. In addition, high-dose folate supplementation may have untoward effects neutralising a beneficial effect of homocysteine lowering. In particular, enhancement of cell proliferation by nurturing the DNA and RNA biosynthesis pathways may stimulate smooth muscle cell and inflammatory cell proliferation in (advanced) atherosclerotic lesions. If so, the role of folate may be more promising in early prevention of atherothrombosis than in the treatment of high-risk, elderly patients.

SUMMARY

In uncomplicated diabetes mellitus, folate status and plasma homocysteine levels are usually comparable to those in subjects without diabetes. Lower plasma homocysteine levels in diabetic subjects have been ascribed to glomerular hyperfiltration and raised concentrations have been associated with subclinical nephropathy and, in some studies, with insulin resistance. Several cross-sectional and prospective studies have shown that hyperhomocysteinaemia is related to micro- and macrovascular disease and death, especially in diabetes. The relationship with diabetic neuropathy is unclear. Although homocysteine is thought to act as a vasculotoxic compound itself, there are no studies that clearly link hyperhomocysteinaemia to oxidative stress, inflammation or endothelial dysfunction in diabetes. Folate treatment may improve vascular function in patients with diabetes, which suggests that homocysteine-independent effects of folate may exist. Additional research is warranted into the less well-explored pathophysiological mechanisms that link altered folate metabolism and vascular disease, such as hypomethylation of DNA and proteins and impaired DNA synthesis and repair.

So far, clinical endpoint trials in high-risk patients, including those with diabetes, have shown that homocysteine lowering treatment is not associated with an improved cardiovascular event rate. However, studies specifically focused on patients with diabetes or at specific diabetic endpoints are lacking. Until the results of such studies become available, there is no evidence base for routine homocysteine lowering therapy using high-dose B vitamins. On the other hand, prevention of folate deficiency is a reasonable target of dietary prescription. Treatment of markedly elevated homocysteine levels (e.g. >20 μmol/l) with moderate doses of folic acid, alone or in combination with other B vitamins, remains a reasonable option.

REFERENCES

1. Rimm EB, Willett WC, Hu FB *et al*. Folate and Vitamin B6 from diet and supplements in relation to risk of coronary heart disease among women. *JAMA* 1998; 279:359–364.
2. Voutilainen S, Virtanen JK, Rissanen TH *et al*. Serum folate and homocysteine and the incidence of acute coronary events: the Kuopio Ischaemic Heart Disease Risk Factor Study. *Am J Clin Nutr* 2004; 80:317–323.
3. Homocysteine Studies Collaboration. Homocysteine and risk of ischemic heart disease and stroke: a meta-analysis. *JAMA* 2002; 288:2015–2022.
4. Mitchell HK, Snell EE, Williams RJ. Concentrations of 'folic acid'. *J Am Chem Soc* 1941; 63:2284.
5. Kelly P, McPartlin J, Goggins M, Weir DG, Scott JM. Unmetabolized folic acid in serum: acute studies in subjects consuming fortified food and supplements. *Am J Clin Nutr* 1997; 65:1790–1795.
6. Nygard O, Refsum H, Ueland PM, Vollset SE. Major lifestyle determinants of plasma total homocysteine distribution: the Hordaland Homocysteine Study. *Am J Clin Nutr* 1998; 67:263–270.
7. Jacques PF, Bostom AG, Wilson PW, Rich S, Rosenberg IH, Selhub J. Determinants of plasma total homocysteine concentration in the Framingham Offspring cohort. *Am J Clin Nutr* 2001; 73:613–621.
8. Ganji V, Kafai MR. Demographic, health, lifestyle, and blood vitamin determinants of serum total homocysteine concentrations in the third National Health and Nutrition Examination Survey, 1988–1994. *Am J Clin Nutr* 2003; 77:826–833.
9. Stam F, van Guldener C, ter Wee PM *et al*. Homocysteine clearance and methylation flux rates in health and end-stage renal disease: association with S-adenosylhomocysteine. *Am J Physiol Renal Physiol* 2004; 287:F215–F223.
10. Smulders YM, Rakic M, Slaats EH *et al*. Fasting and post-methionine homocysteine levels in NIDDM. Determinants and correlations with retinopathy, albuminuria, and cardiovascular disease. *Diabetes Care* 1999; 22:125–132.
11. Stabler SP, Estacio R, Jeffers BW, Cohen JA, Allen RH, Schrier RW. Total homocysteine is associated with nephropathy in non-insulin-dependent diabetes mellitus. *Metabolism* 1999; 48:1096–1101.
12. Mazza A, Motti C, Nulli A *et al*. Lack of association between carotid intima-media thickness and methylenetetrahydrofolate reductase gene polymorphism or serum homocysteine in non-insulin-dependent diabetes mellitus. *Metabolism* 2000; 49:718–723.
13. Pavia C, Ferrer I, Valls C, Artuch R, Colome C, Vilaseca MA. Total homocysteine in patients with type 1 diabetes. *Diabetes Care* 2000; 23:84–87.
14. Targher G, Bertolini L, Zenari L *et al*. Cigarette smoking and plasma total homocysteine levels in young adults with type 1 diabetes. *Diabetes Care* 2000; 23:524–528.
15. Emoto M, Kanda H, Shoji T *et al*. Impact of insulin resistance and nephropathy on homocysteine in type 2 diabetes. *Diabetes Care* 2001; 24:533–538.
16. Kaye JM, Stanton KG, McCann VJ *et al*. Homocysteine, folate, methylenetetrahydrofolate reductase genotype and vascular morbidity in diabetic subjects. *Clin Sci* 2002; 102:631–637.
17. Looker HC, Fagot-Campagna A, Gunter EW *et al*. Homocysteine as a risk factor for nephropathy and retinopathy in type 2 diabetes. *Diabetologia* 2003; 46:766–772.
18. Soedamah-Muthu SS, Chaturvedi N, Teerlink T, Idzior-Walus B, Fuller JH, Stehouwer CD, the Eurodiab Prospective Complications Study Group. Plasma homocysteine and microvascular and

macrovascular complications in type 1 diabetes: a cross-sectional nested case-control study. *J Intern Med* 2005; 258:450–459.

19. Wollesen F, Brattstrom L, Refsum H, Ueland PM, Berglund L, Berne C. Plasma total homocysteine and cysteine in relation to glomerular filtration rate in diabetes mellitus. *Kidney Int* 1999; 55:1028–1035.

20. Veldman BA, Vervoort G, Blom H, Smits P. Reduced plasma total homocysteine concentrations in type 1 diabetes mellitus is determined by increased renal clearance. *Diabet Med* 2005; 22:301–305.

21. Zinneman HH, Nuttall FQ, Goetz FC. Effect of endogenous insulin on human amino acid metabolism. *Diabetes* 1966; 15:5–8.

22. Jacobs RL, House JD, Brosnan ME, Brosnan JT. Effects of streptozotocin-induced diabetes and of insulin treatment on homocysteine metabolism in the rat. *Diabetes* 1998; 47:1967–1970.

23. Ratnam S, Wijekoon EP, Hall BN, Garrow TA, Brosnan ME, Brosnan JT. Effects of diabetes and insulin on betaine-homocysteine S-methyltransferase expression in rat liver. *Am J Physiol Endocrinol Metab* 2006; 290:E933–E939.

24. Wijekoon EP, Hall B, Ratnam S, Brosnan ME, Zeisel SH, Brosnan JT. Homocysteine metabolism in ZDF (type 2) diabetic rats. *Diabetes* 2005; 54:3245–3251.

25. Fonseca VA, Mudaliar S, Schmidt B, Fink LM, Kern PA, Henry RR. Plasma homocysteine concentrations are regulated by acute hyperinsulinemia in nondiabetic but not type 2 diabetic subjects. *Metabolism* 1998; 47:686–689.

26. Tessari P, Coracina A, Kiwanuka E *et al.* Effects of insulin on methionine and homocysteine kinetics in type 2 diabetes with nephropathy. *Diabetes* 2005; 54:2968–2976.

27. Giltay EJ, Hoogeveen EK, Elbers JM, Gooren LJ, Asscheman H, Stehouwer CD. Insulin resistance is associated with elevated plasma total homocysteine levels in healthy, non-obese subjects. *Atherosclerosis* 1998; 139:197–198.

28. Abbasi F, Facchini F, Humphreys MH, Reaven GM. Plasma homocysteine concentrations in healthy volunteers are not related to differences in insulin-mediated glucose disposal. *Atherosclerosis* 1999; 146:175–178.

29. Godsland IF, Rosankiewicz JR, Proudler AJ, Johnston DG. Plasma total homocysteine concentrations are unrelated to insulin sensitivity and components of the metabolic syndrome in healthy men. *J Clin Endocrinol Metab* 2001; 86:719–723.

30. Buysschaert M, Dramais AS, Wallemacq PE, Hermans MP. Hyperhomocysteinemia in type 2 diabetes: relationship to macroangiopathy, nephropathy, and insulin resistance. *Diabetes Care* 2000; 23:1816–1822.

31. Pouwels MJ, den Heijer M, Blom HJ, Tack CJ, Hermus AR. Improved insulin sensitivity and metabolic control in type 2 diabetes does not influence plasma homocysteine. *Diabetes Care* 2003; 26:1637–1639.

32. Gallistl S, Sudi K, Mangge H, Erwa W, Borkenstein M. Insulin is an independent correlate of plasma homocysteine levels in obese children and adolescents. *Diabetes Care* 2000; 23:1348–1352.

33. Bar-On H, Kidron M, Friedlander Y *et al.* Plasma total homocysteine levels in subjects with hyperinsulinemia. *J Intern Med* 2000; 247:287–294.

34. Hoogeveen EK, Kostense PJ, Jager A *et al.* Serum homocysteine level and protein intake are related to risk of microalbuminuria: the Hoorn study. *Kidney Int* 1998; 54:203–209.

35. Wulffele MG, Kooy A, Lehert P *et al.* Effects of short-term treatment with metformin on serum concentrations of homocysteine, folate and Vitamin B12 in type 2 diabetes mellitus: a randomized, placebo-controlled trial. *J Intern Med* 2003; 254:455–463.

36. de Lorgeril M, Salen P, Paillard F, Lacan P, Richard G. Lipid-lowering drugs and homocysteine. *Lancet* 1999; 353:209–210.

37. Lipscombe J, Lewis GF, Cattran D, Bargman JM. Deterioration in renal function associated with fibrate therapy. *Clin Nephrol* 2001; 55:39–44.

38. Chico A, Perez A, Cordoba A *et al.* Plasma homocysteine is related to albumin excretion rate in patients with diabetes mellitus: a new link between diabetic nephropathy and cardiovascular disease? *Diabetologia* 1998; 41:684–693.

39. Vaccaro O, Perna AF, Mancini FP *et al.* Plasma homocysteine and microvascular complications in type 1 diabetes. *Nutr Metab Cardiovasc Dis* 2000; 10:297–304.

40. Cronin CC, McPartlin JM, Barry DG, Ferriss JB, Scott JM, Weir DG. Plasma homocysteine concentrations in patients with type 1 diabetes. *Diabetes Care* 1998; 21:1843–1847.

41. Hofmann MA, Kohl B, Zumbach MS *et al.* Hyperhomocyst(e)inemia and endothelial dysfunction in IDDM. *Diabetes Care* 1998; 21:841–848.

42. Lanfredini M, Fiorina P, Peca MG *et al.* Fasting and post-methionine load homocyst(e)ine values are correlated with microalbuminuria and could contribute to worsening vascular damage in non-insulin-dependent diabetes mellitus patients. *Metabolism* 1998; 47:915–921.

43. Chiarelli F, Pomilio M, Mohn A *et al.* Homocysteine levels during fasting and after methionine loading in adolescents with diabetic retinopathy and nephropathy. *J Pediatr* 2000; 137:386–392.

44. Jager A, Kostense PJ, Nijpels G *et al.* Serum homocysteine levels are associated with the development of (micro)albuminuria: the Hoorn study. *Arterioscler Thromb Vasc Biol* 2001; 21:74–81.

45. Ozmen B, Ozmen D, Turgan N, Habif S, Mutaf I, Bayindir O. Association between homocysteinemia and renal function in patients with type 2 diabetes mellitus. *Ann Clin Lab Sci* 2002; 32:279–286.

46. de Luis DA, Fernanadez N, Arranz ML, Aller R, Izaola O, Romero E. Total homocysteine levels relation with chronic complications of diabetes, body composition, and other cardiovascular risk factors in a population of patients with diabetes mellitus type 2. *J Diabetes Complications* 2005; 19:42–46.

47. Agardh CD, Agardh E, Andersson A, Hultberg B. Lack of association between plasma homocysteine levels and microangiopathy in type 1 diabetes mellitus. *Scand J Clin Lab Invest* 1994; 54:637–641.

48. Davies L, Wilmshurst EG, McElduff A, Gunton J, Clifton-Bligh P, Fulcher GR. The relationship among homocysteine, creatinine clearance, and albuminuria in patients with type 2 diabetes. *Diabetes Care* 2001; 24:1805–1809.

49. Abdella NA, Mojiminiyi OA, Akanji AO, Moussa MA. Associations of plasma homocysteine concentration in subjects with type 2 diabetes mellitus. *Acta Diabetol* 2002; 39:183–190.

50. Hovind P, Tarnow L, Rossing P *et al.* Progression of diabetic nephropathy: role of plasma homocysteine and plasminogen activator inhibitor-1. *Am J Kidney Dis* 2001; 38:1376–1380.

51. Hultberg B, Agardh E, Andersson A *et al.* Increased levels of plasma homocysteine are associated with nephropathy, but not severe retinopathy in type 1 diabetes mellitus. *Scand J Clin Lab Invest* 1991; 51:277–282.

52. Agardh E, Hultberg B, Agardh CD. Severe retinopathy in type 1 diabetic patients is not related to the level of plasma homocysteine. *Scand J Clin Lab Invest* 2000; 60:169–174.

53. Buysschaert M, Jamart J, Dramais AS, Wallemacq P, Hermans MP. Micro- and macrovascular complications and hyperhomocysteinaemia in type 1 diabetic patients. *Diabetes Metab* 2001; 27:655–659.

54. Hoogeveen EK, Kostense PJ, Eysink PE *et al.* Hyperhomocysteinemia is associated with the presence of retinopathy in type 2 diabetes mellitus: the Hoorn study. *Arch Intern Med* 2000; 160:2984–2990.

55. Ambrosch A, Dierkes J, Lobmann R *et al.* Relation between homocysteinaemia and diabetic neuropathy in patients with type 2 diabetes mellitus. *Diabet Med* 2001; 18:185–192.

56. Cohen JA, Jeffers BW, Stabler S, Schrier RW, Estascio R. Increasing homocysteine levels and diabetic autonomic neuropathy. *Auton Neurosci* 2001; 87:268–273.

57. Hoogeveen EK, Kostense PJ, Valk GD *et al.* Hyperhomocysteinaemia is not related to risk of distal somatic polyneuropathy: the Hoorn study. *J Intern Med* 1999; 246:561–566.

58. Spoelstra-de Man AM, Smulders YM, Dekker JM *et al.* Homocysteine levels are not associated with cardiovascular autonomic function in elderly Caucasian subjects without or with type 2 diabetes mellitus: the Hoorn study. *J Intern Med* 2005; 258:536–543.

59. Araki A, Sako Y, Ito H. Plasma homocysteine concentrations in Japanese patients with non-insulin-dependent diabetes mellitus: effect of parenteral methylcobalamin treatment. *Atherosclerosis* 1993; 103:149–157.

60. Hoogeveen EK, Kostense PJ, Beks PJ *et al.* Hyperhomocysteinemia is associated with an increased risk of cardiovascular disease, especially in non-insulin-dependent diabetes mellitus: a population-based study. *Arterioscler Thromb Vasc Biol* 1998; 18:133–138.

61. Tan KC, O K, Chow WS, Ai VH, Siow YL, Lam KS. Hyperhomocysteinemia and impaired vasomotor function in type 2 diabetes mellitus. *Eur J Clin Invest* 2002; 32:328–334.

62. Friedman AN, Hunsicker LG, Selhub J, Bostom AG, Collaborative Study Group. Total plasma homocysteine and arteriosclerotic outcomes in type 2 diabetes with nephropathy. *J Am Soc Nephrol* 2005; 16:3397–3402.

63. Okada E, Oida K, Tada H *et al.* Hyperhomocysteinemia is a risk factor for coronary arteriosclerosis in Japanese patients with type 2 diabetes. *Diabetes Care* 1999; 22:484–490.

64. Passaro A, D'Elia K, Pareschi PL *et al.* Factors influencing plasma homocysteine levels in type 2 diabetes. *Diabetes Care* 2000; 23:420–421.

65. Al-Nozah M, Al-Daghri N, Bartlett WA *et al.* Serum homocysteine concentration is related to diabetes mellitus, but not to coronary heart disease, in Saudi Arabians. *Diabetes Obes Metab* 2002; 4:118–123.

66. Becker A, Kostense PJ, Bos G *et al.* Hyperhomocysteinaemia is associated with coronary events in type 2 diabetes. *J Int Med* 2003; 253:293–300.
67. Soinio M, Marniemi J, Laakso M, Lehto S, Ronnemaa T. Elevated homocysteine level is an independent predictor of coronary heart disease events in patients with type 2 diabetes mellitus. *Ann Intern Med* 2004; 140:94–100.
68. Scaglione L, Gambino R, Rolfo E *et al.* Plasma homocysteine, methylenetetrahydrofolate reductase gene polymorphism and carotid intima-media thickness in Italian type 2 diabetic patients. *Eur J Clin Invest* 2002; 32:24–28.
69. Becker A, Henry RM, Kostense PJ *et al.* Plasma homocysteine and S-adenosylmethionine in erythrocytes as determinants of carotid intima-media thickness: different effects in diabetic and non-diabetic individuals. The Hoorn study. *Atherosclerosis* 2003; 169:323–330. Erratum in: *Atherosclerosis* 2004; 173:153.
70. Ciccarone E, Castelnuovo A, Assanelli D *et al.* Homocysteine levels are associated with the severity of peripheral arterial disease in type 2 diabetic patients. *J Thromb Haemost* 2003; 1:2540–2547.
71. Stehouwer CD, Gall MA, Hougaard P, Jakobs C, Parving HH. Plasma homocysteine concentration predicts mortality in non-insulin-dependent diabetic patients with and without albuminuria. *Kidney Int* 1999; 55:308–314.
72. Kark JD, Selhub J, Bostom A, Adler B, Rosenberg IH. Plasma homocysteine and all-cause mortality in diabetes. *Lancet* 1999; 353:1936–1937.
73. Hoogeveen EK, Kostense PJ, Jakobs C *et al.* Hyperhomocysteinemia increases risk of death, especially in type 2 diabetes: 5-year follow-up of the Hoorn study. *Circulation* 2000; 101:1506–1511.
74. van Guldener C, Stehouwer CD. Hyperhomocysteinemia vascular pathology, and endothelial dysfunction. *Semin Thromb Hemost* 2000; 26:281–289.
75. Becker A, van Hinsbergh VW, Kostense PJ *et al.* Serum homocysteine is weakly associated with von Willebrand factor and soluble vascular cell adhesion molecule 1, but not with C-reactive protein in type 2 diabetic and non-diabetic subjects. *Eur J Clin Invest* 2000; 30:763–770.
76. Jager A, van Hinsbergh VW, Kostense PJ *et al.* Increased levels of soluble vascular cell adhesion molecule 1 are associated with risk of cardiovascular mortality in type 2 diabetes: the Hoorn study. *Diabetes* 2000; 49:485–491.
77. Spijkerman AM, Smulders YM, Kostense PJ *et al.* S-adenosylmethionine and 5-methyltetrahydrofolate are associated with endothelial function after controlling for confounding by homocysteine: the Hoorn study. *Arterioscler Thromb Vasc Biol* 2004; 25:778–784.
78. Shukla N, Thompson CS, Angelini GD, Mikhailidis DP, Jeremy JY. Homocysteine enhances impairment of endothelium-dependent relaxation and guanosine cyclic monophosphate formation in aortae from diabetic rats. *Diabetologia* 2002; 45:1325–1331.
79. Yi P, Melnyk S, Pogribna M, Pogribny IP, Hine RJ, James SJ. Increase in plasma homocysteine associated with parallel increases in plasma S-adenosylhomocysteine and lymphocyte DNA hypomethylation. *J Biol Chem* 2000; 275:29318–29323.
80. Lee ME, Wang H. Homocysteine and hypomethylation. A novel link to vascular disease. *Trends Cardiovasc Med* 1999; 9:49–54.
81. Andreassi MG, Botto N, Cocci F *et al.* Methylenetetrahydrofolate reductase gene C677T polymorphism, homocysteine, Vitamin B12, and DNA damage in coronary artery disease. *Hum Genet* 2003; 112:171–177.
82. Castro R, Rivera I, Struys EA *et al.* Increased homocysteine and S-adenosylhomocysteine concentrations and DNA hypomethylation in vascular disease. *Clin Chem* 2003; 49:1292–1296.
83. Hiltunen MO, Turunen MP, Hakkinen TP *et al.* DNA hypomethylation and methyltransferase expression in atherosclerotic lesions. *Vasc Med* 2002; 7:5–11.
84. Cwikiel M, Eskilsson J, Albertsson M. Stavenow L. The influence of 5-fluorouracil and methotrexate on vascular endothelium. An experimental study using endothelial cells in the culture. *Ann Oncol* 1996; 7:731–737.
85. Lowering blood homocysteine with folic acid based supplements: meta-analysis of randomised trials. Homocysteine Lowering Trialists' Collaboration. *Br Med J* 1998; 316:894–898.
86. Wald DS, Bishop L, Wald NJ *et al.* Randomized trial of folic acid supplementation and serum homocysteine levels. *Arch Intern Med* 2001; 161:695–700.
87. Bellamy MF, McDowell IF, Ramsey MW, Brownlee M, Newcombe RG, Lewis MJ. Oral folate enhances endothelial function in hyperhomocysteinaemic subjects. *Eur J Clin Invest* 1999; 29:659–662.

88. Verhaar MC, Wever RM, Kastelein JJ *et al.* Effects of oral folic acid supplementation on endothelial function in familial hypercholesterolemia. A randomized placebo-controlled trial. *Circulation* 1999; 100:335–338.

89. Doshi SN, McDowell IF, Moat SJ *et al.* Folic acid improves endothelial function in coronary artery disease via mechanisms largely independent of homocysteine lowering. *Circulation* 2002; 105:22–26.

90. van Guldener C, Janssen MJFM, Lambert J *et al.* No change in impaired endothelial function after long-term folic acid therapy of hyperhomocysteinaemia in haemodialysis patients. *Nephrol Dial Transplant* 1998; 13:106–112.

91. Dusitanond P, Eikelboom JW, Hankey GJ *et al.* Homocysteine-lowering treatment with folic acid, cobalamin, and pyridoxine does not reduce blood markers of inflammation, endothelial dysfunction, or hypercoagulability in patients with previous transient ischemic attack or stroke: a randomized substudy of the VITATOPS trial. *Stroke* 2005; 36:144–146.

92. Durga J, van Tits LJ, Schouten EG, Kok FJ, Verhoef P. Effect of lowering of homocysteine levels on inflammatory markers: a randomized controlled trial. *Arch Intern Med* 2005; 165:1388–1394.

93. De Vriese AS, van de Voorde J, Blom HJ, Vanhoutte PM, Verbeke M, Lameire NH. The impaired renal vasodilator response attributed to endothelium-derived hyperpolarizing factor in streptozotocin-induced diabetic rats is restored by 5-methyltetrahydrofolate. *Diabetologia* 2000; 43:1116–1125.

94. Pena AS, Wiltshire E, Gent R, Hirte C, Couper J. Folic acid improves endothelial function in children and adolescents with type 1 diabetes. *J Pediatr* 2004; 144:500–504.

95. van Etten RW, de Koning EJ, Verhaar MC, Gaillard CA, Rabelink TJ. Impaired NO-dependent vasodilation in patients with Type II (non-insulin-dependent) diabetes mellitus is restored by acute administration of folate. *Diabetologia* 2002; 45:1004–1010.

96. Spoelstra-de Man MA, Brouwer CB, Terheggen F, Bollen JM, Stehouwer CD, Smulders YM. No effect of folic acid on markers of endothelial dysfunction or inflammation in patients with type 2 diabetes and mild hyperhomocysteinaemia. *Neth J Med* 2004; 62:246–253.

97. Vermeulen EG, Stehouwer CD, Twisk JW *et al.* Effect of homocysteine-lowering treatment with folic acid plus Vitamin B6 on progression of subclinical atherosclerosis: a randomised, placebo-controlled trial. *Lancet* 2000; 355:517–522.

98. Schnyder G, Roffi M, Pin R *et al.* Decreased rate of coronary restenosis after lowering of plasma homocysteine levels. *N Engl J Med* 2001; 345:1593–1600.

99. Lange H, Suryapranata H, De Luca G *et al.* Folate therapy and in-stent restenosis after coronary stenting. *N Engl J Med* 2004; 350:2673–2681.

100. Liem A, Reynierse-Buitenwerf GH, Zwinderman AH, Jukema JW, van Veldhuisen DJ. Secondary prevention with folic acid: effects on clinical outcomes. *J Am Coll Cardiol* 2003; 41:2105–2113.

101. Toole JF, Malinow MR, Chambless LE *et al.* Lowering homocysteine in patients with ischemic stroke to prevent recurrent stroke, myocardial infarction, and death: the Vitamin Intervention for Stroke Prevention (VISP) randomized controlled trial. *JAMA* 2004; 291:565–575.

102. Bonaa KH, Njolstad I, Ueland PM *et al.* Homocysteine lowering and cardiovascular events after acute myocardial infarction. *N Engl J Med* 2006; 354:1578–1588.

103. The Heart Outcomes Prevention Evaluation (HOPE) 2 Investigators. Homocysteine lowering with folic acid and B vitamins in vascular disease. *N Engl J Med* 2006; 354:1567–1577.

104. Albert CM, Cook NR, Gaziano JM *et al.* Effect of folic acid and B vitamins on risk of cardiovascular events and total mortality among women at high risk for cardiovascular disease: a randomized trial. *JAMA* 2008; 299:2027–2036.

105. Ebbing M, Bleie Ø, Ueland PM *et al.* Mortality and cardiovascular events in patients treated with homocysteine-lowering B vitamins after coronary angiography: a randomized controlled trial. *JAMA* 2008; 300:795–804.

106. Jamison RL, Hartigan P, Kaufman JS *et al.* Effect of homocysteine lowering on mortality and vascular disease in advanced chronic kidney disease and end-stage renal disease: a randomized controlled trial. *JAMA* 2007; 298:1163–1170.

107. Wang X, Qin X, Demirtas H *et al.* Efficacy of folic acid supplementation in stroke prevention: a meta-analysis. Lancet 2007; 369:1876–1882.

13

Medical treatment of symptomatic diabetic neuropathy

E. Salgami, A. J. M. Boulton

INTRODUCTION

Of the many causes of peripheral neuropathy, diabetes mellitus represents the commonest in the Western world today [1]. Diabetes-related neuropathy is estimated to have an annual incidence up to 2% from large studies and was shown to affect up to 50% of older diabetic patients [1–5]. As the global prevalence of diabetes is predicted to rise more than 4% by 2030 [6], it is conceivable that neuropathy will be the most prevalent of all the long-term complications of diabetes. The most common of all of the peripheral neuropathies in diabetes are somatic neuropathies, which affect the lower extremities. The types of distal sensory neuropathy that produce symptoms are discussed below. Detailed reviews of all aspects of these neuropathies were published as a technical review [1], which formed the basis of a recent Position Statement of the American Diabetes Association (ADA) [7]. There are many subgroups of neuropathies and readers are referred to published review papers of the autonomic neuropathies [8] and the mononeuropathies [9].

DEFINITIONS

Members of an International Consensus Meeting on the outpatient diagnosis and management of diabetic peripheral neuropathy (DPN) agreed on a simple definition of neuropathy as *'the presence of symptoms and/or signs of peripheral nerve dysfunction in people with diabetes, after the exclusion of other causes'* [10]. This group also agreed that neuropathy cannot be diagnosed without a careful clinical examination and that absence of symptoms must never be equated with absence of neuropathy. The importance of excluding non-diabetic causes was emphasised in the Rochester Diabetic Neuropathy Study (RDNS) in which 10% of peripheral neuropathy in diabetes was deemed to be of non-diabetic causation [2].

For day-to-day clinical practice, DPN is a clinical diagnosis. It is generally agreed that DPN should not be diagnosed on the basis of one symptom, sign or test alone; a minimum of two abnormalities (i.e. abnormal symptoms and signs) is recommended [1].

Eleanna Salgami, MD, PhD, Clinical Research Fellow, Department of Medicine, University of Manchester, Manchester, UK.

Andrew J. M. Boulton, MD, DSc (Hon), FRCP, Professor of Medicine and Consultant Physician, University of Manchester and Manchester Royal Infirmary, Manchester, UK; Visiting Professor of Medicine, University of Miami, Miami, Florida, USA.

Table 13.1 Clinical classification of diabetic neuropathies

Polyneuropathies	Mononeuropathies

▪ Distal sensory neuropathy
  – Acute sensory (rare)
  – Chronic sensorimotor (common)
▪ Autonomic
▪ Proximal motor (amyotrophy)
▪ Truncal
	Isolated peripheral
	
	Mononeuritis multiplex
	Cranial
	Truncal

EPIDEMIOLOGY

A clinical classification of the diabetic neuropathies is presented in Table 13.1. Of all the various subdivisions, DPN is the most common and may be divided into the following two main types:

1. Acute sensory neuropathy.
2. Chronic sensorimotor neuropathy.

Whereas the former is rare, the latter is very common, although it may be asymptomatic. However, the epidemiology of DPN remains poorly defined, partly because of differing definitions and diagnostic criteria employed in various studies, poor ascertainment and a lack of population-based studies. The population-based study of Kumar and colleagues [4] showed that over 40% of type 2 diabetic patients have neuropathic deficits, with just under half of these having associated symptoms. In a population-based, comparative study of people with and without diabetes, neuropathic symptoms were shown in 16.2% of the diabetic patients and just under 5% of the non-diabetic population in the North West of England [11]. Two of the larger studies from UK and Spain [3, 5], which are clinic- as opposed to population-based, produced similar results with 20–30% showing evidence of neuropathy and/or symptoms. Future studies should probably include a sample of the general population, as non-diabetic symptomatic neuropathy is not uncommon, especially amongst the elderly [12]. The largest published population-based study looking at the prevalence of symptomatic neuropathy reported a prevalence of 21% [13]. In summary, the prevalence of symptomatic neuropathy may be as high as 21%, whereas neuropathic deficits presenting on examination may be found in up to 50% of all diabetic patients.

The peripheral neuropathy in diabetes has been associated with a number of non-modifiable risk factors like age and height and modifiable risk factors, such as degree of hyperglycaemia, diabetes duration, cigarette smoking, hypertension and dyslipidaemia in different studies [1]. However, there are few papers that have addressed potential risk factors for painful diabetic neuropathy per se [14–17]. The strongest evidence on the development and progression of peripheral neuropathy exists for chronic hyperglycaemia in both type 1 and type 2 diabetes [18, 19]. Additional data from follow-up studies suggest that both the duration and severity of hyperglycaemia are related to the severity of distal neuropathy [14, 20]. Interestingly, in asymptomatic patients with impaired glucose tolerance, early small fibre disease confirmed with nerve biopsies was assumed as a result of exposure to hyperglycaemia [21].

In contrast to the many published reports on the prevalence of diabetic neuropathy, there are few on the natural history of this condition, with conflicting results. Whereas a decrease in the intensity of painful symptoms has been associated with worsening of sensory function [22], others have shown that improvement of sensory function might be accompanied with improvement of pain in patients treated with continuous subcutaneous insulin infusion [17]. Similarly, there are inconsistent data on the occurrence of remissions of pain in

Table 13.2 Contrasts between acute sensory and chronic sensorimotor neuropathies

	Acute sensory	*Chronic sensorimotor*
Mode of onset	Relatively rapid	Gradual, insidious
Symptoms	Severe burning pain, aching; weight loss usual	Burning pain, paraesthesiae numbness; weight loss usual
Symptom severity	+++	0 to ++
Signs	Mild sensory in some; motor unusual	Stocking and glove sensory loss; absent ankle reflexes
Other diabetic complications	Unusual	Increased prevalence
Electrophysiological investigations	May be normal or minor abnormalities	Abnormalities unusual in motor and sensory nerves
Natural history	Complete recovery within one year	Symptoms may persist intermittently for years; at risk of foot ulceration

Table 13.3 Typical neuropathic symptoms

Painful	*Non-painful*
Burning pain	Asleep
Knife-like	'Dead'
Electrical sensations	Numbness
Squeezing	Tingling
Constricting	Prickling
Hurting	
Freezing	
Throbbing	
Sharp	

neuropathy. Typically, in chronic diabetic neuropathy, it is considered that a progressive loss of distal nerve fibres lead to disappearance of symptoms and finally complete sensory loss, with the resulting insensate foot *"at risk of ulceration"* [23].

CLINICAL FEATURES OF DIABETIC PERIPHERAL NEUROPATHY

ACUTE SENSORY NEUROPATHY

Acute sensory neuropathy is rare, tends to occur after a period of metabolic instability and is characterised by severely painful symptoms and few findings on neurological examination. Many of the symptoms of acute sensory and chronic sensorimotor neuropathy are similar, although there are differences in the mode of onset, accompanying signs and prognosis. These are summarised in Table 13.2. Table 13.3 lists the typical symptoms, both painful and non-painful. All painful symptoms of the neuropathies tend to be prone to nocturnal exacerbation, with bedclothes irritating hyperaesthetic skin. Acute painful symptoms may occur in patients with a recent episode of ketoacidosis or transient poorly controlled diabetes. Conversely, sudden improvement of blood glucose levels may result in occurrence of symptoms irrespective of the type of treatment. It is assumed that a greater blood glucose flux in persistent hyperglycaemia or excursions to hyper- and hypoglycaemic levels is associated with the pathogenesis of acute neuropathic pain [24]. Clinical examination of the patient with presumed acute sensory neuropathy may be normal, with allodynia (a painful sensation induced by a non-noxious stimulus) on sensory testing, a relatively normal motor examination and occasionally reduced ankle reflexes. The natural history of this rare acute neuropathy is very different from chronic DPN (Table 13.2). Gradual improvement of acute symptoms is achieved with stable glycaemic control followed by a complete resolution, often spontaneously, in less than a year.

CHRONIC SENSORIMOTOR NEUROPATHY

There is little doubt that chronic sensorimotor neuropathy is by far the most common form of DPN. Many patients with this type of neuropathy may actually be asymptomatic, hence the need for a careful clinical examination to diagnose the condition. A neurological deficit may be discovered by chance during a routine neurological examination or after a neuro-pathic complication, such an ulcer in insensitive foot. Because chronic DPN is a length-dependent process, the sensory manifestations are most pronounced in the lower limbs, though in more severe cases, the fingers and hands may also be involved. Chronic symp-toms may vary in intensity over time but remain constant during the history of neuropathy for many years. The symptoms outlined in Table 13.3 tend to be peculiar to the individual patient. Patients often find it very difficult to describe the symptoms because they are dif-ferent from other types of pain they may have previously experienced. It is suggested that interpretation of neuropathic symptoms should be avoided; history taking with recording of the painful experiences, as described by the individual patient, is suggested instead. Many patients have a combination of both positive (painful) and negative (non-painful) symptoms (Table 13.3). Distinguishing positive from negative (e.g. 'dead feet') sensory symptoms could only be semantic as there is no evidence of a different pattern of underlying neuropathology [7]. Further classification of positive sensory symptoms into painful and non-painful categories might be useful in particular cases.

Although not mentioned in older texts, unsteadiness has increasingly been recognised as a manifestation of chronic DPN resulting from disturbed proprioception and probably abnormal muscle sensory function. Such unsteadiness has been quantified and may result in repetitive trauma (i.e. Charcot neuroarthropathy) or falls, especially if combined with postural hypotension due to diabetic autonomic dysfunction. In the most severe cases, with loss of proprioception, patients may demonstrate a positive Romberg's sign. Findings of pronounced motor neuropathy are unlikely to be related to diabetes, especially if asym-metrical. However, motor weakness with small muscle wasting in the feet and hands may be seen in the more advanced stages of distal neuropathy. The chronic sensorimotor neu-ropathy is often accompanied by distal autonomic neuropathy with findings related to auto-nomic dysfunction, such as warm foot, dry skin and calluses at pressure-bearing areas, thus resulting in a foot 'at risk for neuropathic complications' (i.e. ulceration, Charcot foot). Thus, in summary, patients with chronic DPN invariably have a neuropathic deficit on examination and up to 50% may be experiencing symptoms at any one time.

ASSESSMENT OF SYMPTOMATIC NEUROPATHY AND NEUROPATHIC PAIN

In clinical practice, the diagnosis of DPN is accomplished by a careful neurological history and examination supplemented by simple quantitative testing. Testing of neurological parameters (vibration, pressure, pain and temperature perception) usually reveals a symmetrical sensory impairment or loss in a stocking distribution. Ankle reflexes are generally reduced or absent and knee reflexes may also be reduced in some cases. Measurement of the vibration perception threshold (VPT) with an analogue or a digital device is one of the simple to perform among the different tests available. The 10 g nylon monofilament, pressed against the skin until it buckles, is also frequently used to test pressure perception and subsequently assess sensory neuropathy. However, it is important to know that the filaments being used are accurately assessing pres-

Table 13.4 Stages of diabetic peripheral neuropathy

Stage of neuropathy	Characteristics
No neuropathy	No symptoms or signs
Clinical neuropathy	
Chronic painful	Burning, shooting, stabbing pain with or without 'pins and needles'; increased at night; absent sensation to several modalities; reduced/ absent reflexes
Acute painful	Severe symptoms as above (hyperesthesiae common) may follow initiation of insulin in poorly controlled diabetes; signs minor or absent
Painless with complete/partial sensory loss	Numbness/deadness of feet or no symptoms; painless injury; reduced/absent sensation; reduced thermal sensitivity; absent reflexes
Late complications	Foot lesions; neuropathic deformity; non-traumatic amputation

sure at 10 g. Nerve conduction studies are objective, parametric and non-invasive tests in the evaluation of diabetic neuropathy but they are rarely required in routine practice.

Neuropathic pain is the most disturbing symptom of DPN and among the usual reasons for seeking medical advice. Despite its prevalence, it is often under-diagnosed and thus, inadequately treated. Simple self-report scales, such as a 10 cm visual analogue scale (VAS) or 5-point verbal rating scale (VRS) have been used to provide information on the severity of pain. Pain quality can be estimated with the Neuropathic Pain Scale (NPS), the McGill Pain Questionnaire and other scales. It is well recognised that both the symptoms and deficits may have an adverse affect on quality of life (QoL) in diabetic neuropathy [25]. It is increasingly apparent that whereas patients with negative symptoms (i.e. unsteadiness, numbness) tend to be depressed, those with painful symptoms are more likely to be anxious [26, 27]. For the assessment of QoL in diabetic neuropathy, a condition-specific instrument, the NeuroQoL, has been developed and validated: this includes a symptom checklist that may be used as an outcome measure in clinical trials [28].

STAGES OF PERIPHERAL NEUROPATHY

Diabetic peripheral neuropathy is considered a progressive disease that leads to the insensitive foot complications, namely ulceration, neuropathic deformity (i.e. Charcot foot) and even non-traumatic amputation. The clinical stages of sensory diabetic neuropathy have been proposed by an international consensus expert panel [1] and are shown in Table 13.4. Interestingly, the absence of pain is not a sign of resolution of neuropathy. In a painless lower extremity with partial or complete sensory loss, advanced neuropathy is usually present. As it is not clear why diabetic patients are prone to develop painful or non-painful neuropathy initially, the agreed staging of sensory neuropathy does not imply automatic progression to the next stage. The aim of a clinical staging of the severity of DPN is to prevent or even delay late sequelae of neuropathy, often associated with increased morbidity and mortality.

PATHOGENESIS AND MECHANISMS OF NEUROPATHIC PAIN

Pain, which is a submodality of somatic sensation, has an important protective function by providing a warning of injury and potential tissue damage. In contrast, neuropathic pain has no warning role in the natural history of DPN. Pain occurs following neuronal injury and secondary alterations in function, chemistry and structure but diminishes while nerve damage may progress [29]. Thus, in the common chronic DPN, two abnormalities of pain are present:

1. Spontaneous pain that is of no biological benefit.
2. Loss of peripheral pain sensation, which puts the lower limbs at risk of insensitive injury.

Both small and large nerve fibres are involved in painful neuropathy and axonal atrophy may contribute to pain generation [30]. The observation that acute painful neuropathy may follow either periods of unstable glycaemic control or sudden improvement of control on oral or insulin treatment could be explained by alterations in blood glucose flux [24]. Sudden changes in glycaemia may induce endoneurial ischaemia in terms of a 'steal effect' with arteriovenous shunt and, thus, relative hypoxia and axonal atrophy. Pain might arise from ectopic impulses in dorsal root ganglion cells or may even be of spinal or central origin. Further studies are needed to elucidate the pathogenesis of distal sensory neuropathy in diabetes. Currently, research on diabetic neuropathy and advanced glycation end-products (AGE), oxidative stress, insulin-like growth factors, protein kinase C (PKC) and the polyol pathway is ongoing [1].

A number of both peripheral and central mechanisms have been proposed to contribute to the genesis of neuropathic pain. In the periphery, pathogenetic factors include sensitisation, ectopic discharges (neuroma-type properties), collateral sprouting and ephaptic transmission [7]. Central mechanisms include central sensitisation, enhanced facilitation and attenuated inhibition. The characteristic pattern of neuropathic pain that is worse at night, causing sleep disturbance, with various diurnal profiles among individual patients is not elucidated yet. Advances in understanding the chronobiology and mechanisms of neuropathic pain could lead to novel targeted therapies and better patients' outcome.

MANAGEMENT OF SYMPTOMATIC NEUROPATHY

The treatment of symptomatic sensory neuropathy will be considered on the basis of three main areas:

1. Treatments aimed at the underlying pathogenetic mechanisms in the aetiology of diabetic neuropathy.
2. Specific symptomatic treatments.
3. Patient education to avoid the risk of late complications of neuropathy, including foot ulceration.

As can be seen in Table 13.5, optimal and stable glycaemic control and possibly anti-oxidants may fall under both categories. A more detailed discussion of pharmacological agents for symptomatic relief can be found in a number of reviews on this topic [31–33].

PATHOGENETIC THERAPIES

With the exception of stable near-normoglycaemia, most of the agents listed in this section are experimental.

Stable near-normoglycaemia
In addition to the Diabetes Control and Complications Trial (DCCT) [34], three much smaller but long-term prospective studies have confirmed that maintained near-normoglycaemia prevents the development and retards the progression of peripheral neuropathy as assessed

Table 13.5 Potential treatments for chronic sensorimotor neuropathy

Symptomatic/pharmacological	Pathogenetic
Stable glycaemic control	Optimal glycaemic control
Tricyclic drugs	Aldose reductase inhibitors
SSRIs[1]	Anti-oxidants
SNRIs[2]	PKC-β inhibitors
Anticonvulsant drugs	Other agents
Antiarrhythmic drugs	
Opioid/opioid-like drugs	
Other agents	
Physical/topical	**Combination**
Acupuncture	Two agents
Electrical therapies	Pharmacological and topical
Capsaicin	Pharmacological and physical
Vasodilators	
Others	

[1] SSRIs: selective serotonin reuptake inhibitors;
[2] SNRIs: serotonin and norepinephrine reuptake inhibitors.

by electrophysiology. These include the Stockholm Diabetes Intervention Study (SDIS) [35], the Oslo study [36] and, in type 2 diabetes, the Kumomato study [37].

The optimal method of achieving and maintaining normoglycaemia is by pancreas or islet cell transplantation. However, as most published studies are of combined kidney and pancreas transplant and the recipients had generally a long duration of diabetes and established neuropathy, only modest improvements of measures of neuropathy were seen [38]. Nevertheless, achieving near-normoglycaemia should be the primary aim in both the prevention and the initial management of symptomatic DPN.

Aldose-reductase inhibitors (ARI)
Despite the fact that the first trials of ARI in neuropathy took place over 25 years ago, only one agent is available at the time of writing, in one country. As these drugs are primarily disease-modifying agents and are not expected to have an affect on symptomatology, the reader is referred elsewhere for the detailed discussion of such agents [1]. The problems that existed with many of these earlier trials can be summarised as:

- *Too small*: the effect of the drug was inadequate in terms of inhibiting nerve sorbitol accumulation.
- *Too few*: inadequate numbers of subjects were included.
- *Too short*: many trials were only 4 weeks or a few months long for a chronic disease that may be of many years' duration.
- *Too late*: no drug targeting a pathogenetic mechanism is likely to be effective when a complication is well established.

Anti-oxidants
There is accumulating evidence to support the role of oxidative stress in the pathogenesis of neuropathy. Studies with the anti-oxidant α-lipoic acid have provided evidence of potential efficacy for this agent, which may well be beneficial for both neuropathic symptoms and natural history of the neuropathy [39,40].

Table 13.6 Management of symptomatic neuropathy

---

1. Exclude non-diabetic causes:
   - Malignant disease (e.g. bronchogenic carcinoma)
   - Metabolic (e.g. hypothyroidism, uraemia)
   - Haematologic (e.g. Vitamin B_{12} deficiency)
   - Toxic (e.g. alcohol)
   - Infection (e.g. human immunodeficiency virus [HIV] infection)
   - Iatrogenic (e.g. isoniazid, vinca alkaloids)
   - Medication-related (chemotherapy, HIV treatment)
2. Provide explanation, support and information on practical measures, e.g. bed cradle to lift bedclothes off hyperaesthetic skin
3. Assess level of blood glucose control and blood glucose profiles: possibly continuous glucose monitoring
4. Aim for optimal, stable control
5. Consider pharmacological therapy:
   - antidepressants or anticonvulsants
   - opioid or opioid-like drug
   - combination treatment
6. Consider acupuncture, topical or physical therapies (alone or in combination with any pharmacological treatment)
7. Consider pain clinic referral

PKC-β inhibition

Intracellular hyperglycaemia increases diacyl glycerol, which activates PKC formation, leading to multiple pathogenetic consequences. Whereas preliminary data suggested that treatment of peripheral neuropathy with a PKC-β inhibitor might ameliorate measures of nerve function and improve certain symptoms [41], this has not yet been confirmed in larger, longer duration clinical trials [42]. Further investigation of this agent for DPN has thus been halted.

SYMPTOMATIC TREATMENTS

With the exception of optimisation of blood glucose control, the pharmacological and other interventions described in this section are not expected to have any effect on the natural history of diabetic neuropathy or cause changes in objective measures of peripheral nerve function. Moreover, despite differences between acute and chronic sensory neuropathies (Table 13.2), it should be pointed out that the principles of symptomatic management are the same for the two conditions. A logical approach to management is provided in Table 13.6 and might comprise the following:

1. Is this DPN?

It must be remembered that, as noted above, there are many causes of peripheral neuropathy, of which diabetes is the most common. However, exclusion of non-diabetic neuropathies that may also be seen in patients with diabetes, including hypothyroidism, Vitamin B_{12} deficiency and uraemia, is of great importance. In addition, potentially serious conditions, such as malignancies (e.g. small-cell carcinoma presenting as a paraneoplastic syndrome), toxic causes (e.g. alcohol), infections (e.g. HIV), iatrogenic (e.g. isoniazid, vinca alkaloids) and medication-related (chemotherapy, HIV treatment) should be ruled out. In most cases, further investigation such as detailed quantitative sensory testing and electrophysiology, which would require referral to a neurologist, is not necessary. Abnormalities of the above tests simply confirm the presence of peripheral nerve dysfunction without indicating the underlying cause.

2. Initial therapy and counselling

Once a diagnosis is established, giving patients a full explanation of their condition, allaying fears and misconceptions and informing them that pain may resolve in time can be extremely reassuring. Simple physical treatments, such as the use of a bed cradle to lift the bedclothes off hyperaesthetic skin, can be beneficial. In patients with relatively mild pain, common analgesics or anti-inflammatory agents may be sufficient to treat the discomfort.

3. Control of hyperglycaemia

Any change, either short- or long-term, in blood glucose control during a trial might influence painful symptoms, irrespective of any efficacy of the trial agent. A number of small, open-label, uncontrolled studies have suggested that achieving stable near-normoglycaemia is helpful in the management of painful neuropathic symptoms [17, 24]. It therefore appears that the stability of glycaemic control is equally important as the level of achieved control. Whatever the cause, these observations have serious implications for the conduct of clinical trials of potential new agents in the management of painful neuropathy.

4. Pharmacological management

A large number of therapeutic agents have been proposed in the management of painful symptomatology. These are discussed below with a critique of the evidence supporting their use. In management of symptomatic DPN, first-line treatment for neuropathic pain may be either an antidepressant (i.e. amitriptyline) or an anticonvulsant agent (Table 13.6). For refractory cases to the above, chronic opioid treatment could be a safe option if proper guidelines are observed. The effective dose of any agent for neuropathic pain should be individualised according to the patient response and tolerability. It is felt that despite several available pharmacological options, few patients obtain complete pain relief [31]. Certain agents in combination (i.e. an antidepressant with an anticonvulsant) or combined with non-pharmacological therapies (acupuncture, topical and physical therapies) may provide better symptomatic relief with fewer side-effects. There is only limited evidence to support the use of non-steroidal anti-inflammatory drugs (NSAIDs) in DPN. The use of NSAIDs may be required as a rescue therapy when neuropathic painful symptoms are acute and the analgesic action of the long-term regime is expected to start. Such agents, however, should be used with caution in renal impairment that often exists in patients with diabetes.

Tricyclic drugs

The use of the tricyclic drugs in the management of neuropathic pain is supported by several randomised controlled trials and a systematic review, involving ten antidepressants [43–46]. Putative mechanisms by which these drugs relieve pain include inhibition of norepinephrine and/or serotonin reuptake at synapses of central descending pain control systems.

Most experience has been achieved with amitriptyline and imipramine, which are frequently prescribed for neuropathic pain despite their unlicensed use. Imipramine is less sedative than amitriptyline and may be better tolerated. The dosage of both these agents required for symptomatic relief is similar (25–150 mg daily) although daily doses higher than 75 mg may require specialist supervision. In the elderly, it can be useful to start at a dose of 10 mg daily. The long half-life of tricyclic antidepressants allows once-daily administration, hence the compliance of diabetic patients, usually on multiple medications, is expected to be high. In order to avoid undue drowsiness, the dose can be taken in the evening or at bedtime. However, the major problem with all of these agents remains the frequency of adverse reactions, which are predictable in up to 30% of patients. Of these, 4% will have to discontinue a tricyclic drug due to major adverse effects [46]. Although drowsiness and lethargy are common, it is the anticholinergic side-effects, particularly dry mouth, which are most troublesome.

Selective serotonin reuptake inhibitors (SSRIs)
These agents inhibit the presynaptic reuptake of serotonin but not norepinephrine. Studies suggest that treatment with paroxetine and citalopram (both at 40 mg daily) are efficacious in relieving neuropathic pain [47, 48]. Although these agents are felt to be less efficacious in comparison with the tricyclic drugs, troublesome side-effects are generally less common with the SSRIs.

Other newer antidepressants (e.g. duloxetine) for treatment of neuropathic pain are described below.

Anticonvulsants
Anticonvulsant drugs have been used in the management of neuropathic pain for many years [1]. Most trials of the first generation anticonvulsants, including carbamazepine, phenytoin and sodium valproate, have been small single-centre studies. Moreover, many of these agents are associated with significant central adverse events and interfered with blood glucose control [33, 49–51]. However, in recent years, a number of newer agents have been proven to be efficacious in randomised trials and these have been the subject of a recent review [52]. In all anticonvulsant agents, common side-effects such as drowsiness and dizziness could be reduced if low doses are given initially and then gradually increased.

Gabapentin is now widely used for neuropathic symptoms (this agent is structurally related to the neurotransmitter γ-aminobutyric acid, GABA) and was introduced some years ago as an anticonvulsant for complex partial seizures. In a large, randomised controlled trial of gabapentin in symptomatic diabetic neuropathy, significant pain relief together with reduced sleep disturbance was reported using dosages of 900–3600 mg daily [53]. A review of a number of trials of gabapentin for neuropathic pain concluded that dosages of 1800–3600 mg/day of this agent were effective and the side-effect profile appeared to be superior to that of the tricyclic drugs [54]. Although clinical experience suggests that many patients derive some relief from slightly lower dosages, a common failure of management is to give an insufficient dosage for an effective relief of pain.

Pregabalin is structurally related to gabapentin and has been shown in a number of randomised, controlled trials to be effective in decreasing neuropathic pain and well tolerated at dosage up to 600 mg daily [55–57]. In addition, pregabalin was demonstrated to improve sleep disturbance and quality of life as early as first week of treatment, probably due to its anti-anxiety properties [58]. These short- and long-term beneficial effects with a tolerable safety profile were confirmed in a recent review of seven randomised, multicentre trials [59]. Both gabapentin and pregabalin are licensed for the treatment of neuropathic pain in the UK; pregabalin is also licensed for this indication in the USA.

In recent years, controlled trial evidence has also been published for a number of other anticonvulsant drugs, including oxcarbazepine and lamotrigine as monotherapy [60, 61]. However, trials of another anticonvulsant agent, topiramate, have produced differing results regarding its efficacy in painful diabetic neuropathy [62, 63]. Most recently, a small, randomised controlled trial of zonisamide in neuropathy was reported [64]. This pilot study randomised only a small number of patients and has failed to demonstrate any benefit over placebo. Moreover, moderate to severe central side-effects were common with a high number of dropouts in the zonisamide-treated group. In summary, gabapentin and pregabalin appear to have the strongest evidence-base among anticonvulsants drugs used for treating painful neuropathy with the greatest efficacy, tolerability and safety. Although both have a similar pharmacological profile, a recent cost-effectiveness study supported the dominance of pregabalin compared to its predecessor gabapentin in the management of diabetic neuropathic pain [65]. The superior side-effect profile of both of the above to the tricyclic drugs may be associated with a selective binding to the α-2-δ (A2D) protein subunit of voltage-gated calcium channels [59].

Antiarrhythmic agents
The class 1B antiarrhythmic agent, mexiletine, a sodium channel blocker, has been studied in the treatment of painful diabetic neuropathy [66, 67]. The trials of this agent, which is structurally related to lidocaine, used up to 450 mg daily, which is lower than the dose used for cardiac arrhythmias. Remarkably, neither gastrointestinal side-effects, especially nausea, nor serious cardiac arrhythmias have been reported in patients receiving mexiletine at a medium dose. However, regular electrocardiogram monitoring is necessary and the long-term use of this agent cannot be recommended.

Opioid drugs
In the past, there has been reluctance by some physicians, particularly endocrinologists, managing diabetic neuropathy to consider the use of opioids, probably because of the fear of addiction. However, as stated in an editorial [68] *'we must focus urgent attention on the needs of suffering patients'*. It is increasingly apparent that some troublesome neuropathic pain, which is unresponsive to the therapies listed above, may respond to opioids [69]. There is now increasing evidence that opioids and opioid-like drugs can be efficacious in resistant neuropathic pain.

Tramadol is an opioid-like, centrally-acting, synthetic non-narcotic analgesic. The analgesia produced is the combined effect of pure opioid action and enhancement of serotoninergic and adrenergic pathways. Tramadol efficacy in the management of patients with moderate to moderately severe painful neuropathy at an average dose of 210 mg daily was confirmed in a randomised controlled trial [70]. A subsequent follow-up study suggested that the symptomatic relief at a tramadol range 50–400 mg daily could be maintained for at least 6 months [71]. Side-effects are common, however, but are expected to be fewer than other opioids (including less potential for addiction). Modified-release preparations have been designed for once- or twice-daily administration when the individual opioid analgesic requirements are established. Subsequently, two randomised controlled trials have confirmed the efficacy of controlled-release oxycodone (oxycodone CR) for moderate-to-severe neuropathic pain in diabetes with improvement in quality of life [72, 73]. It is advised that opioids such as oxycodone CR should be considered as add-on therapies for patients failing to respond to non-opioid medications. Most recently, there was a suggestion that methadone, a schedule 2, long-acting opioid, might be beneficial in severe neuropathic pain that is refractory to non-opioid treatments [74].

Other agents
Two drugs of the serotonin and norepinephrine reuptake inhibitors class (SNRIs) were recently approved by the FDA for the treatment of painful diabetic neuropathy. Duloxetine has recently been shown in a large randomised controlled trial to be safe, well tolerated and effective in the management of painful diabetic neuropathy [75]. In recent studies, duloxetine 60 mg once- or twice-daily demonstrated a significant treatment effect on neuropathic pain with a rapid course of action that was sustained over 52 weeks and a few significant side-effects [76, 77]. Treatment with duloxetine was associated with modest changes in glycaemia with limited other metabolic changes in a recent study [78].

Venlafaxine is a SNRI agent that lacks the sedative and antimuscarinic effects of the tricyclic drugs. Extended-release venlafaxine has been shown in a large randomized trial to be effective and safe at doses up to 225 mg daily in relieving pain associated with diabetic neuropathy [79]. However, seven patients in the above trial had clinically important electrographic changes during treatment.

Antagonism of N-methyl-D-aspartate (NMDA) receptors was found to affect the glutamate transcription and mediate painful neuropathic symptoms, notably hyperalgesia and allodynia. Preliminary studies using two NMDA antagonists, dextromethorphan and memantine, provide some evidence for the efficacy of these agents regarding neuropathic pain. Dextromethorphan and memantine are currently licensed for use in cough suppression and Alzheimer's disease, respectively. In a small study, dextromethorphan was demonstrated to be effective in selected patients with painful neuropathy [80]. However, evidence of published studies for memantine efficacy in reducing diabetic neuropathic pain is equivocal [80, 81]. This class of drugs may prove to be useful in the treatment of neuropathic pain in the future trials.

Drug combinations
It is unfortunate that there are few published trials either of combinations of agents or of direct comparisons between active drugs for the treatment of diabetic neuropathy. One report assessed the potential combination of morphine and gabapentin in severe neuropathic pain [82]. In this study, the combination of sustained-release morphine and gabapentin achieve better analgesia at lower dosage of each drug than when either was given alone. These observations certainly suggest that out of short-term use, this combination may be useful in selected cases of painful neuropathy.

5. Topical agents
The use of topical agents to treat neuropathic pain offers several theoretical advantages, including minimal systemic side-effects, lack of drug interactions and (usually) no need to titrate dosages. However, few topical agents have been confirmed in appropriately designed randomised controlled trials.

Capsaicin is an extract of chilli peppers that depletes tissue of substance P and reduces chemically-induced pain. There have been a number of controlled studies of capsaicin cream (0.075%) that have resulted in a licensed topical use for symptomatic relief of painful diabetic neuropathy. Although a meta-analysis [83] did suggest overall efficacy from a number of trials, a more recent study failed to confirm any pain relief by this agent [84]. A potential problem with all trials of capsaicin is a difficulty in ensuring that they are truly blinded as topical capsaicin itself gives rise to transient hyperalgesia (usually a mild burning sensation) in many patients.

As a result of confirmed efficacy in randomised controlled trials, the topically applied lidocaine patch is currently approved by the US Food and Drug Administration (FDA) for the treatment of postherpetic neuralgia. In painful diabetic neuropathy, two open-label, multicentre pilot studies with a 5% lidocaine patch for up to 18 hours a day showed significant improvement of pain and quality of life measures with good tolerance [85, 86]. Interestingly, pain relief was maintained over a 5-week active treatment period and allowed tapering of concomitant analgesic therapy [85]. These preliminary data are certainly promising, the main advantage being the lack of adverse events, probably due to topical action without systemic accumulation of lidocaine. However, these observations do need to be confirmed in adequately designed randomised controlled trials.

Nitrate preparations may have a role in DPN as impaired nitric oxide (NO) generation is thought to be involved in the pathogenesis of chronic neuropathic pain. Isosorbide dinitrate spray, a NO donor and potential local vasodilator applied locally to the lower limbs was shown to be effective in relieving overall diabetic neuropathic pain and burning sensation in a crossover trial [87]. More recently, the use of nitrate patches has also been shown to be useful [88]. However, both of these studies were small and single-centre and a multi-centre trial is now indicated for this agent.

6. Acupuncture and physical therapies
Acupuncture
This is generally considered the first-choice therapy of alternative medicine for chronic pain relief. Acupuncture's potential mechanisms of action in the periphery and, recently, a central

modulation of a limbic network including the hypothalamus [89] are currently under investigation. Despite anecdotal evidence, only a few uncontrolled studies report significant benefits of acupuncture in the relief of painful symptomatology. In the most recent of these, a 10-week uncontrolled study of up to six courses of traditional Chinese acupuncture resulted in 77% of patients experiencing significant pain relief [90]. During a follow-up of 1 year, the majority of these patients were able to discontinue or significantly reduce other pain medication. Methodological problems (i.e. finding the correct site for 'sham' acupuncture) are factors influencing the paucity of controlled trials to confirm the efficacy of acupuncture. The effect of Chinese acupuncture on peripheral neuropathy of undefined aetiology assessed by quantitative measures was recently reported in a pilot study [91]. In this study, the subjective improvement of symptoms was correlated with an improvement of nerve conduction. As acupuncture has not been related with interactions, it might be used as a supplemental intervention to conventional pharmacological treatment for painful neuropathy. Despite acupuncture being considered a side-effect-free therapy, the potential dangers of trauma to a painless neuropathic limb in patients with diabetes should be taken into consideration [92].

Other physical therapies
The efficacy of pulsed electrical stimulation through stocking electrodes in the treatment of painful diabetic neuropathy, previously supported in an open-label study, was not confirmed to be efficacious in a randomised crossover trial [93]. A number of other physical therapies have been proposed and do have support from small controlled trials: these include low-intensity laser therapy [94], percutaneous electrical nerve stimulation [95], static magnetic field therapy [96], and monochromatic infrared energy (MIRE) treatment [97]. However, although the latter has been shown to be efficacious in terms of both pain and sensory improvement in one study [97], a further randomised, double-blind, controlled study suggests that the previous claim that it improves sensation may not be true [98]. For patients with the most severe painful neuropathy unresponsive to *any* of the above therapies, the use of electrical spinal cord stimulation was proposed in a small case-series study [99]. In a recent follow-up study of patients, it was suggested that long-term symptomatic relief could be achieved [100]. However, electrical spinal cord stimulation cannot be generally recommended except in very resistant cases as it is invasive, expensive and has not been validated in controlled studies.

PATIENT EDUCATION AND PREVENTION OF LATE NEUROPATHIC COMPLICATIONS

All patients with diabetic neuropathy, whether complicated by painful symptomatology or not, require education in neuropathy and preventative foot care. The vast majority of foot lesions are potentially preventable and many patients require podiatry referral or more frequent follow-up. Patients and physicians should always pay close attention to foot inspection to reinforce the message of the need for regular self-care, since neuropathy is the most important component in the pathway to foot ulceration [101, 102].

SUMMARY

Diabetic peripheral neuropathy (DPN) is among the most common of all long-term complications of diabetes, affecting up to 50% of older type 2 diabetic patients. Neuropathic deficits present on examination may be found in up to 50% of all diabetic patients whereas the prevalence of symptomatic neuropathy may be as high as 21%. In the most common chronic DPN, painful symptoms have no biological effect and diminish while nerve damage may progress. The first step in the management of DPN is to exclude other causes of neuropathy and assess the level of glycaemic control. Approaches to painful or uncomfortable symptoms may target the underlying pathogenetic mechanisms, the specific symptoms and patient education in foot care. Optimising glycaemic control is paramount for modification of the natural history of DPN and improvement of symptomatology. With the exception of near-normoglycaemia, most pathogenetic therapies are experimental. A number of symptomatic pharmacological therapies have been proven to be efficacious in randomised controlled trials. Whereas the tricyclic drugs are still commonly prescribed, their use is limited by troublesome and predictable side-effects. The anticonvulsants gabapentin and pregabalin are now widely used in the management of neuropathic pain as the adverse event profile appears to be superior to the tricyclic agents. Duloxetine was recently approved for the treatment of painful diabetic neuropathy. There is also increasing evidence that opioids and opioid-like agents (i.e. tramadol) may be efficacious in some severe cases that are unresponsive to 'traditional' treatments. Although several treatment options are available, few patients obtain complete pain relief. Combination treatment, including acupuncture, topical and physical therapies, may provide better patient outcome with fewer side-effects. Further studies are necessary to evaluate the efficacy of current treatment modalities and clarify the role of symptomatic treatment in DPN. Ongoing research into the pathogenetic mechanisms of neuropathic pain in diabetes may lead to novel targeted therapies in the future.

REFERENCES

1. Boulton AJM, Malik RA, Arezzo JS et al. Diabetic somatic neuropathies. Diabetes Care 2004; 27:1458–1486.
2. Dyck PM, Katz KM, Karnes JL et al. The prevalence by staged severity of various types of diabetic neuropathy, retinopathy and nephropathy in a population-based cohort: the Rochester Diabetic Neuropathy Study. Neurology 1993; 43:817–824.
3. Young MJ, Boulton AJM, McLeod AF et al. Multicentre study of the prevalence of diabetic peripheral neuropathy in the UK hospital clinic population. Diabetologia 1993; 36:150–156.
4. Kumar S, Ashe HC, Parnell LN et al. The prevalence of foot ulceration and its correlates in type 2 diabetes: a population-based study. Diabet Med 1994; 11:480–484.
5. Cabezas-Cerrato J. The prevalence of diabetic neuropathy in Spain: a study in primary care and hospital clinic groups. Diabetologia 1998; 41:1263–1269.
6. Wild S, Roglic G, Green A et al. Global prevalence of diabetes: estimates for the year 2000 and projections for 2030. Diabetes Care 2004; 27:1047–1053.
7. Boulton AJM, Vinik AI, Arezzo JC et al. Diabetic neuropathies: a statement by the American Diabetes Association. Diabetes Care 2005; 28:956–962.
8. Vinik AI, Maser RE, Mitchell B et al. Diabetic autonomic neuropathy: a technical review. Diabetes Care 2003; 26:1553–1579.
9. Vinik AI, Mehrbyan A, Cohen L et al. Focal entrapment neuropathies in diabetes. Diabetes Care 2004; 27:1783–1788.
10. Boulton AJM, Gries FA, Jervell JA et al. Guidelines for the diagnosis and outpatient management of diabetic peripheral neuropathy. Diabet Med 1998; 15:508–514.
11. Daousi C, MacFarlane IA, Woodward A et al. Chronic painful peripheral neuropathy in an urban community: a controlled comparison of people with and without diabetes. Diabet Med 2004; 21:976–982.
12. Garrow AP, Silman AJ, MacFarlane GJ. The Cheshire Foot Pain and Disability Survey: a population survey assessing prevalence and associations. Pain 2004; 110:378–384.
13. Abbott CA, Carrington AL, Ashe H et al. The North-West Diabetes Foot Care Study: incidence of and risk factors for new diabetic foot ulceration in a community-based cohort. Diabet Med 2002; 19:377–384.
14. Partanen J, Niskanen L, Lehtinen J et al. Natural history of peripheral neuropathy in patients with non-insulin dependent diabetes. N Engl J Med 1995; 333:39–84.
15. Sorensen L, Molyneaux L, Yue DK. Insensate versus painful diabetic neuropathy: the effects of height, gender, ethnicity and glycaemic control. Diabetes Res Clin Pract 2002; 57:45–51.
16. Harris M, Eastman R, Cowie C. Symptoms of sensory neuropathy in adults with NIDDM in the U.S. population. Diabetes Care 1993; 16:1446–1452.

17. Boulton AJM, Drury J, Clarke B et al. Continuous subcutaneous insulin infusion in the management of painful diabetic neuropathy. Diabetes Care 1982; 5:386–390.
18. The effect of intensive diabetes therapy on the development and progression of neuropathy. The Diabetes Control and Complications Trial Research Group. Ann Intern Med 1995; 122:561–568.
19. Intensive blood-glucose control with sulphonylureas or insulin compared with conventional treatment and risk of complications in patients with type 2 diabetes (UKPDS 33). UK Prospective Diabetes Study (UKPDS) Group. Lancet 1998; 352:837–853.
20. Dyck PJ, Davies JL, Wilson DM et al. Risk factors for severity of diabetic polyneuropathy: intensive longitudinal assessment of the Rochester Diabetic Neuropathy Study cohort. Diabetes Care 1999; 22:1479–1486.
21. Boulton AJ. Treatment of prediabetic neuropathy. Curr Diab Rep 2006; 6:415–416.
22. Benbow SJ, Chan AW, Bowsher D et al. A prospective study of painful symptoms, small-fibre function and peripheral vascular disease in chronic painful diabetic neuropathy. Diabet Med 1994; 11:17–21.
23. Boulton AJ, Malik RA. Diabetic neuropathy. Med Clin North Am 1998; 82:909–929.
24. Oyibo S, Prasad YD, Jackson NJ et al. The relationship between blood glucose excursions and painful diabetic peripheral neuropathy: a pilot study. Diabet Med 2002; 19:870–873.
25. Vileikyte L. Psychological aspects of diabetic peripheral neuropathy. Diabetes Rev 1999; 7:387–394.
26. Vileikyte L, Rubin RR, Leventhal H. Psychological aspects of diabetic neuropathic foot complications: an overview. Diabetes Metab Res Rev 2004; 20:S13–S18.
27. Vileikyte L, Leventhal H, Gonzalez JS et al. Diabetic peripheral neuropathy and depressive symptoms: the association revisited. Diabetes Care 2005; 28:2378–2383.
28. Vileikyte L, Peyrot M, Bundy C et al. The development and validation of a neuropathy and foot ulcer specific quality of life rate. Diabetes Care 2003; 26:2549–2555.
29. Woolf CJ, Mannion RJ. Neuropathic pain: aetiology, symptoms, mechanisms, and management. Lancet 1999; 353:1959–1964.
30. Boulton AJ. What causes neuropathic pain? J Diabetes Complications 1992; 6:58–63.
31. Corbett CF. Practical management of patients with painful diabetic neuropathy. Diabetes Educator 2005; 31:523–524.
32. Adriaensen H, Plaghki L, Mathieu C et al. Critical review of oral drug treatments for diabetic neuropathic pain-clinical outcomes based on efficacy and safety data from placebo-controlled and direct comparative studies. Diabetes Metab Res Rev 2005; 21:231–240.
33. Freeman R. Newer agents for the treatment of painful diabetic peripheral neuropathy. Curr Diab Rep 2005; 5:409–416.
34. DCCT Research Group. The effect of intensive diabetes therapy on the development and progression of neuropathy. Ann Int Med 1995; 122:561–568.
35. Reichard P, Nilsson BY, Rosenqvist CL. The effect of long-term intensified insulin treatment on the development of microvascular complications of diabetes. N Engl J Med 1993; 329:304–309.
36. Amthor KF, Dahl-Jorgensen K, Berg TJ et al. The effect of 8 years of strict glycaemic control on peripheral nerve function in IDDM patients: the Oslo study. Diabetologia 1994; 37:579–586.
37. Ohkubo Y, Kishikawa H, Araki E et al. Intensive insulin therapy prevents the progression of diabetic microvascular complications in Japanese patients with non-insulin dependent diabetes: a randomized prospective 6-year study. Diabetes Res Clin Pract 1995; 28:103–117.
38. Kennedy WR, Navarro X, Goetz FC et al. Effects of pancreas transplantation on diabetic neuropathy. N Engl J Med 1990; 322:1031–1037.
39. Ziegler D, Reljanovic M, Mehnert H et al. Alpha-lipoic acid in the treatment of diabetic polyneuropathy in Germany: current evidence from clinical trials. Exp Clin Endocrinol Diabetes 1999; 107:421–430.
40. Ametov AS, Barinov A, Dyck PJ et al., SYDNEY Trial Study Group: The sensory symptoms of diabetic polyneuropathy are improved with a-lipoic acid: the SYDNEY trial. Diabetes Care 2003; 26:770–776.
41. Vinik A, Tesfaye S, Zhang D et al. LY333531 treatment improves diabetic peripheral neuropathy with symptoms (Abstract). Diabetes 2002; 51(suppl 2):A79.
42. Vinik AI, Bril V, Kempler P et al. Treatment of symptomatic diabetic peripheral neuropathy with the PKC-β inhibitor roboxistaurin during a 1-year randomised placebo-controlled, double-blind clinical trial. Clin Ther 2005; 27:1164–1180.
43. Max, MB, Lynch SA, Muir J et al. Effects of desipramine, amitriptyline and fluoxetine on pain relief in diabetic neuropathy. N Engl J Med 1992; 326:1250–1256.
44. Watson CP. The treatment of neuropathic pain: antidepressants and opioids. Clin J Pain 2000; 16:S49–S55.

45. Mendell JR, Sahenk Z. Painful sensory neuropathy. *N Engl J Med* 2003; 248:1243–1255.

46. McQuay H, Tramer M, Nye BA. A systemic review of antidepressants in neuropathic pain. *Pain* 1996; 68:217–227.

47. Sindrup SH, Gram LF, Brosen K *et al*. The SSRI paroxetine is effective in the treatment of diabetic neuropathy symptoms. *Pain* 1990; 42:135–144.

48. Sindrup SH, Bjerre U, Dejgaard A *et al*. The selective serotonin reuptake inhibitor citalopram relieves the symptoms of diabetic neuropathy. *Clin Pharmacol Ther* 1992; 53:547–552.

49. Rull JA, Quibrera R, Gonzalez-Millan H *et al*. Symptomatic treatment of peripheral diabetic neuropathy with carbamazepine (Tegretol): double blind crossover trial. *Diabetologia* 1969; 5:215–218.

50. Saudek CD, Werns S, Reidenberg MM. Phenytoin in the treatment of diabetic symmetrical polyneuropathy. *Clin Pharmacol Ther* 1977; 22:196–199.

51. Kochar DK, Jain N, Agarwal RP *et al*. Sodium valproate in the management of painful neuropathy in type 2 diabetes – a randomized placebo controlled study. *Acta Neurol Scand* 2002; 106:248–252.

52. Vinik AI. Use of antiepileptic drugs in the treatment of chronic painful diabetic neuropathy. *J Clin Endocrinol Metab* 2005; 90:4936–4945.

53. Backonja M, Beydoun A, Edwards KR *et al*. Gabapentin for the symptomatic treatment of painful neuropathy in patients with diabetes mellitus: a randomized controlled trial. *JAMA* 1998; 280:1831–1836.

54. Backonja M, Glazman RL. Gabapentin dosing for neuropathic pain: evidence from randomized placebo controlled clinical trials. *Clin Ther* 2003; 25:81–104.

55. Rosenstock J, Tuchman M, LaMoreaux L *et al*. Pregabalin for the treatment of painful diabetic peripheral neuropathy: a double-blind, placebo-controlled trial. *Pain* 2004; 110:628–638.

56. Richter RW, Portenoy R, Sharma U *et al*. Relief of painful diabetic peripheral neuropathy with pregabalin: a randomized, placebo-controlled trial. *J Pain* 2005; 6:253–260.

57. Freynhagen R, Strojek K, Griesing T *et al*. Efficacy of pregabalin in neuropathic pain evaluated in a 12-week, randomized, double-blind, multicentre, placebo-controlled trial of flexible- and fixed-dose regimens. *Pain* 2005; 115:254–263.

58. Lesser H, Sharma U, LaMoreaux L *et al*. Pregabalin relieves symptoms of painful diabetic neuropathy: a randomized controlled trial. *Neurology* 2004; 63:2104–2110.

59. Freeman R, Durso-Decruz E, Emir B. Efficacy, safety and tolerability of pregabalin treatment for painful diabetic peripheral neuropathy: findings from seven randomized, controlled trials across a range of doses. *Diabetes Care* 2008; 31:1448–1454.

60. Dogra S, Beydoun S, Mazzola J *et al*. Oxcarbazepine in painful diabetic neuropathy: a randomized, placebo-controlled study. *Eur J Pain* 2005; 9:543–554.

61. Eisenberg E, Luri Y, Braker C *et al*. Lamotrigine reduces painful diabetic neuropathy: a randomized, controlled study. *Neurology* 2001; 57:505–509.

62. Thienel U, Neto W, Schwabe SK *et al*. Topiramate in painful diabetic polyneuropathy: findings from three double-blind placebo-controlled trials. *Acta Neurol Scand* 2004; 110:221–231.

63. Raskin P, Donofrio PD, Rosenthal NR *et al*. Topiramate vs. placebo in painful diabetic neuropathy: analgesic and metabolic effects. *Neurology* 2004; 63:865–873.

64. Atli A, Dogra S. Zonisamide in the treatment of painful diabetic neuropathy: a randomized, double-blind, placebo-controlled, pilot study. *Pain Med* 2005; 6:225–234.

65. Tarride JE, Gordon A, Vera-Llonch M *et al*. Cost-effectiveness of pregabalin for the management of neuropathic pain associated with diabetic peripheral neuropathy and postherpetic neuralgia: a Canadian perspective. *Clin Ther* 2006; 28:1922–1934.

66. Stracke H, Meyer UE, Schumacher HE *et al*. Mexiletine in the treatment of diabetic neuropathy. *Diabetes Care* 1992; 15:1550–1555.

67. Jarvis B, Coukell AJ. Mexiletine: a review of its therapeutic use in painful diabetic neuropathy. *Drugs* 1998; 56:691–707.

68. Foley KM. Opioids and chronic neuropathic pain. *N Engl J Med* 2003; 348:1279–1281.

69. Boulton AJM. Opioids for painful diabetic neuropathy. *Curr Diabet Rep* 2005; 5:407–408.

70. Harati Y, Gooch C, Swenson M *et al*. Double-blind randomized trial of tramadol for the treatment of the pain of diabetic neuropathy. *Neurology* 1998; 50:1842–1846.

71. Harati Y, Gooch C, Swenson M *et al*. Maintenance of the long-term effectiveness of tramadol in treatment of the pain of diabetic neuropathy. *J Diabetes Compl* 2000; 14:65–70.

72. Gimbel JS, Richards P, Portenoy RK. Controlled-release oxycodone for pain in diabetic neuropathy: a randomized controlled trial. *Neurology* 2003; 60:927–934.

73. Watson CPN, Moulin D, Watt-Watson J et al. Controlled-release oxycodone relieves neuropathic pain: a randomized controlled trial in painful diabetic neuropathy. *Pain* 2003; 105:71–78.
74. Hays L, Reid C, Doran M et al. Use of methadone for the treatment of diabetic neuropathy. *Diabetes Care* 2005; 28:485–487.
75. Goldstein DJ, Lu Y, Detke MJ et al. Duloxetine vs placebo in patients with painful diabetic neuropathy. *Pain* 2005; 116:109–118.
76. Wernicke JF, Pritchett YL, D'Souza DN et al. A randomized controlled trial of duloxetine in diabetic peripheral neuropathic pain. *Neurology* 2006; 67:1411–1420.
77. Sultan A, Gaskell H, Derry S et al. Duloxetine for painful diabetic neuropathy and fibromyalgia pain: a systematic review. *BMC Neurol* 2008; 1:8–29.
78. Hardy T, Sachson R, Shen S et al. Does treatment with duloxetine for neuropathic pain impact glycemic control? *Diabetes Care* 2007; 30:21–26.
79. Rowbotham MC, Goli V, Kunz NR et al. Venlafaxine extended release in the treatment of painful diabetic neuropathy: a double-blind, placebo-controlled study. *Pain* 2004; 110:697–706.
80. Sang CN, Booher S, Gilron I et al. Dextromethorphan and memantine in painful diabetic neuropathy and postherpetic neuralgia: efficacy and dose-response trials. *Anesthesiology* 2002; 96:1053–1061.
81. Kirby LC. Memantine in the treatment of diabetic patients with painful peripheral neuropathy: a double-blind placebo-controlled phase IIB trial. *Pain Med* 2002; 3:182–185.
82. Gilron I, Bailey JM, Tu D et al. Morphine, gabapentin, or their combination for neuropathic pain. *N Engl J Med* 2005; 352:1324–1334.
83. Zhang WY, Wan Po AL. The effectiveness of topically applied capsaicin: a meta-analysis. *Eur J Clin Pharmacol* 1994; 45:517–522.
84. Low PA, Opfer-Gehrking TL, Dyck PJ et al. Double-blind, placebo-controlled study of the application of capsaicin cream in chronic distal painful polyneuropathy. *Pain* 1995; 62:163–168.
85. Barbano RL, Herrmann DN, Hart-Gouleau S et al. Effectiveness, tolerability, and impact on quality of life of the 5% lidocaine patch in diabetic polyneuropathy. *Arch Neurol* 2004; 61:914–918.
86. Argoff CE, Galer BS, Jensen MP et al. Effectiveness of the lidocaine patch 5% on pain qualities in three chronic pain states: assessment with the Neuropathic Pain Scale. *Curr Med Res Opin* 2004; 20: S21–S28.
87. Yuen KC, Baker NR, Rayman G. Treatment of chronic painful diabetic neuropathy with isosorbide dinitrate spray: a double-blind placebo-controlled cross-over study. *Diabetes Care* 2002; 25:1699–1703.
88. Rayman G, Baker NR, Krishnan ST. Glyceryl trinitrate patches as an alternative to isosorbide dinitrate spray in the treatment of chronic painful diabetic neuropathy. *Diabetes Care* 2003; 26:2697–2698.
89. Napadow V, Ketter N, Liu J et al. Hypothalamus and amygdala response to acupuncture stimuli in carpal tunnel syndrome. *Pain* 2007; 130:254–266.
90. Abusaisha BB, Constanzi JB, Boulton AJM. Acupuncture for the treatment of chronic painful diabetic neuropathy: a long-term study. *Diabetes Res Clin Pract* 1998; 39:115–121.
91. Schroder S, Liepert J, Remppis A et al. Acupuncture treatment improves nerve conduction in peripheral neuropathy. *Eur J Neurol* 2007; 14:276–281.
92. Ewins DL, Bakker K, Young MJ et al. Alternative medicine: potential dangers for the diabetic foot. *Diabet Med* 1993; 10:980–982.
93. Oyibo SO, Breislin K, Boulton AJ. Electrical stimulation therapy through stocking electrodes for painful diabetic neuropathy: a double blind, controlled crossover study. *Diabet Med* 2004; 21:940–944.
94. Zinman LH, Ngo M, Ng ET et al. Low-intensity laser therapy for painful symptoms of diabetic sensorimotor polyneuropathy: a controlled trial. *Diabetes Care* 2004; 27:921–924.
95. Hamza MA, White PF, Craig WF et al. Percutaneous electrical nerve stimulation: a novel analgesic therapy for diabetic neuropathic pain. *Diabetes Care* 2000; 23:365–370.
96. Weintraub MI, Wolfe GI, Barohn RA et al. Static magnetic field therapy for symptomatic diabetic neuropathy: a randomized, double-blind, placebo-controlled trial. *Arch Phys Med Rehabil* 2003; 86:736–746.
97. Leonard DR, Farooqi MH, Myers S. Restoration of sensation, reduced pain, and improved balance in subjects with diabetic peripheral neuropathy: a double-blind, randomized, placebo-controlled study with monochromatic near-infrared treatment. *Diabetes Care* 2004; 27:168–172.
98. Clifft JK, Kasser RJ, Newton TS et al. The effect of monochromatic infrared energy on sensation in patients with diabetic peripheral neuropathy: a double-blind, placebo-controlled study. *Diabetes Care* 2005; 28:2896–2900.
99. Tesfaye S, Watt J, Benbow SJ et al. Electrical spinal-cord stimulation for painful diabetic peripheral neuropathy. *Lancet* 1996; 348:1698–1701.

100. Daousi C, Benbow SJ, MacFarlane IA. Electrical spinal cord stimulation in the long-term treatment of chronic painful diabetic neuropathy. *Diabet Med* 2005; 22:393–398.
101. Boulton AJ, Kirsner RS, Vileikyte L. Neuropathic diabetic foot ulcers. *N Engl J Med* 2004; 351:48–55.
102. Boulton AJ. The diabetic foot: from art to science. The 18th Camillo Golgi lecture. *Diabetologia* 2004; 47:1343–1353.

Abbreviations

4S	Scandinavian Simvastatin Survival Study
4T	Treating To Target in Type 2 diabetes
5-MTHF	5-methyltetrahydrofolate
A2D	α-2-δ
A to Z	Aggrastat to Zocor
ABCD	Appropriate Blood pressure Control in Diabetes
ABCD-HT	Appropriate Blood pressure Control in Diabetes on Hypertensive Patients
ABCD-NT	Appropriate Blood pressure Control in Diabetes on Normotensive Patients
ABP	ambulatory blood pressure
ABPM	ambulatory blood pressure monitoring
ACC	acetyl-CoA carboxylase
ACCORD	Action to Control Cardiovascular Risk in type 2 Diabetes
ACE	angiotensin converting enzyme
ACEI	angiotensin-converting enzyme inhibitors
ACS	acute coronary syndromes
ADA	American Diabetes Association
ADMA	asymmetric dimethylarginine
AdoHcy	S-adenosylhomocysteine
AdoMet	S-adenosylmethionine
ADOPT	A Diabetes Outcome Progression Trial
ADP	adenosine diphosphate
ADVANCE	Action in Diabetes and Vascular Disease: Preterax and Diamicorn MR Controlled Evaluation
AERx® iDMS	Insulin Diabetes Management System
AF	activating function
AFCAPS/TexCAPS	Air Force/Texas Coronary Atherosclerosis Prevention Study
AGE	advanced glycosylated end-products
AHA	American Heart Association
AIIRA	angiotensin II receptor antagonsist
ALLHAT-LLT	Antihypertensive and Lipid-Lowering Treatment to Prevent Heart Attack Trial

AMP	adensosine monophosphate
AMPK	AMP-activated protein kinase
AMPK	AMP-activated protein kinase
apoCIII	apolipoprotein CIII
ARB	angiotensin II receptor blocker
ARI	Aldose-reductase inhibitors
ARR	aldosterone–renin ratio
ASCEND	A Study of Cardiovascular Events in Diabetes
ASCOT	Anglo-Scandinavian Cardiac Outcomes Trial
ASCOT-LLA	Anglo-Scandinavian Cardiac Outcomes Trial–Lipid Lowering Arm
ASPEN	Atorvastatin Study for Prevention of Coronary Heart Disease Endpoints in Non-Insulin-Dependent Diabetes Mellitus
ASTERIOD	A Study To Evaluate the Effect of Rosuvastatin on Intravascular Ultrasound-Derived Coronary Atheroma Burden
ATP	adenosine triphosphate
AUC	area under curve
BBLT	Blood Pressure Lowering Treatment Trialists'
bd	twice a day
BENEDICT	Bergamo Nephrologic Diabetes Complications Trial
BHS	British Hypertension Society
BIP	Bezafibrate Infarction Prevention study
BMI	body mass index
BP	blood pressure
BTG	β-thromboglobulin
CABG	coronary artery bypass graft
CALM	Candesartan and Lisinopril Microalbuminuria trial
cAMP	cyclic adenosine monophosphate
CARDS	Collaborative AtoRvastatin Diabetes Study
CARE	Cholesterol and Recurrent Events
CB_1	cannabinoid receptor-1
CBGM	continuous blood glucose monitoring
CDC	Centers for Disease Control and Prevention
CDKAL1	cyclin dependent kinase 5 (CDK5) regulatory subunit associated protein 1-like 1
CEMACH	Confidential Enquiry into Maternal and Child Health
CH_2	methylene
CH_3	methyl
CHARISMA	Clopidogrel for High Atherothrombotic Risk and Ischemic Stabilization, Management and Avoidance
CHD	coronary heart disease
CHO	formyl
CI	confidence interval
CII	continuous insulin infusion
CIPII	continuous intraperitoneal insulin infusion
CoA	coenzyme A

CORAL	Cardiovascular Outcomes in Renal Atherosclerotic Lesions trial
CORALL	cholesterol-lowering effects of rosuvastatin compared with atorvastatin in patients with type 2 diabetes
COX	cyclo-oxygenase
CR	controlled release
CRP	C-reactive protein
CSII	continuous subcutaneous insulin infusion
CT	computed tomography
CTT	Cholesterol Treatment Trialists' Collaborators
CV	cardiovascular
CVD	cardiovascular disease
DAIS	Diabetes Atherosclerosis Intervention Study
DAVID	Drug Evaluation in Artherosclerotic Vascular Disease in Diabetes study
DBD	DNA binding domain
DBP	diastolic blood pressure
DCCT	Diabetes Control and Complications Trial
DETAIL	Diabetics Exposed to Telmisartan and Enalapril study
DHA	docosahexaenoic acid
DIGAMI-2	Diabetes and Insulin-Glucose Infusion in Acute Myocardial Infarction-2 study
DKD	diabetic kidney disease
DLCO	diffusing capacity
DM	diabetes mellitus
DNA	deoxyribonucleic acid
DPN	diabetic peripheral neuropathy
DPP	Diabetes Prevention Program
DPP	dipeptidyl peptidase
DRASTIC	Dutch Renal Artery Stenosis Intervention Cooperative
EASD	European Association for the Study of Diabetes
ECG	electrocardiogram
ELISA	enzyme-linked immunosorbent assay
eNOS	endothelial nitric oxide synthase
EPA	eicosapentaenoic acid
ESC	European Society of Cardiology
ESH-ESC	European Society of Hypertension – European Society of Cardiology
ESRD	end-stage renal disease
ETDRS	Early Treatment in Diabetic Retinopathy Study
EUCLID	EURODIAB Controlled trial of Lisinoprilin Insulin-dependent Diabetes
EUROPA	European Trial on Reduction of Cardiac Events with Perindopril in Stable Coronary Artery Disease
EVADIAC	Evaluation dans le Diabète du Traitement par Implants Actifs
EVIDENS	Evidence in Diabetes Enquiry Stem Research Group

FA	fatty acid
FAS	fatty acid synthetase
FDA	US Food and Drug Administration
FEV$_1$	forced expiratory volume in one second
FFA	free fatty acid
FH	familial hypercholesterolaemia
FIELD	Fenofibrate Intervention and Event Lowering in Diabetes study
FPG	fasting plasma glucose
FTO	fat mass and obesity
GABA	γ-aminobutyric acid,
GFR	glomerular filtration rate
GI	gastrointestinal
GIP	gastric inhibitory polypeptide
GIP	glucose-dependent insulinotropic polypeptide
GIPR	GIP receptor
GLP-1	glucagon-like peptide-1
GLUT1	glucose transporter 1
GLUT2	glucose transporter 2
GLUT4	glucose transporter 4
GP	glycoprotein
GREACE	GREek Atorvastatin Coronary heart disease Evaluation study
GRPP	glicentin-related pancreatic peptide
HbA1c	glycosylated haemoglobin
HDL	high-density lipoprotein
HDL-C	high density lipoprotein-cholesterol
HHS	Helsinki Heart Study
HIV	human immunodeficiency virus
HMG	3-hydroxy-3-methyl-glutaryl
HNF-1α	hepatocyte nuclear factor 1α
HOMA	homeostasis model assessment
HOME	Hyperinsulinemia: the Outcome of its Metabolic Effects
HOPE	Heart Outcomes Prevention Evaluation study
HOT	Hypertension Optimal Treatment study
HPS	Heart Protection Study
HR	hazard ratio
hsCRP	high-sensitivity C-reactive protein
HTA	Health Technology Assessment
Hum-R	regular human insulin
IDEAL	Incremental Decrease in End Points through Aggressive Lipid Lowering trial
IDF	International Diabetes Federation
IDNT	Irbesartan in Diabetic Nephropathy Trial
IFG	impaired fasting glucose
IFG	impaired fasting glycaemia
IGF2BP2	insulin-like growth factor binding protein two

IGT	impaired glucose tolerance
IHD	ischaemic heart disease
IL	interleukin
IM	intramuscular
IP	intraperitoneal
IR	insulin resistance
IRAS	Insulin Resistance Atherosclerosis study
IRMA-2	Irbesartan in Patients with Type 2 Diabetes and Microalbuminuria trial
IU	international unit
IV	intravenous
IVUS	intravascular ultrasound
JBS	Joint British Societies
JPAD	Low-Dose Aspirin for Primary Prevention of Atherosclerotic Events in Patients with type 2 Diabetes trial
K_{ATP}	ATP-sensitive potassium channel
LADA	latent autoimmune diabetes in adults
LAR	long-acting release
LBD	ligand binding domain
LDL	low-density lipoprotein
LDL-C	low-density lipoprotein-cholesterol
LEAD	Liraglutide Effect and Action in Diabetes
LIFE	Losartan Intervention For Endpoint Reduction in Hypertension study
LIPID	Long-Term Intervention with Pravastatin in Ischaemic Disease
LIPS	Lescol Intervention Prevention Study
LKB	alias of serine-threonine kinase 11
LPL	lipoprotein lipase
LTSS	long-term sensor system
MAGE	mean amplitude of glycaemic excursions
MARVEL	Microalbuminuria Reduction with Valsartan study
MDI	multiple daily injection
MI	myocardial infarction
MICRO-HOPE	Heart Outcomes Prevention Evaluation substudy
MIRE	monochromatic infrared energy
MIP	MiniMed Implantable Pump
MMAD	mass media aerodynamic diameter
MMP9	matrix metalloproteinase 9
MODY3	maturity-onset diabetes of the young,
MTHFR	methylenetetrahydrofolate reductase
NAD(P)H	nicotinamide adenine dinucleotide phosphate
NCEP ATPIII	third Adult Treatment Panel of the National Cholesterol Education Program
NCOR	nuclear receptor corepressor
NGT	normal glucose tolerance

NHANES	National Health and Nutrition Examination Survey
NICE	National Institute for Clinical Excellence
NMDA	N-methyl-D-aspartate
NNT	numbers needed to treat
NO	nitric oxide
NOS	nitric oxide synthase
NPH	Neutral Protamine Hagedorn
NPS	Neuropathic Pain Scale
NSAID	non-steroidal anti-inflammatory drug
OAD	oral antidiabetic(s)
OCP	oral contraceptive pill
OCT	organic cation transporter
od	once a day
OGTT	oral glucose tolerance text
OR	odds ratio
PAD	peripheral arterial disease
PAI-1-ag	type 1 plasminogen activator inhibitor antigen
PC	prohormone convertase
PCI	percutaneous coronary intervention
PCOS	polycystic ovary syndrome
PDE	phosphodiesterase
PDGF	platelet-derived growth factor
PEACE	Prevention of Events with Angiotension Converting Enzyme inhibition
PF-4	platelet factor-4
PGC-1α	peroxisome proliferator activated receptor γ coactivator 1α
PIMS	programmable implantable medication system
PKA	protein kinase A
PKC	protein kinase C
POPADAD	The Prevention of Progression of Arterial Disease and Diabetes trial
Post-CABG	Post Coronary Artery Bypass Graft
PPAR	peroxisome proliferator-activated receptor
PPP	Primary Prevention Project
PPP	Prospective Pravastatin Pooling (Project)
PPRE	PPAR responsive element
PROactive	PROspective pioglitAzone Clinical Trial In macroVascular Events
PROGRESS	Perindopril Protection against Recurrent Stroke Study
PROSPER	Prospective Study of Pravastatin in the Elderly at Risk
PROVE-IT TIMI 22	Pravastatin or Atorvastatin Evaluation and Infection Therapy – Thrombolysis in Myocardial Infarction 22
PSGL-1	P-selectin glycoprotein ligand
PTCA	transluminal coronary angioplasty
PVD	peripheral vascular disease
PYY	peptide tyrosine tyrosine

qd	four times a day
QoL	quality of life
RA-IA	rapid acting insulin analogues
RAS	renal artery stenosis
RDNS	Rochester Diabetic Neuropathy Study
RECORD	Rosiglitazone Evaluated for Cardiac Outcomes and Regulation of Glycaemia in Diabetes
RENAAL	Reduction of Endpoints in Noninsulin-dependent diabetes mellitus with the Angiotensin II Antagonist Losartan
RESULT	Rosiglitazone Early versus SULphonylurea Titration
RIA	radio-immunoassay
RIAD	Risk Factor in Impaired Glucose Tolerance for Atherosclerosis and Diabetes
RIO	Rimonabant In Obesity
RNA	ribonucleic acid
ROADMAP	Randomised Olmesartan and Diabetes Microalbuminuria Prevention trial
ROS	reactive oxygen species
RR	relative risk
RXR	retinoic X receptor
SBP	self blood pressure
SBPM	self blood pressure monitoring
SC	subcutaneous
SCR-1	steroid receptor coactivator-1
SD	standard deviation
SDIS	Stockholm Diabetes Intervention Study
sdLDL	small dense low-density lipoprotein
SE	standard error
SEM	standard error of the mean
SENDCAP	St Mary's, Ealing, Northwick Park Diabetes Cardiovascular Disease Prevention study
SHEP	Systolic Hypertension in the Elderly Program
sICAM-1	soluble intercellular adhesion molecule-1
SIGN	Scottish Intercollegiate Guidelines Network
SLC30a8	pancreatic β-cell zinc transporter
SMBG	self-monitoring of blood glucose
SPARCL	Stroke Prevention by Aggressive Reduction in Cholesterol Levels
SNP	single nucleotide polymorphism
SNRI	serotonin and norepinephrine reuptake inhibitor
SPPARM	selective PPAR modulator
SREBP1	sterol regulatory element binding protein-1
SSRI	selective serotonin reuptake inhibitor
STK11	serine-threonine kinase 11
STOP-NIDDM	Study to Prevent Non-Insulin-Dependent Diabetes Mellitus
SU	sulfonylurea

SUR1	sulphonylurea receptor
sVCAM-1	soluble vascular cell adhesion molecule-1
Syst-Eur	Systolic Hypertension in Europe trial
t-PA-ag	tissue-type plasminogen activator antigen
T2D	type 2 diabetes
TA	technology appraisal
TC	total cholesterol
TCF7L2	transcription factor 7-like 2 gene
TG	triglycerides
TIA	transient ischaemic attack
T1DM	type 1 diabetes mellitus
TNF-α	tumour necrosis factor-alpha
TNT	Treatment to New Targets study
TORC2	target of rapamycin complex 2
TXA2	thromboxane A2
TZD	thiazolidenedione
UAER	urinary albumin excretion rate
UKPDS	United Kingdom Prospective Diabetes Study
URANUS	Use of Rosuvastatin versus Atorvastatin in Type 2 Diabetes Mellitus
USPHS	US Physicians' Health Study
USPSTF	US Preventive Services Task Force
VA	Veterans Affairs
VA-HIT	Veterans Affairs High-Density Lipoprotein Cholesterol Intervention Trial
VALIANT	Valsartan in Acute Myocardial Infarction Trial
VAS	visual analogue scale
VHA	Veterans Health Administration
VISP	Vitamin Intervention for Stroke Prevention
VLDL	very low-density lipoprotein
VLDL-C	very low-density lipoprotein-cholesterol
VPT	vibration perception threshold
VRS	verbal rating scale
VSMC	vascular smooth muscle cell
vWf	von Willebrand factor
WCH	white coat hypertenisives
WOSCOPS	West of Scotland Coronary Prevention Study

Index